ACUTE ISCHEMIC STROKE

Edited by **Julio César García Rodríguez**

Acute Ischemic Stroke
Edited by Julio César García Rodríguez

Published by InTech
Janeza Trdine 9, 51000 Rijeka, Croatia

Publishing Process Manager Vana Persen

Technical Editor Teodora Smiljanic

Cover Designer InTech Design Team

Additional hard copies can be obtained from orders@intechopen.com

Acute Ischemic Stroke, Edited by Julio César García Rodríguez
p. cm.
ISBN 978-953-307-983-7

For EU product safety concerns:
IN TECH d.o.o., Prolaz Marije Krucifikse Kozulić 3, 51000 Rijeka, Croatia,
info@intechopen.com or visit our website at intechopen.com.

Meet the editor

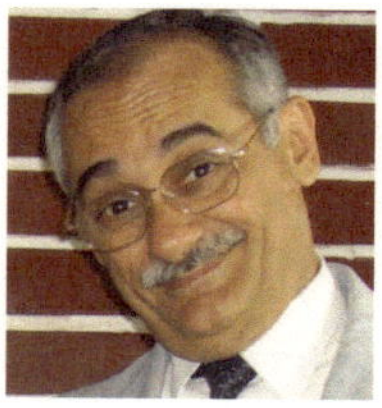

Dr Julio César García Rodríguez graduated in Biochemistry from Havana University in 1979. He obtained the PhD in 2002, the Titular Professor Grade in 2005, and Biotechnologist of Second Level in 2007. He is Titular Professor of the Havana Medical University where his focus is within the fields of basic Neuroprotection and clinical trial. Fundamentally, his results are in experimental models of stroke using erythropoietin (EPO) as neuroprotectant. He has authored more than 75 scientific publications and several books chapters. He is a pioneer in the use of EPO with low sialic acid content (Neuro-EPO) by nasal way – an innovative new procedure which could have significant, positive consequences for those undergoing treatment for neurodegenerative disorders in the 21st century. He is member of the Society of Neuroscience of Cuba and received three prizes from the Academy of Sciences of Cuba (ACC). Among other distinctions, he has the Order Juan Thomas Roig from ACC and the "San Jorge" Medal from the Academic of Sciences of Ukraine.

Contents

Preface

We've arrived at the second decade of the XXI century of the modern era with 7 billion human beings on our planet. Average life expectancy is 69 years of age, but for the *industrialized countries* it stands at 80 years, while for the called *developing countries* and for those denominated as less *developed* countries is only of 67 and 57 years respectively. With this overview of the world's population ages, the illness vascular brain increases gradually in the industrialized countries. Among them, it is the stroke that is of more incidences in the population. It is the third leading cause of death and the most common cause of disability. Indeed, stroke is a big global health problem affecting millions of people every year. This whole health problem has been increasingly growing and has not only negative impact in the labor productivity – such as in health expenses of, being repealed many human resources and financial with a relatively low impact; but also in the prevention and in the recovery of the patients.

In this somber panorama, it would be necessary to wonder: How can the neurosciences contribute in the XXI century? Indeed, significant progress has been made on stroke molecular aspects and neuroprotection in acute phase of this disease. This information is scattered throughout the literature in original research papers, reviews, and some recently edited books. However, until now there hasn't been a book which summarizes in a comprehensible way, for the specialized readers as well as for the ones simply interested on the topic – the main achieved advances and challenges outlined in the preclinical research, the diagnosis, and treatment of the stroke.

This book is not only addressed at students and under-graduate and postgraduate professors, avid to know and to fertilize with new knowledge, but it also seeks to be an useful tool to investigators, doctors, nursing, occupational therapist, physiotherapist, family members, and social workers that professionally fight against this neurodegenerative wants.

For the thematic organization of this book, we have thought of exposing the reader the following order: the physiopathology of the illness, those more outstanding aspects of the preclinical research, the different treatments, and to conclude, the complications of the acute ischemic stroke. In a very brief synthesis, we can say that: Chapter 1 describes the pathophysiology that leads to expansion of the infarct into surrounding peri-infarct tissue, diaschisis and degeneration in distal but anatomically connected regions, and the adaptive changes that occur distal to the infarct after focal stroke. Chapter 2 explains the molecular aspects of the exitotoxicity and oxidative stress in acute ischemic stroke (AIS). Chapter 3 explains a novel preclinical neuroprotective therapy in AIS using Neuro-EPO by nasal way. Chapter 4 outlines the association of dysphagia and other risk factors in the development of respiratory infections in AIS patients. Chapter 5 describes the involvement of serum lipids and Statin treatment during AIS. Chapter 6 describes the endovascular management of AIS. Chapter 7 explains the microemboli monitoring in AIS. Chapter 8 provides a cursory review each of the major established methods of AIS recanalization therapy, followed by a detailed review of intracranial stenting. Chapter 9 discusses the surgical treatment of AIS patients using decompressive craniectomy. Chapter10 makes a critical revision of our understanding of the dynamics, persistence, and regulation of collateral blood flow and expanding on studies evaluating the mechanisms and efficacy of collateral therapeutics and improved strategies for AIS. In Chapter 11, the authors make a critical analysis and explain the role of both vertebral or vertebrobasilar size in AIS, and finally, Chapter 12 deals with the hyperbaric oxygen for Stroke.

This Editor expects that the efforts carried out in this book to integrate and to consolidate the molecular, clinical and therapeutic knowledge of AIS, and the neuroprotection in this illness will contribute in accelerating the search of more effective and safer therapeutic alternatives for the more than five million people that currently suffer AIS in our planet.

I truly want to express my gratitude and my personal satisfaction to all the authors, other highly qualified people, and real experts in their field; that have worked in this book preparation.

Prof. Julio César García Rodríguez
Life Science and Nanosecurity, Scientific Advisor's Office, State Council,
Cuba

1

Diaschisis, Degeneration, and Adaptive Plasticity After Focal Ischemic Stroke

Bernice Sist, Sam Joshva Baskar Jesudasan and Ian R. Winship
Centre for Neuroscience and Department of Psychiatry, University of Alberta, Canada

1. Introduction

Focal stroke refers to sudden brain dysfunction due to an interruption of blood supply to a particular region of the brain. An ischemic stroke (~80% of focal strokes) occurs due to a blockage of a blood vessel, typically by a blood clot, whereas a haemorrhagic stroke results from rupture of a cerebral blood vessel and the resulting accumulation of blood in the brain parenchyma. Symptoms of stroke will vary depending on the size and location of the tissue damaged by the reduced blood flow (the infarct), but common symptoms include sudden weakness of the limbs or face, trouble speaking or understanding speech, impaired vision, headache and dizziness. According to the World Health Organization (WHO), more than 15 million people suffer a stroke each year, of which five million people will die. Stroke is a leading cause of chronic adult disability worldwide, and the majority of those who survive their stroke (more than five million people per year) are left with permanent sensorimotor disabilities, which may include loss of strength, sensation, coordination or balance (with the nature and severity of disability depending on the location and size of the lesion).

Despite the significant societal and personal cost of stroke, treatment options remain limited. Currently, only recombinant tissue-type plasminogen activator (rtPA), a serine proteinase, has proved effective in treating ischemic stroke in clinical trials (NINDS, 1995). Thrombolysis after rtPA administration occurs as a result of plasminogen being converted to plasmin by rtPA. The plasmin then participates in the degradation of fibrin to restore blood flow to territories downstream of the occlusion. Unfortunately, few patients are treated with rtPA, in part due to it short therapeutic window of 4.5 hours (relative to delays in symptom recognition, transport, and triaging) after ischemic onset (Lansberg et al., 2009; Kaur et al., 2004; Clark et al., 1999; Del Zoppo et al., 2009). Moreover, rtPA is ineffective for many patients treated within its therapeutic window, particularly with respect to middle cerebral artery occlusion (MCAo), the most common cause of focal ischemic stroke (Kaur et al., 2004; Seitz et al., 2011). Given the limited treatment options for stroke, an improved understanding of its pathophysiology and the brains endogenous mechanisms for neuroprotection, brain repair and neuroanatomical rewiring is important to developing new strategies and improving stroke care.

While death and disability due to stroke can be predicted based on the size and location of the infarct, damage due to stroke extends beyond the ischemic territories. Moreover, while treatment options remain limited, partial recovery after stroke occurs due to adaptive changes (plasticity) in brain structure and function that allow uninjured brain regions to adopt the function of neural tissue destroyed by ischemia (Winship and Murphy, 2009; C.E. Brown and Murphy, 2008). While pathological and adaptive changes that occur in peri-infarct cortex have been well characterized, less research has examined adaptive and maladaptive changes distal to the infarct. In this chapter, we will review the pathophysiology that leads to expansion of the infarct into surrounding peri-infarct tissue, diaschisis and degeneration in distal but anatomically connected regions, and the adaptive changes that occur distal to the infarct after focal stroke.

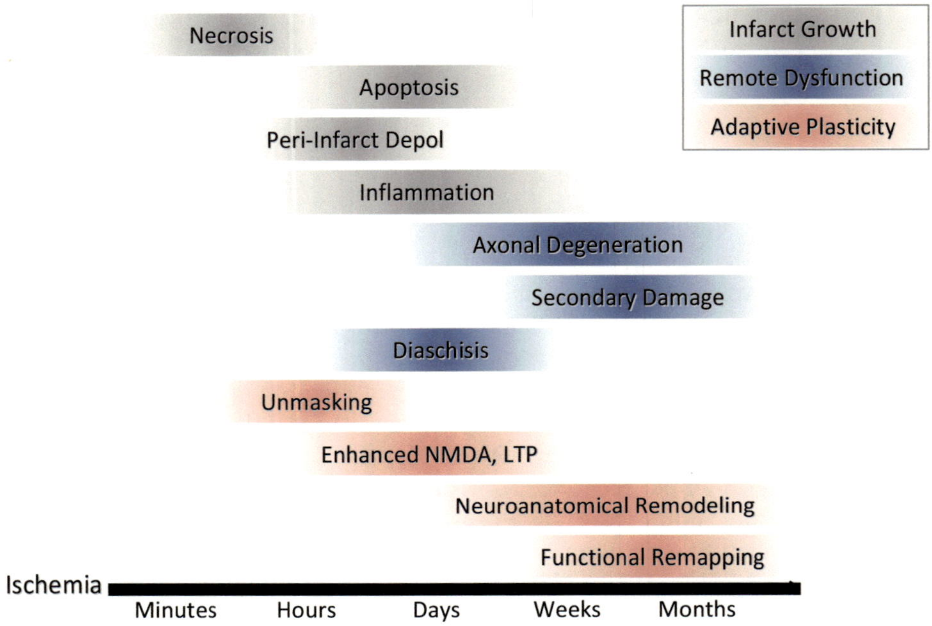

Fig. 1. Timeline of stroke-induced degeneration, dysfunction and adaptive plasticity. During ischemia, several processes lead to development of an infarct core and expansion of this core into penumbral tissue (grey bars). Metabolic failure in the core of the ischemic territory leads to rapid and irreversible cell death (necrosis), while inflammation and peri-infarct depolarizations can induce delayed cell death (through apoptosis) in cells in the penumbra over the following days and weeks. Focal stroke can also induce degeneration and dysfunction in regions far from the infarct (blue bars). Brain dysfunction distal to the stroke (diaschisis) can appear soon after ischemia and persist for weeks, and includes changes in blood flow, metabolism, and altered inhibitory neurotransmission remote from the infarct. Similarly, remote to the site of injury, axons from neurons in the infarct core degenerate, inducing inflammation that can trigger secondary damage and atrophy in structures with neuroanatomical links to the infarct. Finally, adaptive plasticity induced by the stroke can occur immediately following ischemia and persist for months (red bars). Functional unmasking of existing connections can lead to rapid redistribution of some function lost to the infarct, and changes in glutamatergic transmission and long-term potentiation have been reported in peri-infarct cortex and beyond in the first week after stroke. Neuroanatomical rewiring to compensate for lost connections starts days after ischemia and persists for months, allowing functional representations lost to stroke to remap to new locations in the weeks and months after this initial insult.

2. Mechanisms of cell death and infarct growth after ischemic stroke

At the centre of the stroke, the "ischemic core", brain damage is fast and irreversible as reduced blood flow leads to the activation of proteolytic enzymes, degradation of the cytoskeleton, cytotoxic swelling, and peroxidation of membrane lipids (Witte et al., 2000).
As blood flow within the core drops below 20% of normal flow rates, metabolic failure leads to anoxic depolarization and activation of the "ischemic cascade" that triggers neuronal death beginning within minutes of ischemic onset (Dirnagl et al., 1999; Hossmann, 1994; Witte et al., 2000). Reduced blood flow decreases delivery of oxygen and glucose to the brain, which leads to reduced production of adenosine triphosphate (ATP) and failure of energy dependent membrane receptors, ion channels and ionic pumps. These failures lead to collapse of transmembrane potential as ions such as sodium (Na+), potassium (K+) and calcium (Ca^{2+}) flow freely down their concentration gradients, leading to anoxic depolarization and the release of additional excitatory neurotransmitters (primarily glutamate). The resulting excitotoxicity is potentiated by the disruption of energy dependent glutamate reuptake from the synaptic cleft, and the ensuing activation of the glutamatergic N-methyl-D-amino (NMDA) receptor and the alpha-amino-3-hydroxy-5-methyl-4-isoxazole-propionic acid (AMPA) receptor lead to further depolarization and excitotoxicity. Water begins to enter the cells in response to change in ion concentrations, producing cytotoxic oedema, a pathophysiological marker of ischemia.
Intracellular increases in Ca^{2+} concentration are particularly important regulators of cell death in the ischemic core due to the role Ca^{2+} plays as a second messenger. Ca^{2+}increases activate multiple signalling pathways that contribute to cell death, including enhancing the production of nitric oxide (NO). NO is an intracellular messenger important for the normal physiology of an organism, with a well-characterized role in regulating circulation (Huang, 1994; Dirnagl et al., 1999). NO production is regulated by nitric oxide synthase (NOS), a Ca^{2+} dependent enzyme. Following ischemia, increased activation of NOS can lead to neurotoxic levels of NO (A.T. Brown et al., 1995; Dirnagl et al., 1999; Danton and Dietrich, 2003). During initial stages of ischemia, NO produced by endothelial NOS triggers arterial dilation near the region of occlusion, thereby increasing blood flow and increases the chance of survival of the penumbra. However, NO can react with a superoxide anion to form the highly reactive species peroxynitrite, which can react with and damage virtually any cellular component (Mergenthaler et al., 2004). Increases in NO can initiate cell death by inducing lipid oxidation chain reactions, which disrupt the lipid membranes of the mitochondria (Burwell and Brookes, 2008), or by causing energy failures by acting as an electron acceptor and thereby disrupting cellular respiration in the mitochondria (Bolaños et al., 1997; Brookes et al., 1999; Burwell and Brookes, 2008; Dirnagl et al., 1999). Moreover, these reactive species lead to peroxidation of the plasma, nuclear, and mitochondrial membranes, inducing DNA damage and cell lysis. Beyond their direct effects on cell death, increased levels of reactive oxygen and nitrogen species also induce release of pro-inflammatory factors from immune cells, leading to inflammation and expansion of the stroke core (discussed further in Section 2.2) (Lai and Todd, 2006; Jin et al., 2010; Vila et al., 2000, 2003).
Surrounding the stroke core is a band of tissue referred to as the penumbra, in which blood flow is partially preserved due to redundant collateral circulation. While this tissue is somewhat ischemic, neurons here can be saved from death by reperfusion or neuroprotective treatments soon after ischemic onset. The brain maintains independent thresholds for functional integrity and structural integrity, thereby keeping a gradient of cell

viability after ischemic insults. The threshold for functional integrity and that of structural integrity are governed by two key factors: the residual flow rate of blood and duration of reduced flow (Heiss and Graf, 1994). Since the threshold for functional integrity is higher than that for structural integrity, the neurons in the penumbra are electrically silent but still able to maintain ion homeostasis and structural integrity (Astrup et al., 1981; Ferrer and Planas, 2003; Heiss and Graf, 1994; Symon, 1975; Hossmann, 1994). However, viability in the penumbra is variable and time dependent, and a number of processes lead to cell death and expansion of the infarct core into the penumbra. Three of these factors, peri-infarct depolarizations, inflammation, and apoptosis, are discussed below.

2.1 Peri-infarct depolarizations

Excitotoxicity and anoxic depolarizations caused by ischemia increase extracellular glutamate and potassium levels in the stroke core, which may then diffuse into penumbral regions and trigger depolarization of the resident neurons and glia (Mergenthaler et al., 2004). A propagating wave of depolarization moving away from the core is initiated and places additional stress on the metabolically compromised cells in the penumbra. These depolarizations can occur several times per hour during acute stroke (Busch et al., 1996; Wolf et al., 1997). Since there are fluctuations in blood flow which compromise oxygen and glucose supply, depolarizations within the peri-infarct cortex contribute to energy failure and cell death, leading to the growth of the infarct core over time (Back et al., 1996). Recent data from animal models suggests that ischemic depolarizations are accompanied by intracellular Ca^{2+} accumulation and a loss of synaptic integrity (Murphy et al., 2008). Murphy et al. (2008) demonstrated that ischemic depolarizations and increases in intracellular calcium were glutamate receptor independent and suggested that these depolarizations were the major ionic event associated with the degeneration of synaptic structure early after ischemic onset. Notably, persistent depolarizations resembling anoxic depolarization and transient depolarizations resembling recurrent peri-infarct depolarizations emerge not only in cortex, but also occur in striatal gray matter, suggesting that infarct expansion due to peri-infarct depolarization extends beyond the cortex (Umegaki et al., 2005).

2.2 Inflammation and infarct growth

Inflammation is a non-specific physiological response to infection or injury. The central nervous system is often labeled as "immune privileged" due to the presence of a blood brain barrier that separates it from the periphery and prevents entry of most infectious materials into the brain. However, inflammation after brain injury is characterized by the infiltration and proliferation of immune cells in an attempt to eliminate cellular debris and pathogens, and the secretion of chemokines and pro- and/or anti-inflammatory cytokines. After stroke, the inflammatory response contributes to cell death and infarct growth for days after ischemic onset (Dirnagl et al., 1999). Leukocytes, monocytes, neurons, and glial cells (microglia and astrocytes) all participate in the inflammatory response to stroke. During ischemia, leukocytes aggregate and adhere to the vascular endothelium, in part due to increased release of chemokines such as monocyte chemo attractant protein 1 (MCP1) and adhesion molecules such as selectins in ischemic territories (Danton and Dietrich, 2003; Mergenthaler et al., 2004). Following ischemia, endothelial cells increase their expression of selectin, which promotes cellular interactions with leukocytes and aggregates of leukocytes that accumulate platelets and fibrin and thereby occlude vessels, reduce perfusion and contribute to the expansion of the infarct (Ritter, 2000; Danton and Dietrich, 2003).

Glial cells are major contributors to post-stroke inflammation. As the resident immune cells of the brain, microglia serve to monitor the brain microenvironment for injury or infection. After stroke, microglia become activated and migrate to the stroke penumbra. Therein, they assume an activated morphology and participate (along with leukocytes, neurons, and astrocytes) in modulating inflammation through the secretion of pro- and anti-inflammatory cytokines.

Cytokines are small glycoproteins and able to trigger multiple signaling pathways relevant to cell death. Cytokines are important mediators of apoptosis (programmed cell death) during stroke. In the hours following stroke, microglia transform from surveying the microenvironment in a ramified "resting state" into an amoeboid phagocytotic state, scavenging for debris and secreting cytotoxic and pro-inflammatory factors such as interleukin-1 (IL-1), interleukin-6 (IL-6) and tumor necrosis factor alpha (TNF-α) (Danton and Dietrich, 2003; J.J. Legos et al., 2000; E. Tarkowski et al., 1999). Within the first 24 hours after stroke, amoeboid microglia and macrophages expressing high levels of interleukin-1 beta (IL-1β) accumulate at the border of the infarct area (Clausen et al., 2008; Mabuchi et al., 2000). The interleukin-1 family of cytokines has multiple members that mediate degeneration following ischemic stroke. Evidence for the importance of interleukin-1 alpha (IL-1α) and IL-1β has been confirmed by studies that demonstrate that deleting both cytokines can reduce infarct volume (Boutin et al., 2001). IL-1α is an important modulator of cerebrovascular inflammation and induces activation of endothelial cells and expression of adhesion molecules, allowing leukocytes and neutrophils to enter the central nervous system and increase secretion of pro-inflammatory cytokines and production of reactive oxygen species (Jin et al., 2010; Thornton et al., 2010). TNF-α released by immune cells binds to the TNF type 1 receptor, inducing the recruitment of adaptor proteins that influence multiple distinct signaling pathways. These adaptor proteins can enhance inflammation or lead to apoptosis by increasing the adhesion of leukocytes and elevating release of IL-1, NO, or other inflammatory mediators (Hallenbeck, 2002; Lykke et al., 2009). Conversely, the same signaling pathways can lead to the transduction of a cell survival signal, perhaps in response to activation at different receptor subtypes (Hallenbeck, 2002; Lykke et al., 2009). Similarly, activated immune cells also secrete anti-inflammatory cytokines (TNF-β1, IL-10) under some conditions, reinforcing the complexity of the inflammatory response as it relates to cell death (Mergenthaler et al., 2004).

2.3 Apoptosis

Following cerebral ischemia, both necrotic and apoptotic cell death contribute to ultimate lesion volume. Necrosis is a passive process confined to the ischemic core where cell death is fast and characterized by the loss of membrane integrity, abnormal morphology of organelles and cellular swelling (Bredesen, 2000; Ferrer and Planas, 2003). Programmed cell death, or apoptosis, is an energy dependent process that occurs in cells distributed throughout the penumbra that involves translation of proteins to facilitate an "orderly" cell death process. Apoptosis is the systematic degradation of a cell in response to injury and is characterized by the condensation of chromatin, nuclear fragmentation, preserved membrane integrity and blebbing of the plasma membrane (apoptotic bodies) (Bredesen, 2000).

Apoptosis can be triggered through an intrinsic pathway or an extrinsic pathway. The intrinsic apoptotic signaling pathway is due to the disruption of mitochondrial transmembrane potential and integrity, which can be induced through multiple pro-apoptotic pathways (Ferri and Kroemer, 2001). The mitochondria produce reactive oxygen species after injury or excessive Ca^{2+} influx, such as might occur due to excitoxicity or persistent NMDA receptor activation (Zipfel et al., 2000), causing disruption to the membrane permeability (Burwell and Brookes, 2008; Lewen et al., 2000; Zipfel et al., 2000). Changes in mitochondrial membrane permeability increase the release of pro-apoptotic factors including cytochrome c (Bredesen, 2000; Ferri and Kroemer, 2001; Garrido et al., 2006; Saelens et al., 2004; Vaux, 2011). The release of cytochrome c disrupts metabolism and energy production within the mitochondria, further exacerbating free radical production and release of cytochrome c (Burwell and Brookes, 2008; Lewen et al., 2000). High levels of oxidative stress will push cells towards necrosis while moderate levels will trigger apoptosis (Lewen et al., 2000). The release of cytochrome c into the cytosol also stimulates the assembly of apoptosomes, protein complexes that serve to activate cysteine-dependent aspartic acid proteases (caspases) (Ferri and Kroemer, 2001).

Caspases are the major regulators of apoptosis and have been categorized based on their function (Alnemri et al., 1996; Graham and Chen, 2001). Initiator caspases (caspase-2, -8, -9, -10) cleave the inactive pro-forms of effector caspases (caspase-3, -6, -7), allowing them to trigger apoptosis by cleaving multiple protein substrates and degrade DNA by activating nucleases (Fujimura et al., 1998; Enari et al., 1998; Lewen et al., 2000; Mergenthaler et al., 2004). Caspases 1, 3, 8, and 9 are involved in inducing apoptosis during stroke, with caspase-1 involved in the early activation of cytokine release and caspase-3 central to the apoptotic signaling cascade (Mergenthaler et al., 2004; Ferrer and Planas, 2003). Blockage of caspase-3 function is associated with robust neuroprotection in animal models of stroke (Hara et al., 1997; Le et al., 2002).

The extrinsic apoptotic pathway also acts through the activation of caspases. The TNF class of cytokines are the major mediators of the extrinsic apoptotic pathway. Binding at the TNF receptors leads to caspase activation via the TNF receptor-associated death domain (TRADD) and the Fas-associated death domain protein (FADD) (Bredesen, 2000; Ferrer and Planas, 2003). Accordingly, elevated TNF-α signaling increases caspase-3 mediated neuronal apoptosis and infarct volume after ischemic stroke (Emsley and Tyrell, 2002; Pettigrew et al., 2008). Conversely, blockade of TNF-α via TNF-binding proteins has been demonstrated to be neuroprotective during cerebral ischemia (Nawashiro et al., 1997).

3. Diaschisis and degeneration distal to the infarct

While the size and location of the stroke core and the expansion of the infarct accounts for much of the death and disability due to stroke, focal ischemia induces widespread changes in the brain, even in non-ischemic territories. In this section, we will examine dysfunction and degeneration induced by focal stroke in regions that are anatomically connected but distal to the infarct.

3.1 Diaschisis after stroke

Diaschisis is defined as brain dysfunction in a region of the brain distal to a site of injury that is anatomical connected to the damaged area. While functional deafferentiation is thought to be the primary mechanism of diaschisis (Finger et al., 2004), it is influenced by a number of factors. In stroke, brain swelling and spreading depression as well as neuroanatomical disconnection contribute to diaschisis that can manifest as altered neuronal excitability or neurotransmitter receptor expression, hypometabolism, and/or hypoperfusion in areas not directly damaged by ischemia.

Both cytotoxic and vasogenic oedema are induced by stroke, and persistent water accumulation occurs in the brain over the days following ischemia in animal models and human stroke patients (Witte et al., 2000). Oedema remote to the infarct can occur and may result from the migration of extravasated fluid and protein (Izumi et al., 2002). In the case of large strokes such as MCAo, acute brain swelling can directly compress the contralesional hemisphere and remote ipsilesional regions (O'brien et al., 1974; Izumi et al., 2002). The effects of widespread brain swelling are multifold, inducing secondary damage directly through physical compression and inducing secondary hypoperfusion and ischemia due to compression of low resistance vasculature (Witte et al., 2000).

Reductions in cerebral blood flow on the side of the brain opposite of an ischemic insult have been reported in stroke patients since the 1960s (Kempinsky et al., 1961; Hoedt-Rasmussen and Skinhoj, 1964). Local measurement of cerebral blood flow confirmed this reduction in perfusion in sites remote from the infarct, including the contralesional hemisphere, and demonstrated a progressive decline in blood flow in both hemispheres during the first week after infarction in most stroke patients (Slater et al., 1977). Based on this progressive decline, Slater et al. (1977) suggested that diaschisis in the contralesional hemisphere involved a process more complex than simple destruction of axonal afferents, and proposed that a combination of decreased neuronal stimulation, loss of cerebral autoregulation, release of vasoactive compounds, and oedema, as well as other factors, led to the widespread and long-lasting changes in cerebral blood flow. Transhemispheric reductions in cerebral oxygen metabolism and cerebral blood flow have been confirmed using positron emission tomography (PET) and shown to correlate with the patients' level of consciousness (Lenzi et al., 1982). Moreover, approximately 50% of patients exhibit "mirror diaschisis" during the first two weeks after stroke, as indicated by a decrease in oxygen metabolism and blood flow in the contralateral brain regions homotypical to the infarct (Lenzi et al., 1982). In addition to regional changes in blood flow, animal models have suggested that vasoreactivity (measured in response to hypercapnia) is impaired even in non-infarcted, non-penumbral brain regions (Dettmers et al., 1993).

Not surprisingly, in light of the changes in cerebral blood flow discussed above, widespread hypometabolism has been reported in human patients and animal models after focal stroke. In patients measured acutely and three weeks after MCAo, oxygen consumption measured by PET decreased throughout the ipsilesional hemisphere (including the thalamus and remote, non-ischemic tissue) between imaging sessions (Iglesias et al., 2000). Similarly, using small cortical strokes in rats, Carmichael et al. (2004) demonstrated impaired glucose metabolism (a direct reflection of neuronal activity) one day after stroke throughout ipsilesional cortex, striatum, and thalamus that was not associated with reductions in blood flow. The affected cortex was approximated 13X larger than the infarct and incorporated functionally related areas in the sensorimotor cortex. By eight days post-stroke, hypometabolism in the thalamus and striatum had resolved, but persisted in this ipsilesional cortex.

In addition to diffuse changes in the cerebral cortices, region specific diaschisis has been identified in the ipsilesional thalamus and contralateral cerebellum after stroke (Iglesias et al., 2000; De Reuck et al., 1995; Nagasawa et al., 1994; Baron et al., 1981). Decreased blood flow and metabolism in the contralateral cerebellum (typically called crossed cerebellar diaschisis, CCD) has been reported via a number of modalities (computed tomography (CT) and single photon emission CT, PET, and magnetic resonance imaging) after cerebral hemispheric infarction. CCD occurs within 6 hours of ischemic onset (Kamouchi et al., 2004) and persists into the chronic phase of stroke recovery. In the acute phase (approximately 16 hours after onset) of stroke, CCD is not correlated with clinical outcome (Takasawa et al., 2002). However, CCD in the subacute period (approximately 10 days after stroke) is significantly correlated with performance on the Scandinavian Stroke Scale and Barthel Index (Takasawa et al., 2002). CCD varies according to the size and location of the cerebral infarction. Infarcts incorporating temporal association cortex and pyramidal tract of the corona radiata were correlated with CCD in the medial zone of the cerebellum, whereas lesions of the primary and supplementary motor cortex, premotor cortex, primary somatosensory cortex, and posterior limb of the internal capsule were associated with CCD in the intermediate cerebellum (Z. Liu et al., 2007). Finally, infarcts occupying the primary motor cortex, supplementary motor cortex, premotor cortex and genu of the internal capsule were associated with CCD in the lateral cerebellum (Z. Liu et al., 2007). Notably, CCD in the lateral and intermediate were found to be better predictors of clinical outcome.

As discussed in Section 2.1, peri-infarct depolarizations place tremendous metabolic stress on neurons in the penumbra and contribute to delayed cell death and infarct expansion. However, it is important to note that, at least in animal models, these depolarizations travel into healthy brain tissue throughout the ipsilesional hemisphere as waves of spreading depression (SD). SD moves through cortex at ~2-5 mm/minute and is characterized by local suppression of electrical activity and a large direct current (DC) shift associated with the redistribution of ions between the intracellular and extracellular space (Chuquet et al, 2007; Somjen, 2001). Even in non-ischemic regions, these waves induce significant metabolic stress, with an initial increase in brain metabolism followed by profound hypometabolism and transient changes in the expression of a number of neurotrophic and inflammatory cytokines and molecular signalling cascades (Witte et al., 2007). In vivo calcium imaging has demonstrated the SD is associated with calcium waves propagating through both neurons and astrocytes, and that these waves elicit vasoconstriction sufficient to stop capillary blood flow in affected cortex (Chuquet et al., 2007). Chuquet et al. (2007) suggest that SD propagation is driven by neuronal signals, while astrocyte waves are responsible for hemodynamic failure after SD.

In addition to changes in metabolism and blood flow, diaschisis is also reflected by direct changes in neuronal activity in regions of the brain remote to the ischemic infarct. While task-evoked blood oxygen level dependent (BOLD) signals (an indirect measure of neuronal activation) detected during functional magnetic resonance imaging (fMRI) are normal in areas of diaschisis (Fair et al., 2009), synaptic signalling and sensory-evoked activity may be impaired. For example, in patients with stroke affecting the striate cortex, visual activation (evidenced by fMRI BOLD signals) was reduced or absent in extrastriate cortex in the first 10 days after stroke (Brodtmann et al., 2007). Visually evoked activation was restored in these regions six months after infarction.

Numerous reports have identified significant changes in neuronal excitability throughout the brain after stroke. Mechanisms responsible for changes in electrical properties within the peri-infarct cortex have included fluctuations in cerebral blood flow (Dietrich et al., 2010) and disrupted balance of excitatory and inhibitory membrane receptors (Jolkkonen et al., 2003; Qü et al., 1998; Que et al., 1999; Schiene et al., 1996; Clarkson et al., 2010). Focal stroke produces a long-lasting impairment in gamma-aminobutyric acid (GABA) transmission in peri-infarct and contralesional cortex (Buchkremer-Ratzmann et al., 1996; Domann et al., 1993; Schiene et al., 1996; Wang, 2003). A massive upregulation of $GABA_A$ receptor mRNA has been reported throughout the ipsilesional hemisphere in rats (Neumann-Haefelin et al., 1999) after targeted cortical stroke. Translation of the $GABA_A$ receptor is impaired, however, such that $GABA_A$ receptor protein and binding are reduced and GABAergic inhibition (measured by paired pulse inhibition) is impaired in both cerebral hemispheres (Neumann-Haefelin et al., 1999; Buchkremer-Ratzmann et al., 1996, 1998; Buchkremer-Ratzmann and Witte, 1997a,b). This $GABA_A$ dysfunction would lead to cortical hyperexcitability, an assertion supported by in vivo recordings that identified increased spontaneous activity in neurons near the infarct (Schiene et al., 1996). Notably, long-lasting disinhibition of both the ipsi- and contralesional hemispheres has been reported in human stroke patients (Butefisch et al., 2003; Manganotti et al., 2008). This hyperexcitability may explain epileptic-like electrical activity often observed after ischemic stroke (Back et al., 1996). However, alterations in GABAergic inhibition appear to be more complex than a simple loss of GABA activity. Cortical GABAergic signalling contains both synaptic and extrasynaptic components, and these components are responsible for phasic and tonic inhibition, respectively (Clarkson et al., 2010). Reduced paired pulse inhibition would reflect a change in phasic inhibition, while more recent studies suggest that $GABA_A$ -mediated tonic (extrasynaptic) inhibition may be potentiated for at least two weeks after stroke, likely due to impaired function of GABA transporters (GAT-3/GAT-4) (Clarkson et al., 2010). Moreover, selectively blocking tonic inhibition produces an early and sustained restoration of sensorimotor function, suggesting that counteracting heightened tonic inhibition after stroke may promote recovery in stroke patients (Clarkson et al., 2010).

3.2 Degeneration of areas distal to infarct

Regions that participate in post-stroke plasticity (to be discussed further in Section 4) typically share an anatomical connection with the brain region damaged by stroke. In a similar manner, focal damage in one area of the brain can lead to dysfunction and degeneration in neuroanatomically related brain areas.

Diffusion tensor imaging (DTI) (Basser et al., 1994) and tractography (Jones et al., 1999; Mori et al., 1999) are powerful new tools for evaluating white matter structure in human stroke patients in vivo. Changes in fractional anisotropy (FA), a DTI-derived measure of white matter microstructure (Beaulieu, 2002) can be used to map Wallerian and retrograde degeneration (Pierpaoli et al., 2001; Werring et al., 2000) or measure potentially beneficial changes in white matter structure (Crofts et al., 2011). DTI is a type of magnetic resonance imaging developed in the 1980s and involves the measurement of water diffusion rate and directionality, combined together to give what is called a tensor (Le Bihan et al., 2001). Tractography or fibre tracking is achieved by combining tensors mathematically. Since water preferentially diffuses along the orientation of white matter tracts, tractography can be used to assess the integrity of major white matter tracts such as the CST. DTI may be useful for predicting motor impairments early after an ischemic event, since changes in water diffusion are observable early after ischemic onset (Moseley, 1990; Le Bihan et al., 2001).

A recent study using DTI and computational network analysis revealed widespread changes in "communicability" based on white matter degeneration in stroke patients (Crofts et al., 2011). Communicability represents a measure of the integrity of both direct and indirect white matter connections between regions. Not surprisingly, reduced communicability was found in the ipsilesional hemisphere. However, communicability was also reduced in homotypical locations in the contralesional hemisphere, a finding that Croft et al. (2011) interpreted as evidence of secondary degeneration of white matter pathways in remote regions with direct or indirect connections with the infarcted territory. Notably, the authors also identified regions with increased communicability indicative of adaptive plasticity.

Thalamic atrophy has also been reported in the months following infarct in human stroke patients (Tamura et al., 1991). The thalamus is a main relay station for sensory afferents from multiple sensory modalities ascending to the cortex. Within the ventral nuclear group of the thalamus are the ventroposteromedial nucleus, a primary relay station for facial somatosensation, as well as the ventroposterolateral nucleus, the relay station somatosensation of the limbs and the body (Platz, 1994 and Steriade, 1988; Binkofski et al., 1996). After stroke, the ipsilesional thalamus exhibits hypometabolism and atrophy, likely due to a loss of cortical afferents and efferents (Binkofski et al., 2004; Fujie et al., 1990; Tamura et al., 1991). Dependent upon lesion size and location, one or both nuclei may contain neurons with shrunken cytoplasm and abnormal nuclei as well as elevated infiltration of microglia (Dihne et al., 2002; Iizuka et al., 1990). Although the majority of excitatory and inhibitory receptors lost originate from the ischemic core, a small but significant number of receptors are also lost in the retrogradely affected thalamic nuclei (Qü et al., 1998). Receptor densities are not affected in the contralateral thalamic nuclei (Qü et al., 1998). Thalamic degeneration after stroke appears to be progressive. Two weeks after MCAo in rats, ipsilesional thalamic volume is 87% of the contralateral thalamus, and falls to 77% at one month, 54% at three and six months (Fujie et al., 1990). This progressive atrophy likely results from degeneration of corticothalamic and thalamocortical pathways linking the thalamus to the infarcted cortex (Fujie et al., 1990; Iizuka et al., 1990; Tamura et al., 1991; Qü et al., 1998). Interestingly, vascular remodelling and neurogenesis in thalamic nuclei is enhanced in response to the secondary thalamic damage due to a cortical infarct (Ling et al., 2009).

3.3 Degeneration in the spinal cord

Following spinal cord injury, the inflammatory response leads to cell death and scar formation and damage of previously healthy tissue by cytotoxic inflammatory by-products (Hagg and Oudega, 2006; Weishaupt et al., 2010). As such, spinal cord injury is followed by degeneration of axons below the site of injury that are disconnected from their cell bodies. This is termed Wallerian degeneration (WD) as first described in 1850 by Waller. WD exhibits the following stereotypical course: (i) degeneration of axonal structures in the days following injury, (ii) infiltration of macrophages and degradation of myelin and (iii) gradual fibrosis and atrophy of fibre tracts. WD can affect many tracts including the corticothalamic tract, thalamocortical tract, descending corticospinal tract (CST) and ascending sensory fibre tracts, depending on the location of the injury. As described above, changes in white matter connectivity suggestive of WD have been reported in the contralesional cortex after stroke (Crofts et al., 2011).

The pathological time course of WD, including the degeneration of the axons and the degeneration of myelin in regions such as the CST, can be analyzed based on distinct DTI image characteristics acquired at different time points during stroke recovery (DeVetten et al., 2010; X. Liu et al., 2011; Yu et al., 2009). However, the heterogeneity of the stroke population has made clear inferences on the role of CST degeneration in sensorimotor disability difficult to make. The use of DTI in the first 3 days after stroke may not be useful for prognosis as WD in the spinal cord may not be detectable. However, DTI at 30 days post-stroke appear useful in defining prognosis and response to rehabilitation (Binkofski et al., 1996; Puig et al., 2010). Dynamic changes in WD can first be detected in the CST using DTI in the first two weeks following stroke and begin to stabilize by 3 months after injury (DeVetten et al., 2010; Puig et al., 2010; Yu et al., 2009). DTI studies suggest that sparing and integrity of the ipsilesional and contralesional CST can aid in prognosis for motor recovery after stroke (Binkofski et al., 1996; DeVetten et al., 2010; Lindenberg et al., 2009, 2011; (Xiang) Liu et al., 2010; Madhavan et al., 2011; Puig et al., 2010; Schaechter et al., 2006; Thomalla et al., 2004; Yu et al., 2009). While patients that did not recover well from stroke had reduced FA in both corticospinal tracts relative to healthy controls, patients that exhibited good functional recovery had elevated FA in these same tracts (Schaechter et al., 2006).

Histological assessment in animal models has confirmed that focal stroke damaging the sensorimotor cortex induces secondary degeneration of the descending CST (Weishaupt et al., 2010). Damage to motor neurons in the forelimb motor cortex induces degeneration of their descending axons and activation of immune cells near their terminals in the cervical spinal cord. In the weeks following cortical injury, secondary damage extends past the cervical cord and progressive and delayed degeneration of descending CST fibres is observed in the thoracic spinal cord. An increased population of microglia was also observed in the cervical spinal cord within one week of infarction, and Weishaupt et al. (2010) suggest that this initial infiltration of microglia and concomitant release of pro-inflammatory and cytotoxic proteins is the likely mechanism of secondary damage to CST fibres terminating below the cervical cord.

4. Reactive plasticity after stroke

4.1 Plasticity in peri-infarct cortex

Stroke-induced impairments in motor, sensory and cognitive function improve over time, likely due to adaptive rewiring (plasticity) of damaged neural circuitry. Post-stroke plasticity includes physiological and anatomical changes that facilitate remapping of lost function onto surviving brain tissue through the expression of growth-promoting genes in peri-infarct cortex (Carmichael et al., 2005). These altered patterns of gene expression induce long-lasting increases in neuronal excitability (Centonze et al., 2007; Mittmann et al., 1998; Buchkremer-Ratzmann et al., 1996; Domann et al., 1993; Schiene et al., 1996; Butefisch et al., 2003; Manganotti et al., 2008; Hagemann et al., 1998). In addition to altered GABAergic transmission (discussed in Section 3.1), studies using animal models of focal stroke have demonstrated that NMDA receptor-mediated and non-NMDA receptor-mediated glutamate transmission are potentiated for four weeks after MCAo (Centonze et al., 2007; Mittmann et al., 1998). Long-term potentiation is also facilitated in peri-lesional cortex for seven days after focal cortical stroke (Hagemann et al., 1998), providing a favorable environment for functional rewiring of lost synaptic connections.

Moreover, stroke induces considerable neuronanatomical remodeling with elevated axonal sprouting, dendritic remodeling, and synaptogenesis persisting for weeks after stroke (Brown et al., 2007; Brown et al., 2009; Carmichael et al., 2001; Carmichael and Chesselet, 2002; Li et al., 1998; Stroemer et al., 1995). Changes in gene expression patterns of growth promoting and inhibiting factors occur early after ischemic onset and persist for months after injury, facilitating axonal growth and rewiring of injured tissue (Carmichael et al., 2005; Zhang et al., 2000). Growth-associated protein-43 (GAP-43) is an essential component of the growth cones of extending axons that is up regulated during development and after neuronal injury. mRNA expression for GAP-43 shows a two-fold increase as early as 3 days after stroke and remains up-regulated 28 days after injury (Carmichael et al., 2005). During long-term (months) recovery, a progression from axonal sprouting to synaptogenesis is suggested by increased synaptophysin (a presynaptic component of mature synapses) levels and a return to baseline GAP-43 levels (Stroemer et al., 1995; Carmichael, 2003). The expression of growth inhibiting genes such as ephrin-A5 and brevican also fluctuate during recovery. For example, brevican mRNA increases slowly over time before peaking 28 days after stroke (Carmichael et al., 2005). It is therefore the balance of the expression profiles of growth promoting and growth inhibiting genes that govern adaptive plasticity after ischemic insult.

Adaptive plasticity includes significant neuroanatomical remodelling of the peri-infarct cortex. Neuroanatomical tract tracing has shown that this axonal sprouting leads to rewiring of local and distal intracortical projections (Brown et al., 2009; Carmichael et al., 2001; Dancause et al., 2005) with enhanced interhemispheric connectivity that correlates with improved sensorimotor function (van der Zijden et al., 2007; van der Zijden et al., 2008). Anatomical remodeling is also apparent in the dendritic trees of peri-infarct neurons. As the locus for the majority of excitatory synapses in the brain, dendritic spines provide the anatomical framework for excitatory neurotransmission. These spines show significant alterations to their structural morphology during the acute and chronic phases of stroke, including reversible dendritic blebbing, changes in spine length, dendritic spine retraction, and enhanced spine turnover in response to injury (Brown et al., 2007, 2008; Li and Murphy, 2008; Risher et al., 2010; Zhang et al., 2005, 2007). Dendritic spines are dynamic yet resilient during acute stroke. In cases where reperfusion of the ischemic area occurs within 60 minutes, dendritic blebbing and retraction cease and neuroanatomical structure is restored (Li and Murphy, 2008). Additionally, spines are highly dynamic during long-term stroke recovery. It has been suggested that dynamic changes in spine morphology are important during learning and adaptive plasticity (Majewska et al., 2006). Repeated imaging studies show an initial loss of dendritic spines in the hours after stroke followed by increased spine turnover (formation and elimination) during the weeks that follow (Brown et al., 2008). Because the degree of tissue reperfusion in the peri-infarct cortex varies with distance from the infarct core, greater perfusion rates further from the core are associated with greater spine densities after long-term recovery (Mostany et al., 2010). While dendritic arbors themselves are stable over several weeks in non-stroke animals, dendritic arbor remodeling, including both dendritic tip growth and retraction, is up-regulated within the first two weeks after stroke (Brown et al., 2010). However, this phenomenon appears restricted to the peri-infarct cortex, as dendrites farther from the stroke do not appear to exhibit large-scale structural plasticity (Mostany and Portera-Cailliau, 2011).

These physiological and anatomical changes facilitate functional reorganization of the cortex after stroke (Winship and Murphy, 2009). Reorganization of the motor cortex following focal stroke has been investigated in animal models and human patients using motor-mapping techniques.(Castro-Alamancos and Borrel, 1995; Friel et al., 2000; Frost et al., 2003; Remple et al., 2001; Kleim et al., 2003; Gharbawie et al., 2005; Nudo and Milliken, 1996; Traversa et al., 1997; Cicinelli et al., 1997) These studies show that ablation of the remapped cortex reinstates behavioural impairments (Castro-Alamancos and Borrel, 1995) and physical therapy induces an increase in motor map size that correlates with significant functional improvement (Liepert et al., 1998; Liepert et al., 2000).

Functional imaging has been used to demonstrate that patients with stroke-induced sensorimotor impairments show a reorganization of cortical activity evoked by stimulation of the stroke-affected limbs after stroke (Calautti and Baron, 2003; Carey et al., 2006; Chollet et al., 1991; Cramer et al., 1997; Cramer and Chopp, 2000; Herholz and Heiss, 2000; Jaillard et al., 2005; Nelles et al., 1999a; Nelles et al., 1999b; Seitz et al., 1998; Ward et al., 2003b; Ward et al., 2003ab; Ward et al., 2006; Weiller et al., 1993). Strikingly, increased activity in novel ipsilesional sensorimotor areas has been correlated with improved recovery in human stroke patients (Fridman et al., 2004; Johansen-Berg et al., 2002b; Johansen-Berg et al., 2002a; Schaechter et al., 2006). A number of studies in animal models have used in vivo imaging to map regional reorganization of functional representations after stroke (van der Zijden et al., 2008; Dijkhuizen et al., 2001; Dijkhuizen et al., 2003; Weber et al., 2008). Winship and Murphy (2008) showed that small strokes damaging the forelimb somatosensory cortex resulted in posteromedial remapping of the forelimb representation. Moreover, the authors showed that adaptive re-mapping is initiated at the cellular level by surviving neurons adopting new roles in addition to their usual function. Later in recovery, these "multitasking" neurons become more selective to a particular stimulus, which may reflect a transitory phase in the progression from involvement in one sensorimotor function to a new function that replaces processing lost to stroke (Winship and Murphy, 2009). Increases in the receptive field size of peri-infarct neurons in the somatosensory cortex have also been reported using sensory-evoked electrophysiology (Jenkins & Merzenich, 1987; Reinecke et al., 2003) after focal lesions. Regional remapping has also been confirmed with voltage sensitive dye imaging (Brown et al., 2009). Eight weeks after targeted forelimb stroke, forelimb-evoked depolarizations reemerged in surviving portions of forelimb cortex and spread horizontally into neighboring peri-infarct motor and hindlimb areas. Notably, forelimb-evoked depolarization persisted 300-400% longer than controls, and was not limited to the remapped peri-infarct zone as similar changes were observed in the posteromedial retrosplenial cortex located millimeters from the stroke. More recent studies using voltage sensitive dyes suggests that forelimb-specific somatosensory cortex activity can be partially redistributed within one hour of ischemic damage, likely through unmasking of surviving ancillary pathways (Murphy et al., 2008; Sigler et al., 2009).

4.2 Contralesional cortical plasticity

While increased activity in novel ipsilesional sensorimotor areas has been correlated with improved recovery in human stroke patients, (Fridman et al., 2004; Johansen-Berg et al., 2002b; Johansen-Berg et al., 2002a; Schaechter et al., 2006) elevated contralesional activity has generally been associated with extensive infarcts and, as such, poor recovery (Calautti and Baron, 2003; Schaechter, 2004). Recruitment of the contralesional motor cortex in patients with extensive injury has been confirmed using transmagnetic stimulation and functional magnetic resonance imaging (Bestmann et al., 2010), suggesting that remote regions of the brain can participate in recovery from stroke under these conditions. Positron emission tomography (PET) scans have been used to demonstrate bilateral activation during movement (Bestmann et al., 2010; Cao et al., 1998; Chollet et al., 1991). Clinical observations also show that patients who have a second stroke in the contralesional hemisphere will have greater sensorimotor deficits and lose functional recovery of previously impaired abilities (Ago, 2003, Fisher, 1992 and Song, 2005 as cited by Riecker et al., 2010).

In some respects, clinical studies are in agreement with studies in animal models that have used a variety of imaging and electrophysiological assays and found altered patterns of somatosensory activation in both ipsilesional and contralesional cortex during recovery from stroke (Brown et al., 2009; Dijkhuizen et al., 2001; Dijkhuizen et al., 2003; Weber et al., 2008; Winship and Murphy, 2008; Wei et al., 2001; Abo et al., 2001). However, contralesional activation is not always observed (Weber et al., 2008) and, as in human stroke patients, good recovery from stroke-induced sensorimotor impairment is associated with the emergence or restoration of peri-lesional activity (Dijkhuizen et al., 2001; Dijkhuizen et al., 2003; Weber et al., 2008).

Functional recruitment of the contralesional cortex has been suggested by changes neuronal excitability electrical activity, receptor densities, and dendritic structure in the days and weeks following ischemic insult in animal models. Biernaskie and Corbett (2001) showed that an enriched environment paired with a task-specific physical rehabilitation could elicit plasticity in dendritic arbors in the contralesional motor cortex that correlates with improved functional recovery on a skilled reaching task. Increases in NMDA receptor density in the homotypical motor cortex contralateral to a focal ischemic insult have been reported as early as two days after stroke and may persist for at least 24 days (Adkins et al., 2004; Hsu and Jones, 2006; Luhmann et al., 1995). Takatsuru and colleagues (2009) have recently identified adaptive changes in the structure and function of the homotypical contralateral cortex after focal stroke in sensorimotor cortex. Their data demonstrated that stimulus-evoked neuronal activity in the contralesional hemisphere was transiently potentiated two days after focal stroke. At four weeks post-stroke, behavioural recovery was complete and novel patterns of circuit activity were found in the intact contralateral hemisphere. Takatsuru et al. (2009) found anatomical correlates of this contralesional functional remapping using in vivo two-photon microscopy that identified a selective increase in the turnover rate of mushroom-type dendritic spines one week after stroke.

Recently, Mohanjeran et al. (2011) investigated the effect of targeted strokes on contralateral sensory-evoked activity during the first two hours after occlusion using voltage-sensitive dye imaging. Blockade of a single surface arteriole in the mouse forelimb somatosensory cortex reduced the sensory-evoked response to contralateral forelimb stimulation. However, in the contralesional hemisphere, significantly enhanced sensory responses were evoked by stimulation of either forelimb within 30-50 min of stroke onset. Notably, acallosal mice showed similar rapid interhemispheric redistribution of sensory processing after stroke, and pharmacological thalamic inactivation before stroke prevented the contralateral changes in sensory-evoked activity. Combined, these data suggest that existing subcortical connections and not transcallosal projections mediate rapid redistribution of sensory-evoked activity.

4.3 Spinal plasticity after cortical injury

Previous sections have established that neuroanatomically connected regions distal to the infarct exhibit both degenerative and adaptive changes during recovery. As the host for the afferent somatosensory fibres and the efferent CST that control voluntary movement and somatosensation, plasticity in the spinal cord is ideally situated to play a role in functional recovery after stroke. The spontaneous regenerative capacity of the CST in the adult system after spinal cord injury was previously thought to be negligible. However, in recent years research has shown that even in the absence of intervention, the CST is able to spontaneously regenerate after partial lesion (Lundell et al., 2011). After an incomplete spinal cord injury, spared fibres are able to sprout and circumvent the injury site (Rosenzweig et al., 2010; Steward et al., 2008).

Recently, several studies have investigated axonal sprouting in the spinal cord induced by stroke in the brain, and its relation to stroke treatment or spontaneous recovery. Neuroanatomical tracers have been used to demonstrated that CST axons that originate in the uninjured hemisphere exhibit increased midline crossing and innervation of spinal grey matter that has been denervated by stroke (LaPash Daniels et al., 2009; Liu et al., 2009). Liu et al. (2009) used transynaptic retrograde tracers injected into the forepaw to show that spontaneous behavioural recovery after focal stroke was associated with an increase in retrogradely labelled axons in the stroke-affected cervical spinal cord one month after stroke. Notably, transynaptic retrograde labelling of neuronal somata in the ischemic hemisphere was significantly reduced 11 days after MCAo, but a significant increase in retrograde labelling (relative to 11 days post) in both the injured and uninjured hemisphere was found one month after stroke. Similarly, plasticity-enhancing treatments that improve functional recovery often increases the number of CST fibres originating in the uninjured sensorimotor cortex that cross the midline and innervate the stroke-affected side of the cervical spinal cord. For example, treatment of focal stroke with bone marrow stromal cells (Z. Liu et al., 2007, 2008, 2011), anti-Nogo antibody infusion (Weissner et al., 2003; Tsai et al., 2007), and inosine (Zai et al., 2011) are all associated with improved functional recovery and increased innervation of the stroke-affected spinal cord by the unaffected CST originating contralateral to the stroke. While the role of axonal sprouting from the ipsilesional cortex is less defined, enhanced axonal sprouting in corticorubral and corticobulbar tracts originating in both the contralesional and ipsilesional cortex has been reported at the level of the brainstem after MCAo in mice (Reitmeir et al., 2011).

5. Summary

Permanent disabilities after ischemic stroke are dependent on the size and location of the infarct, and the pathophysiology through which the ischemic core expands into the vulnerable penumbral tissue has been well characterized. In the peri-infarct cortex, the relative contributions of excitotoxicity, peri-infarct depolarizations, inflammation and apoptosis are well characterized as they relate to infarct growth during ischemia (Dirnagl et al., 1999; Witte et al., 2000). However, degeneration and dysfunction is not confined to the infarct core and the surrounding peri-infarct cortex. Areas that are remote but neuroanatomically linked to the infarct, including the contralateral cortex, thalamus, and spinal cord exhibit altered neuronal excitability, blood flow, and metabolism after stroke. Moreover, degeneration of afferent or efferent connections with the infracted territory can lead to atrophy and secondary damage in distal structures. Similarly, while the functional reorganization of peri-infarct cortex is well correlated with behavioural recovery, these distal but anatomically related regions also exhibit physiological and anatomical plasticity that may contribute to the resolution of stroke-induced impairments. An understanding of the adaptive plasticity and stroke-induced dysfunction in these remote areas may be important in developing and evaluating delayed strategies for neuroprotection and rehabilitation after stroke.

6. References

Abo M., Chen Z., Lai L.J., Reese T., Bjelke B. (2001) Functional recovery after brain lesion--contralateral neuromodulation: An fMRI study. *Neuroreport*, Vol. 12, pp: (1543-1547).

Adkins, D. L., Voorhies, A. C., & Jones, T. A. (2004). Behavioral and neuroplastic effects of focal endothelin-1 induced sensorimotor cortex lesions. *Neuroscience*, Vol. 128, No. 3, pp. (473-486).

Alnemri, E. S., Livingston, D. J., Nicholson, D. W., Salvesen, G., Thornberry, N. A., Wong, W. W., et al. (1996). Human ICE/CED-3 protease nomenclature. *Cell*, Vol. 82, No. 2, pp. (171).

Astrup, J., Siesjo, B.K., Symon, L. (1981) Threshold in cerebral ischemia- the ischemic penumbra. *Stroke*, Vol. 12, pp. (723-725).

Back, T., Ginsberg, M. D., Dietrich, W D, & Watson, B. D. (1996). Induction of spreading depression in the ischemic hemisphere following experimental middle cerebral artery occlusion: effect on infarct morphology *Journal of cerebral blood flow and metabolism : official journal of the International Society of Cerebral Blood Flow and Metabolism*, Vol.16, No. 2, pp: (202–213).

Baron, J. C., Bousser, M. G., Comar, D., & Castaigne, P. (1981). "Crossed cerebellar diaschisis" in human supratentorial brain infarction. *Transactions of the American Neurological Association*, Vol.105, pp. (459-461).

Beaulieu, C. (2002). The basis of anisotropic water diffusion in the nervous system - a technical review. *NMR in Biomedicine*, Vol. 15, No. 7-8, pp. (435-455).

Bestmann, S., Swayne, O., Blankenburg, F., Ruff, C. C., Teo, J., Weiskopf, N., et al. (2010). The role of contralesional dorsal premotor cortex after stroke as studied with concurrent TMS-fMRI. *The Journal of Neuroscience : The Official Journal of the Society for Neuroscience*, Vol. 30, No. 36, pp. (11926-11937).

Biernaskie, J., & Corbett, D. (2001). Enriched Rehabilitative Training Promotes Improved Forelimb Motor Function and Enhanced Dendritic Growth after Focal Ischemic Injury, 1–9.

Binkofski, F., Seitz, R. J., Arnold, S., Classen, J., Benecke, R., & Freund, H. J. (1996). Thalamic metbolism and corticospinal tract integrity determine motor recovery in stroke. *Annals of neurology*, Vol. 39, No. 4, pp. (460–470).

Bolaños, J. P., Almeida, A., Stewart, V., Peuchen, S., Land, J. M., Clark, J. B., & Heales, S. J. (1997). Nitric oxide-mediated mitochondrial damage in the brain: mechanisms and implications for neurodegenerative diseases. *Journal of Neurochemistry*, Vol. 68, No. 6, pp. (2227–2240).

Boutin, H., LeFeuvre, R. A., Horai, R., Asano, M., Iwakura, Y., & Rothwell, N. J. (2001). Role of IL-1alpha and IL-1beta in ischemic brain damage. *Journal of Neuroscience*, Vol. 21, No.15, pp. (5528–5534).

Bredesen, D. E. (2000). Apoptosis: Overview and signal transduction pathways. *Journal of Neurotrauma*, Vol. 17, No. 10, pp. (801-810).

Brodtmann, A., Puce, A., Darby, D., & Donnan, G. (2007). fMRI demonstrates diaschisis in the extrastriate visual cortex. *Stroke; a Journal of Cerebral Circulation*, Vol. 38, No. 8, pp. (2360-2363).

Brookes, P. S., Bolaños, J .P., & Heales, S. J. (1999). The assumption that nitric oxide inhibits mitochondrial ATP synthesis is correct. *FEBS letters*, Vol. 446, No. 2-3, pp. (261–263).

Brown C.E. & Murphy T.H. (2008a) Livin' on the edge: Imaging dendritic spine turnover in the peri-infarct zone during ischemic stroke and recovery. *Neuroscientist*, Vol. 14, pp. (139-146).

Brown, C. E., Aminoltejari, K., Erb, H., Winship, I. R., & Murphy, T H. (2009a). In Vivo Voltage-Sensitive Dye Imaging in Adult Mice Reveals That Somatosensory Maps Lost to Stroke Are Replaced over Weeks by New Structural and Functional Circuits with Prolonged Modes of Activation within Both the Peri-Infarct Zone and Distant Sites. *Journal of Neuroscience*, Vol. 29, No. 6, pp. (1719–1734).

Brown, C. E., Boyd, Jamie D, & Murphy, Timothy H. (2009b). Longitudinal in vivo imaging reveals balanced and branch-specific remodeling of mature cortical pyramidal dendritic arbors after stroke. *Journal of Cerebral Blood Flow & Metabolism*, Vol. 30, No. 4, pp. (783–791).

Brown, C. E., Li, P, Boyd, J D, Delaney, K. R., & Murphy, T H. (2007). Extensive Turnover of Dendritic Spines and Vascular Remodeling in Cortical Tissues Recovering from Stroke. *Journal of Neuroscience*, Vol. 27, No. 15), pp. (4101–4109).

Brown, C. E., Wong, C., & Murphy, T H. (2008b). Rapid Morphologic Plasticity of Peri-Infarct Dendritic Spines After Focal Ischemic Stroke. *Stroke*, Vol. 39, No. 4, pp. (1286–1291).

Brown, G. C., Bolaños, J P, Heales, S. J., & Clark, J. B. (1995). Nitric oxide produced by activated astrocytes rapidly and reversibly inhibits cellular respiration. *Neuroscience Letters*, Vol. 193, No. 3, pp. (201–204).

Buchkremer-Ratzmann, I., August, M., Hagemann, G., & Witte, O. W. (1996). Electrophysiological transcortical diaschisis after cortical photothrombosis in rat brain. *Stroke; a Journal of Cerebral Circulation*, Vol.27, No. 6, pp. (1105-9).

Buchkremer-Ratzmann, I., & Witte, O. W. (1997). Extended brain disinhibition following small photothrombotic lesions in rat frontal cortex. *Neuroreport*, Vol. 8, No. 2, pp. (519-522).

Burwell, L. S., & Brookes, Paul S. (2008). Mitochondria as a target for the cardioprotective effects of nitric oxide in ischemia-reperfusion injury. *Antioxidants & redox signaling*, Vol. 10, No. 3, pp. (579–599).

Busch, A. E., Quester, S., Ulzheimer, J. C., Waldegger, S., Gorboulev, V., Arndt, P., et al. (1996). Electrogenic properties and substrate specificity of the polyspecific rat cation transporter rOCT1. *The Journal of Biological Chemistry*, Vol. 271, No. 51, pp. (32599-32604).

Butefisch, C. M., Netz, J., Wessling, M., Seitz, R. J., & Homberg, V. (2003). Remote changes in cortical excitability after stroke. *Brain : A Journal of Neurology*, Vol. 126, No. 2, pp. (470-481).

Calautti, C., Jones, P. S., Naccarato, M., Sharma, N., Day, D. J., Bullmore, E. T., Warburton, E. A., et al. (2010). The relationship between motor deficit and primary motor cortex hemispheric activation balance after stroke: longitudinal fMRI study. *Journal of Neurology, Neurosurgery & Psychiatry*, Vol. 81, No. 7, pp. (788–792).

Cao, Y., George, K. P., Ewing, J. R., Vikingstad, E. M., & Johnson, A. F. (1998). Neuroimaging of language and aphasia after stroke. *Journal of Stroke and Cerebrovascular Diseases : The Official Journal of National Stroke Association*, Vol. 7, No. 4, pp. (230-233).

Carmichael S.T. & Chesselet M.F. (2002) Synchronous neuronal activity is a signal for axonal sprouting after cortical lesions in the adult. *Journal of Neuroscience*, Vol 22, pp. (6062-6070).

Carmichael S.T., Wei L., Rovainen C.M., Woolsey T.A. (2001) New patterns of intracortical projections after focal cortical stroke. *Neurobiology of Disease*, Vol. 8, pp. (910-922).

Carmichael, S.T. (2003) Plasticity of cortical projections after stroke. *Neuroscientist*, Vol 9, pp. (64-75).

Carmichael, S. T., Tatsukawa, K., Katsman, D., Tsuyuguchi, N., & Kornblum, H. I. (2004). Evolution of diaschisis in a focal stroke model. *Stroke; a Journal of Cerebral Circulation*, Vol. 35, No. 3, pp. (758-763).

Carmichael, S., Archibeque, I., Luke, L., Nolan, T., Momiy, J., & Li, S. (2005). Growth-associated gene expression after stroke: evidence for a growth-promoting region in peri-infarct cortex. *Experimental Neurology*, Vol. 193, No. 2, pp. (291–311).

Carey J.R., Greer K.R., Grunewald T.K., Steele J.L., Wiemiller J.W., Bhatt E., Nagpal A., Lungu O., Auerbach E.J. (2006) Primary motor area activation during precision-demanding versus simple finger movement. *Neurorehabilitation and Neural Repair*, Vol. 20, pp. (361-370).

Castro-Alamancos M.A., Borrel J. (1995) Functional recovery of forelimb response capacity after forelimb primary motor cortex damage in the rat is due to the reorganization of adjacent areas of cortex. *Neuroscience*, Vol.68, pp. (793-805).

Centonze D., Rossi S., Tortiglione A., Picconi B., Prosperetti C., De Chiara V., Bernardi G., Calabresi P. (2007) Synaptic plasticity during recovery from permanent occlusion of the middle cerebral artery. *Neurobiology of Disease*, Vol. 27, pp. (44-53).

Chollet F., DiPiero V., Wise R.J., Brooks D.J., Dolan R.J., Frackowiak R.S. (1991) The functional anatomy of motor recovery after stroke in humans: A study with positron emission tomography. *Annals of Neurology*, Vol. 29, pp. (63-71).

Chuquet, J., Hollender, L., & Nimchinsky, E. A. (2007). High-resolution in vivo imaging of the neurovascular unit during spreading depression. *The Journal of Neuroscience : The Official Journal of the Society for Neuroscience*, Vol. 27, No. 15, pp. (4036-4044).

Cicinelli P., Traversa R., Rossini P.M. (1997) Post-stroke reorganization of brain motor output to the hand: A 2-4 month follow-up with focal magnetic transcranial stimulation. *Electroencephalography and Clinical Neurophysiology*, Vol. 105, pp. (438-450).

Clark, W. M., Wissman, S., Albers, G. W., Jhamandas, J. H., Madden, K. P., & Hamilton, S. (1999). Recombinant tissue-type plasminogen activator (Alteplase) for ischemic stroke 3 to 5 hours after symptom onset. The ATLANTIS Study: a randomized controlled trial. Alteplase Thrombolysis for Acute Noninterventional Therapy in Ischemic Stroke. *JAMA : the journal of the American Medical Association*,Vol. 282, No. 21, pp. (2019–2026).

Clarkson, A. N., Huang, B. S., Macisaac, S. E., Mody, I., & Carmichael, S. T. (2010). Reducing excessive GABA-mediated tonic inhibition promotes functional recovery after stroke. *Nature*, Vol. 468, No. 7321, pp. (305-309).

Clausen, B. H., Lambertsen, K. L., Babcock, A. A., Holm, T. H., Dagnaes-Hansen, F., & Finsen, B. (2008). Interleukin-1beta and tumor necrosis factor-alpha are expressed by different subsets of microglia and macrophages after ischemic stroke in mice. *Journal of neuroinflammation*,Vol. 5, pp. 46.

Cramer, S. C. (2008). Repairing the human brain after stroke: I. mechanisms of spontaneous recovery. *Annals of Neurology*, Vol. 63, No. 3, pp. (272-287).

Cramer S.C. & Chopp M. (2000) Recovery recapitulates ontogeny. *Trends in Neuroscience*, Vol. 23, pp. (265-271).

Cramer S.C., Nelles G., Benson R.R., Kaplan J.D., Parker R.A., Kwong K.K., Kennedy D.N., Finklestein S.P., Rosen B.R. (1997) A functional MRI study of subjects recovered from hemiparetic stroke. *Stroke*, Vol. 28, pp. (2518-2527).

Crofts, J. J., Higham, D. J., Bosnell, R., Jbabdi, S., Matthews, P. M., Behrens, T. E., et al. (2011). Network analysis detects changes in the contralesional hemisphere following stroke. *NeuroImage*, Vol. 54, No. 1, pp. (161-169).

Dancause N., Barbay S., Frost S.B., Plautz E.J., Chen D., Zoubina E.V., Stowe A.M., Nudo R.J. (2005) Extensive cortical rewiring after brain injury. *Journal of Neuroscience*, Vol. 25, pp. (10167-10179).

Danton, G.H. & Dietrich, W.D. (2003). Inflammatory mechanisms after ischemia and stroke. *Journal of Neuropathology and Experimental Neurology*, Vol. 62, No. 2, pp. 127-136.

Del Zoppo, G. J., Saver, J. L., Jauch, E. C., Adams, H. P.,Jr, & American Heart Association Stroke Council. (2009). Expansion of the time window for treatment of acute ischemic stroke with intravenous tissue plasminogen activator: A science advisory from the american heart Association/American stroke association. *Stroke; a Journal of Cerebral Circulation,* Vol. 40, No. 8, pp. (2945-2948).

De Reuck, J., Decoo, D., Lemahieu, I., Strijckmans, K., Goethals, P., & Van Maele, G. (1995). Ipsilateral thalamic diaschisis after middle cerebral artery infarction. *Journal of the Neurological Sciences,* Vol. 134, No. 1-2, pp. (130-135).

DeVetten, G., Coutts, S. B., Hill, M. D., Goyal, M., Eesa, M., O'Brien, B., Demchuk, A. M., et al. (2010). Acute Corticospinal Tract Wallerian Degeneration Is Associated With Stroke Outcome. *Stroke,* Vol. 41, No. 4, pp. (751–756).

Dettmers, C., Young, A., Rommel, T., Hartmann, A., Weingart, O., & Baron, J. C. (1993). CO2 reactivity in the ischaemic core, penumbra, and normal tissue 6 hours after acute MCA-occlusion in primates. *Acta Neurochirurgica,* Vol. 125, No. 1-4, pp. (150-155).

Dietrich, W. Dalton, Feng, Z.-C., Leistra, H., Watson, B. D., & Rosenthal, M. (2010). Photothrombotic infarction triggers multiple episodes of cortical spreading depression in distant brain regions. *Journal of Cerebral Blood Flow and Metabolism,* Vol. 14, pp. (20–28).

Dihne, M., Grommes, C., Lutzenburg, M., Witte, O. W., & Block, F. (2002). Different Mechanisms of Secondary Neuronal Damage in Thalamic Nuclei After Focal Cerebral Ischemia in Rats. *Stroke,* Vol. 33, No. 12, pp. (3006–3011).

Dijkhuizen R.M., Singhal A.B., Mandeville J.B., Wu O., Halpern E.F., Finklestein S.P., Rosen B.R., Lo E.H. (2003) Correlation between brain reorganization, ischemic damage, and neurologic status after transient focal cerebral ischemia in rats: A functional magnetic resonance imaging study. *Journal of Neuroscience,* Vol. 23, pp. (510-517).

Dijkhuizen R.M., Ren J., Mandeville J.B., Wu O., Ozdag F.M., Moskowitz M.A., Rosen B.R., Finklestein S.P. (2001) Functional magnetic resonance imaging of reorganization in rat brain after stroke. *Proceedings of the National Academy of Sciences of the United States of America,* Vol. 98, pp. (12766-12771).

Dirnagl, U., & Iadecola, C., Moskowitz M.A. (1999). Pathobiology of ischaemic stroke: an integrated view. *Trends in neurosciences.*

Domann, R., Hagemann, G., Kraemer, M., Freund, H. J., & Witte, O. W. (1993). Electrophysiological changes in the surrounding brain tissue of photochemically induced cortical infarcts in the rat. *Neuroscience Letters,* Vol. 155, No. 1, pp. (69-72).

Emsley, H. C., & Tyrrell, P. J. (2002). Inflammation and infection in clinical stroke. *Journal of Cerebral Blood Flow and Metabolism : Official Journal of the International Society of Cerebral Blood Flow and Metabolism,* Vol. 22, No. 12, pp. (1399-1419).

Fair, D. A., Snyder, A. Z., Connor, L. T., Nardos, B., & Corbetta, M. (2009). Task-evoked BOLD responses are normal in areas of diaschisis after stroke. *Neurorehabilitation and Neural Repair,* Vol. 23, No. 1, pp. (52-57).

Ferrer I., Planas A.M. (2003) Signaling of cell death and cell survival following focal cerebral ischemia: Life and death struggle in the penumbra. *Journal of Neuropathology and Experimental Neurology,* Vol. 62, pp. (329-339).

Ferri, K. F., & Kroemer, G. (2001). Organelle-specific initiation of cell death pathways. *Nature Cell Biology,* Vol. 3, No. 11, pp. (E255-63).

Finger, S., Koehler, P. J., & Jagella, C. (2004). The monakow concept of diaschisis: Origins and perspectives. *Archives of Neurology,* Vol. 61, No. 2, pp. (283-288).

Fridman E.A., Hanakawa T., Chung M., Hummel F., Leiguarda R.C., Cohen L.G. (2004) Reorganization of the human ipsilesional premotor cortex after stroke. *Brain,* Vol. 127, pp. (747-758).

Friel K.M., Heddings A.A., Nudo R.J. (2000) Effects of postlesion experience on behavioral recovery and neurophysiologic reorganization after cortical injury in primates. *Neurorehabilitation and Neural Repair,* Vol. 14, pp. (187-198).

Frost S.B., Barbay S., Friel K.M., Plautz E.J., Nudo R.J. (2003) Reorganization of remote cortical regions after ischemic brain injury: A potential substrate for stroke recovery. *Journal of Neurophysiology,* Vol. 89, pp. (3205-3214).

Fujie, W., Kirino, T., Tomukai, N., Iwasawa, T., & Tamura, A. (1990). Progressive shrinkage of the thalamus following middle cerebral artery occlusion in rats. *Stroke; a Journal of Cerebral Circulation,* Vol. 21, No. 10, pp. (1485-1488).

Fujimura, M., Morita-Fujimura, Y., Murakami, K., Kawase, M., & Chan, P. H. (1998). Cytosolic redistribution of cytochrome c after transient focal cerebral ischemia in rats. *Journal of Cerebral Blood Flow and Metabolism : Official Journal of the International Society of Cerebral Blood Flow and Metabolism,* Vol. 18, No. 11, pp. (1239-1247).

Fukui, K., Iguchi, I., Kito, A., Watanabe, Y., & Sugita, K. (1994). Extent of pontine pyramidal tract Wallerian degeneration and outcome after supratentorial hemorrhagic stroke. *Stroke,* Vol. 25, No. 6, pp. (1207–1210).

Garrido, C., Galluzzi, L., Brunet, M., Puig, P. E., Didelot, C., & Kroemer, G. (2006). Mechanisms of cytochrome c release from mitochondria. *Cell Death and Differentiation,* Vol. 13, No. 9, pp. (1423-1433).

Graham, S. H., & Chen, J. (2001). Programmed cell death in cerebral ischemia. *Journal of Cerebral Blood Flow and Metabolism : Official Journal of the International Society of Cerebral Blood Flow and Metabolism,* Vol. 21, No. 2, pp. (99-109).

Gharbawie O.A., Gonzalez C.L., Williams P.T., Kleim J.A., Whishaw I.Q. (2005) Middle cerebral artery (MCA) stroke produces dysfunction in adjacent motor cortex as detected by intracortical microstimulation in rats. *Neuroscience,* Vol. 130, pp. (601-610).

Hagemann G., Redecker C., Neumann-Haefelin T., Freund H.J., Witte O.W. (1998) Increased long-term potentiation in the surround of experimentally induced focal cortical infarction. *Annals of Neurology,* Vol. 44, pp. (255-258).

Hallenbeck, J. M. (2002). The many faces of tumor necrosis factor in stroke. *Nature Medicine,* Vol. 8, No. 12, pp. (1363-1368).

Hara H., Friedlander R.M., Gagliardini V., Ayata C., Fink K., Huang Z., Shimizu-Sasamata M., Yuan J., Moskowitz M.A. (1997) Inhibition of interleukin 1beta converting enzyme family proteases reduces ischemic and excitotoxic neuronal damage. *Proceedings of the National Academy of Sciences of the United States of America,* Vol. 94, pp. (2007-2012).

Heiss, W. D., & Graf, R. (1994). The ischemic penumbra. *Current Opinion in Neurology,* Vol. 7, No. 1, pp. (11-19).

Herholz K. & Heiss W.D. (2000) Functional imaging correlates of recovery after stroke in humans. *Journal of Cerebral Blood Flow and Metabolism,* Vol. 20, pp. (1619-1631).

Hirata, K., Kuge, Y., Yokota, C., Harada, A., Kokame, K., Inoue, H., Kawashima, H., et al. (2011). Gene and protein analysis of brain derived neurotrophic factor expression in relation to neurological recovery induced by an enriched environment in a rat stroke model. *Neuroscience Letters,*Vol. 495, No. 3, pp. (210–215).

Hoedt-Rasmussen, K. & Skinhoj, E. (1964). Transneural depression of the cerebral hemispheric metabolism in man. *Acta Neurologica Scandinavica,* Vol. 40, pp. (41-46).

Hossmann, K. A. (1994). Viability thresholds and the penumbra of focal ischemia. *Annals of Neurology,* Vol. 36, No. 4, pp. (557-565).

Hsu, J. E., & Jones, T. A. (2006). Contralesional neural plasticity and functional changes in the less-affected forelimb after large and small cortical infarcts in rats. *Experimental Neurology,* Vol. 201, No. 2, pp. (479-494).

Iglesias, S., Marchal, G., Viader, F., & Baron, J. C. (2000). Delayed intrahemispheric remote hypometabolism. correlations with early recovery after stroke. *Cerebrovascular Diseases,* Vol. 10, No. 5, pp. (391-402).

Iizuka, H., Sakatani, K., & Young, W. (2005). Neural damage in the rat thalamus after cortical infarcts. *Stroke,* pp. (1-6).

Izumi, Y., Haida, M., Hata, T., Isozumi, K., Kurita, D., & Shinohara, Y. (2002). Distribution of brain oedema in the contralateral hemisphere after cerebral infarction: Repeated MRI measurement in the rat. *Journal of Clinical Neuroscience : Official Journal of the Neurosurgical Society of Australasia,* Vol. 9, No. 3, pp. (289-293).

Jaillard A., Martin C.D., Garambois K., Lebas J.F., Hommel M. (2005) Vicarious function within the human primary motor cortex? A longitudinal fMRI stroke study. *Brain,* Vol. 128, pp. (1122-1138).

Jenkins, W. M., & Merzenich, M. M. (1987). Reorganization of neocortical representations after brain injury: A neurophysiological model of the bases of recovery from stroke. *Progress in Brain Research,* Vol. 71, pp. (249-266).

Jin, R., Yang, G., & Li, G. (2010). Inflammatory mechanisms in ischemic stroke: role of inflammatory cells. *Journal of Leukocyte Biology,* Vol. 87, No. 5, pp. (779–789).

Johansen-Berg H., Dawes H., Guy C., Smith S.M., Wade D.T., Matthews P.M. (2002a) Correlation between motor improvements and altered fMRI activity after rehabilitative therapy. *Brain,* Vol. 125, pp. (2731-2742).

Johansen-Berg H., Rushworth M.F., Bogdanovic M.D., Kischka U., Wimalaratna S., Matthews P.M. (2002b) The role of ipsilateral premotor cortex in hand movement after stroke. *Proceedings of the National Academy of Sciences of the United States of America,* Vol. 99, pp. (14518-14523).

Jolkkonen, J., Gallagher, N. P., Zilles, Karl, & Sivenius, J. (2003). Behavioral deficits and recovery following transient focal cerebral ischemia in rats: glutamatergic and GABAergic receptor densities. *Behavioural brain research,* Vol. 138, No. 2, pp. (187–200).

Jones, D. K., Simmons, A., Williams, S. C., & Horsfield, M. A. (1999). Non-invasive assessment of axonal fiber connectivity in the human brain via diffusion tensor MRI. *Magnetic Resonance in Medicine : Official Journal of the Society of Magnetic Resonance in Medicine / Society of Magnetic Resonance in Medicine,* Vol. 42, No. 1, pp. (37-41).

Jones, T. A., Allred, R. P., Adkins, D. L., Hsu, J. E., O'Bryant, A., & Maldonado, M. A. (2009). Remodeling the brain with behavioral experience after stroke. *Stroke; a Journal of Cerebral Circulation,* Vol. 40, No. 3.

Kamouchi, M., Fujishima, M., Saku, Y., Ibayashi, S., & Iida, M. (2004). Crossed cerebellar hypoperfusion in hyperacute ischemic stroke. *Journal of the Neurological Sciences,* Vol. 225, No. 1-2, pp. (65-69).

Kaur J., Zhao Z., Klein G.M., Lo E.H., Buchan A.M. (2004) The neurotoxicity of tissue plasminogen activator? *Journal of Cerebral Blood Flow and Metabolism,* Vol. 24, pp. (945-963).

Kempinsky, W.H., Boniface W.R., Keating, J.B., & Morgan, P.P. (1961). Serial hemodynamic study of cerebral infarction in man. *Circulation Research,* Vol. 9, pp. (1051-1058).

Kleim J.A., Bruneau R., VandenBerg P., MacDonald E., Mulrooney R., Pocock D. (2003) Motor cortex stimulation enhances motor recovery and reduces peri-infarct dysfunction following ischemic insult. *Neurological Research,* Vol. 25, pp. (789-793).

Lai, A. Y., & Todd, K. G. (2006). Microglia in cerebral ischemia: molecular actions and interactions. *Canadian journal of physiology and pharmacology*, Vol. 84, No. 1, pp. (49–59).

Lansberg M.G., Bluhmki E., Thijs V.N. (2009) Efficacy and safety of tissue plasminogen activator 3 to 4.5 hours after acute ischemic stroke: A metaanalysis. *Stroke*, Vol. 40, pp. (2438-2441).

LaPash Daniels, C. M., Ayers, K. L., Finley, A. M., Culver, J. P., & Goldberg, M. P. (2009). Axon sprouting in adult mouse spinal cord after motor cortex stroke. *Neuroscience Letters*, Vol. 450, No. 2, pp. (191–195).

Le D.A., Wu Y., Huang Z., Matsushita K., Plesnila N., Augustinack J.C., Hyman B.T., Yuan J., Kuida K., Flavell R.A., Moskowitz M.A. (2002) Caspase activation and neuroprotection in caspase-3- deficient mice after in vivo cerebral ischemia and in vitro oxygen glucose deprivation. *Proceedings of the National Academy of Sciences of the United States of America*, Vol. 99, pp. (15188-15193).

Le Bihan, D., Mangin, J. F., Poupon, C., Clark, C. A., Pappata, S., Molko, N., et al. (2001). Diffusion tensor imaging: Concepts and applications. *Journal of Magnetic Resonance Imaging : JMRI*, Vol. 13, No. 4, pp. (534-546).

Legos, J. J., Whitmore, R. G., Erhardt, J. A., Parsons, A. A., Tuma, R. F., & Barone, F. C. (2000). Quantitative changes in interleukin proteins following focal stroke in the rat. *Neuroscience Letters*, Vol. 282, No. 3, pp. (189-192).

Lenzi, G. L., Frackowiak, R. S., & Jones, T. (1982). Cerebral oxygen metabolism and blood flow in human cerebral ischemic infarction. *Journal of Cerebral Blood Flow and Metabolism : Official Journal of the International Society of Cerebral Blood Flow and Metabolism*, Vol. 2, No. 3, pp. (321-335).

Lewén, A., Matz, P., & Chan, P H. (2000). Free radical pathways in CNS injury. *Journal of neurotrauma*, Vol. 17, No. 10, pp. (871–890).

Li Y., Jiang N., Powers C., Chopp M. (1998) Neuronal damage and plasticity identified by microtubule-associated protein 2, growth-associated protein 43, and cyclin D1 immunoreactivity after focal cerebral ischemia in rats. *Stroke*, Vol. 29, pp. (1972-80).

Li, P. and Murphy, T.H. (2008). Two-photon imaging during prolonged middle cerebral artery occlusion in mice reveals recovery of dendritic structure after reperfusion. *Journal of Neuroscience*, Vol. 28, No. 46, pp. (11970–11979).

Liepert J., Bauder H., Wolfgang H.R., Miltner W.H., Taub E., Weiller C. (2000) Treatment-induced cortical reorganization after stroke in humans. *Stroke*, Vol. 31, pp. (1210-1216).

Liepert J., Miltner W.H., Bauder H., Sommer M., Dettmers C., Taub E., Weiller C. (1998) Motor cortex plasticity during constraint-induced movement therapy in stroke patients. *Neuroscience Letters*, Vol. 250, pp. (5-8).

Lindberg, P. G., Bensmail, D., Bussel, B., Maier, M. A., & Feydy, A. (2010). Wallerian Degeneration in Lateral Cervical Spinal Cord Detected with Diffusion Tensor Imaging in Four Chronic Stroke Patients. *Journal of Neuroimaging*, Vol. 21, No. 1, pp. (44–48).

Lindenberg, R., Zhu, L. L., Rüber, T., & Schlaug, G. (2011). Predicting functional motor potential in chronic stroke patients using diffusion tensor imaging. *Human brain mapping*.

Ling, L., Zeng, J., Pei, Z., Cheung, R. T., Hou, Q., Xing, S., & Zhang, S. (2009). Neurogenesis and angiogenesis within the ipsilateral thalamus with secondary damage after focal cortical infarction in hypertensive rats, Vol. 29, No. 9, pp. (1538–1546).

Liu, K., Lu, Y., Lee, J. K., Samara, R., Willenberg, R., Sears-Kraxberger, I., Tedeschi, A., et al. (2010). PTEN deletion enhances the regenerative ability of adult corticospinal neurons. *Nature Neuroscience*, Vol. 13, No. 9, pp. (1075–1081).

Liu, X., Tian, W., Qiu, X., Li, J., Thomson, S., Li, L., & Wang, H. Z. (2011). Correlation Analysis of Quantitative Diffusion Parameters in Ipsilateral Cerebral Peduncle during Wallerian Degeneration with Motor Function Outcome after Cerebral Ischemic Stroke. *Journal of Neuroimaging*,

Liu, Y., Liu, X.-J., & Dandan, S. (2009a). Ion transporters and ischemic mitochondrial dysfunction. *Cell Adhesion & Migration*, Vol. 3, No. 1, pp. (94–98).

Liu, Z., Li, Y., Qu, R., Shen, L., Gao, Q., Zhang, X., Lu, M., et al. (2007). Axonal sprouting into the denervated spinal cord and synaptic and postsynaptic protein expression in the spinal cord after transplantation of bone marrow stromal cell in stroke rats. *Brain Research*, Vol. 1149, pp. (172–180).

Liu, Z., Li, Y, Zhang, R. L., Cui, Y., & Chopp, M. (2011). Bone Marrow Stromal Cells Promote Skilled Motor Recovery and Enhance Contralesional Axonal Connections After Ischemic Stroke in Adult Mice. *Stroke*, Vol. 42, No. 3, pp. (740–744).

Liu, Z., Li, Y., Zhang, X., Savant-Bhonsale, S., & Chopp, Michael. (2008). Contralesional axonal remodeling of the corticospinal system in adult rats after stroke and bone marrow stromal cell treatment. *Stroke*, Vol. 39, No. 9, pp. (2571–2577).

Liu, Z., Zhang, R. L., Li, Y, Cui, Y., & Chopp, M. (2009). Remodeling of the Corticospinal Innervation and Spontaneous Behavioral Recovery After Ischemic Stroke in Adult Mice. *Stroke*, Vol. 40, No. 7, pp. (2546–2551).

Liu, X., Tian, W., Li, L., Kolar, B., Qiu, X., Chen, F., & Dogra, V. S. (2011). Hyperintensity on diffusion weighted image along ipsilateral cortical spinal tract after cerebral ischemic stroke: A diffusion tensor analysis. *European Journal of Radiology*,

Liu, Y., Karonen, J. O., Nuutinen, J., Vanninen, E., Kuikka, J. T., & Vanninen, R. L. (2007). Crossed cerebellar diaschisis in acute ischemic stroke: A study with serial SPECT and MRI. *Journal of Cerebral Blood Flow and Metabolism : Official Journal of the International Society of Cerebral Blood Flow and Metabolism*, Vol. 27, No. 10, pp. (1724-1732).

Luhmann, H. J., Mudrick-Donnon, L. A., Mittmann, T., & Heinemann, U. (1995). Ischaemia-induced long-term hyperexcitability in rat neocortex. *The European Journal of Neuroscience*, Vol. 7, No. 2, pp. (180-191).

Lundell, H., Christensen, M. S., Barthélemy, D., Willerslev-Olsen, M., Biering-Sørensen, F., & Nielsen, J. B. (2011). Cerebral activation is correlated to regional atrophy of the spinal cord and functional motor disability in spinal cord injured individuals. *NeuroImage*, Vol. 54, No. 2, pp. (1254-1261).

Mabuchi, T., Kitagawa, K., Ohtsuki, T., Kuwabara, K., Yagita, Y., Yanagihara, T., Hori, M., et al. (2000). Contribution of microglia/macrophages to expansion of infarction and response of oligodendrocytes after focal cerebral ischemia in rats. *Stroke*, Vol. 31, No. 7, pp. (1735–1743).

Madhavan, S., Krishnan, C., Jayaraman, A., Rymer, W. Z., & Stinear, J. W. (2011). Corticospinal tract integrity correlates with knee extensor weakness in chronic stroke survivors. *Clinical neurophysiology*, pp. (1–7).

Majewska, A. K. (2006). Remodeling of Synaptic Structure in Sensory Cortical Areas In Vivo. *Journal of Neuroscience*, Vol. 26, No. 11, pp. (3021–3029).

Manganotti, P., Acler, M., Zanette, G. P., Smania, N., & Fiaschi, A. (2008). Motor cortical disinhibition during early and late recovery after stroke. *Neurorehabilitation and Neural Repair*, Vol. 22, No. 4, pp. (396-403).

Mergenthaler P., Dirnagl U., Meisel A. (2004) Pathophysiology of stroke: Lessons from animal models. *Metabolic Brain Disease*, Vol. 19, pp. (151-167).

Minnerup, J., Kim, J. B., Schmidt, A., Diederich, K., Bauer, H., Schilling, M., Strecker, J. K., et al. (2011). Effects of Neural Progenitor Cells on Sensorimotor Recovery and Endogenous Repair Mechanisms After Photothrombotic Stroke. *Stroke*, Vol. 42, No. 6, pp. (1757–1763).

Mittmann T., Qu M., Zilles K., Luhmann H.J. (1998) Long-term cellular dysfunction after focal cerebral ischemia: In vitro analyses. *Neuroscience*, Vol. 85, pp. (15-27).

Mohajerani, M. H., Aminoltejari, K., & Murphy, T. H. (2011). Targeted mini-strokes produce changes in interhemispheric sensory signal processing that are indicative of disinhibition within minutes. *Proceedings of the National Academy of Sciences of the United States of America*, Vol. 108, No. 22, pp. (E183-91).

Mori, S., Crain, B. J., Chacko, V. P., & van Zijl, P. C. (1999). Three-dimensional tracking of axonal projections in the brain by magnetic resonance imaging. *Annals of Neurology*, Vol. 45, No. 2, pp. (265-269).

Mostany, R., Chowdhury, T. G., Johnston, D. G., Portonovo, S. A., Carmichael, S. T., & Portera-Cailliau, C. (2010). Local Hemodynamics Dictate Long-Term Dendritic Plasticity in Peri-Infarct Cortex. *Journal of Neuroscience*, Vol. 30, No. 42, pp. (14116–14126).

Mostany, R., & Portera-Cailliau, C. (2011). Absence of Large-Scale Dendritic Plasticity of Layer 5 Pyramidal Neurons in Peri-Infarct Cortex. *Journal of Neuroscience*, Vol. 31, No. 5, pp. (1734–1738).

Murphy, Timothy H, & Corbett, D. (2009). Plasticity during stroke recovery: from synapse to behaviour. *Nature Reviews Neuroscience*, Vol. 10, No. 12, pp. (861–872).

Murphy, T. H., Li, P., Betts, K., & Liu, R. (2008). Two-photon imaging of stroke onset in vivo reveals that NMDA-receptor independent ischemic depolarization is the major cause of rapid reversible damage to dendrites and spines. *Journal of Neuroscience*, Vol. 28, No. 7, pp. (1756–1772).

Nagasawa, H., Kogure, K., Fujiwara, T., Itoh, M., & Ido, T. (1994). Metabolic disturbances in exo-focal brain areas after cortical stroke studied by positron emission tomography. *Journal of the Neurological Sciences*, Vol. 123, No. 1-2, pp. (147-153).

Nawashiro H., Martin D., Hallenbeck J.M. (1997) Neuroprotective effects of TNF binding protein in focal cerebral ischemia. *Brain Research*, Vol. 778, pp. (265-271).

Nelles G., Spiekramann G., Jueptner M., Leonhardt G., Muller S., Gerhard H., Diener H.C. (1999a) Evolution of functional reorganization in hemiplegic stroke: A serial positron emission tomographic activation study. *Annals of Neurology*, Vol. 46, pp. (901-909).

Nelles G., Spiekermann G., Jueptner M., Leonhardt G., Muller S., Gerhard H., Diener H.C. (1999b) Reorganization of sensory and motor systems in hemiplegic stroke patients. A positron emission tomography study. *Stroke*, Vol. 30, pp. (1510-1516).

Neumann-Haefelin, T., Hagemann, G., & Witte, O. W. (1995). Cellular correlates of neuronal hyperexcitability in the vicinity of photochemically induced cortical infarcts in rats in vitro. *Neuroscience Letters*, Vol. 193, No. 2, pp. (101-104).

Neumann-Haefelin, T., Bosse, F., Redecker, C., Muller, H. W., & Witte, O. W. (1999). Upregulation of GABAA-receptor alpha1- and alpha2-subunit mRNAs following ischemic cortical lesions in rats. *Brain Research*, Vol. 816, No. 1, pp. (234-237).

Niizuma, K., Endo, H., & Chan, Pak H. (2009). Oxidative stress and mitochondrial dysfunction as determinants of ischemic neuronal death and survival. *Journal of Neurochemistry*, Vol. 109, pp. (133–138).

NINDS Tissue plasminogen activator for acute ischemic stroke. the national institute of neurological disorders and stroke rt-PA stroke study group. (1995) *New England Journal of Medicine*, Vol. 333, pp. (1581-1587).

Nudo R.J. & Milliken G.W. (1996) Reorganization of movement representations in primary motor cortex following focal ischemic infarcts in adult squirrel monkeys. *Journal of Neurophysiology,* Vol. 75, pp. (2144-2149).

O'Brien, M. D., Waltz, A. G., & Jordan, M. M. (1974). Ischemic cerebral edema. distribution of water in brains of cats after occlusion of the middle cerebral artery. *Archives of Neurology,* Vol. 30, No. 6, pp. (456-460).

Pettigrew, L. C., Kindy, M. S., Scheff, S., Springer, J. E., Kryscio, R. J., Li, Y., et al. (2008). Focal cerebral ischemia in the TNFalpha-transgenic rat. *Journal of Neuroinflammation,* Vol. 5, pp. (47).

Pierpaoli, C., Barnett, A., Pajevic, S., Chen, R., Penix, L. R., Virta, A., et al. (2001). Water diffusion changes in wallerian degeneration and their dependence on white matter architecture. *NeuroImage,* Vol. 13, No. 6, pp. (1174-1185).

Platz, T., Denzler, P., Kaden, B., & Mauritz, K. H. (1994). Motor learning after recovery from hemiparesis. *Neuropsychologia,* Vol. 32, No. 10, pp. (1209-1223).

Puig, J., Pedraza, S., Blasco, G., Daunis-I-Estadella, J., Prats, A., Prados, F., Boada, I., et al. (2010). Wallerian degeneration in the corticospinal tract evaluated by diffusion tensor imaging correlates with motor deficit 30 days after middle cerebral artery ischemic stroke. *AJNR. American journal of neuroradiology,* Vol. 31, No. 7, pp. (1324–1330).

Que, M., Schiene, K., Witte, O. W., & Zilles, K. (1999). Widespread up-regulation of N-methyl-D-aspartate receptors after focal photothrombotic lesion in rat brain. *Neuroscience Letters,* Vol. 273, No. 2, pp. (77–80).

Qü, M., Mittmann, T., Luhmann, H. J., Schleicher, A., & Zilles, K. (1998). Long-term changes of ionotropic glutamate and GABA receptors after unilateral permanent focal cerebral ischemia in the mouse brain. *Neuroscience,* Vol.85, No. 1, pp. (29–43).

Reinecke, S., Dinse, H. R., Reinke, H., & Witte, O. W. (2003). Induction of bilateral plasticity in sensory cortical maps by small unilateral cortical infarcts in rats. *The European Journal of Neuroscience,* Vol. 17, No. 3, pp. (623-627).

Reitmeir, R., Kilic, E., Kilic, U., Bacigaluppi, M., ElAli, A., Salani, G., Pluchino, S., et al. (2011). Post-acute delivery of erythropoietin induces stroke recovery by promoting perilesional tissue remodelling and contralesional pyramidal tract plasticity. *Brain : a journal of neurology,* Vol.134, No. 1, pp. (84–99).

Remple M.S., Bruneau R.M., VandenBerg P.M., Goertzen C., Kleim J.A. (2001) Sensitivity of cortical movement representations to motor experience: Evidence that skill learning but not strength training induces cortical reorganization. *Behavioral Brain Research,* Vol. 123, pp. (133-141).

Riecker, A., Gröschel, K., Ackermann, H., Schnaudigel, S., Kassubek, J., & Kastrup, A. (2010). The role of the unaffected hemisphere in motor recovery after stroke. *Human brain mapping,* Vol. 31, No. 7, pp. (1017–1029).

Ritter, L. S., Orozco, J. A., Coull, B. M., McDonagh, P. F., & Rosenblum, W. I. (2000). Leukocyte accumulation and hemodynamic changes in the cerebral microcirculation during early reperfusion after stroke. *Stroke; a Journal of Cerebral Circulation,* Vol. 31, No. 5, pp. (1153-1161).

Rosenzweig, E. S., Courtine, G., Jindrich, D. L., Brock, J. H., Ferguson, A. R., Strand, S. C., Nout, Y. S., et al. (2010). Extensive spontaneous plasticity of corticospinal projections after primate spinal cord injury. *Nature Neuroscience,* Vol. 13, No. 12, pp. (1505–1510).

Schaechter J.D. (2004) Motor rehabilitation and brain plasticity after hemiparetic stroke. *Progress in Neurobiology,* Vol. 73, pp. (61-72).

Schaechter J.D., Moore C.I., Connell B.D., Rosen B.R., Dijkhuizen R.M. (2006) Structural and functional plasticity in the somatosensory cortex of chronic stroke patients. *Brain,* Vol. 129, pp. (2722-2733).

Schiene, K., Bruehl, C., Zilles, K., Qü, M., Hagemann, G., Kraemer, M., & Witte, O. W. (1996). Neuronal hyperexcitability and reduction of GABAA-receptor expression in the surround of cerebral photothrombosis. *Journal of cerebral blood flow and metabolism : official journal of the International Society of Cerebral Blood Flow and Metabolism,* Vol. 16, No. 5, pp. (906–914).

Seitz R.J., Hoflich P., Binkofski F., Tellmann L., Herzog H., Freund H.J. (1998) Role of the premotor cortex in recovery from middle cerebral artery infarction. *Archives of Neurology,* Vol. 55, pp. (1081-1088).

Sigler, A., Mohajerani, M. H., & Murphy, T. H. (2009). Imaging rapid redistribution of sensory-evoked depolarization through existing cortical pathways after targeted stroke in mice. *Proceedings of the National Academy of Sciences of the United States of America,* Vol. 106, No. 28, pp. (11759-11764).

Slater, R., Reivich, M., Goldberg, H., Banka, R., & Greenberg, J. (1977). Diaschisis with cerebral infarction. *Stroke; a Journal of Cerebral Circulation,* Vol. 8, No. 6, pp. (684-690).

Somjen, G. G. (2001). Mechanisms of spreading depression and hypoxic spreading depression-like depolarization. *Physiological Reviews,* Vol. 81, No. 3, pp. (1065-1096).

Steriade, M., & Llinas, R. R. (1988). The functional states of the thalamus and the associated neuronal interplay. *Physiological Reviews,* Vol. 68, No. 3, pp. (649-742).

Steward, O., Zheng, B., Tessier-Lavigne, M., Hofstadter, M., Sharp, K., & Yee, K. M. (2008). Regenerative Growth of Corticospinal Tract Axons via the Ventral Column after Spinal Cord Injury in Mice. *Journal of Neuroscience,* Vol. 28, No. 27, pp. (6836–6847).

Stroemer, R. P., Kent, T. A., & Hulsebosch, C. E. (1995). Neocortical neural sprouting, synaptogenesis, and behavioral recovery after neocortical infarction in rats. *Stroke,* Vol. 26, No. 11, pp. (2135–2144).

Takasawa, M., Watanabe, M., Yamamoto, S., Hoshi, T., Sasaki, T., Hashikawa, K., . . . Kinoshita, N. (2002). Prognostic value of subacute crossed cerebellar diaschisis: Single-photon emission CT study in patients with middle cerebral artery territory infarct. *AJNR.American Journal of Neuroradiology,* Vol. 23, No. 2, pp. (189-193).

Takatsuru, Y., Fukumoto, D., Yoshitomo, M., Nemoto, T., Tsukada, H., & Nabekura, J. (2009). Neuronal Circuit Remodeling in the Contralateral Cortical Hemisphere during Functional Recovery from Cerebral Infarction. *Journal of Neuroscience,* Vol. 29, No. 32, pp. (10081–10086).

Tamura, A., Tahira, Y., Nagashima, H., Kirino, T., Gotoh, O., Hojo, S., & Sano, K. (1991). Thalamic atrophy following cerebral infarction in the territory of the middle cerebral artery. *Stroke,* Vol. 22, No. 5, pp. (615–618).

Thomalla, G., Glauche, V., Koch, M., Beaulieu, C., Weiller, C., & Rother, J. (2004). Diffusion tensor imaging detects early Wallerian degeneration of the pyramidal tract after ischemic stroke. *NeuroImage,* Vol. 22, No. 4, pp. (1767–1774).

Thornton, P., McColl, B. W., Greenhalgh, A., Denes, A., Allan, S. M., & Rothwell, N. J. (2010). Platelet interleukin-1alpha drives cerebrovascular inflammation. *Blood,* Vol. 115, No. 17, pp. (3632-3639).

Traversa R., Cicinelli P., Bassi A., Rossini P.M., Bernardi G. (1997) Mapping of motor cortical reorganization after stroke. A brain stimulation study with focal magnetic pulses. *Stroke,* Vol. 28, pp. (110-117).

Tsai, S. Y., Markus, T. M., Andrews, E. M., Cheatwood, J. L., Emerick, A. J., Mir, A. K., et al. (2007). Intrathecal treatment with anti-nogo-A antibody improves functional recovery in adult rats after stroke. *Experimental Brain Research.Experimentelle Hirnforschung.Experimentation Cerebrale,* Vol. 182, No. 2, pp. (261-266).

Umegaki, M. (2005). Peri-Infarct Depolarizations Reveal Penumbra-Like Conditions in Striatum. *Journal of Neuroscience,* Vol. 25, No. 6, pp. (1387–1394).

van der Zijden J.P., van der Toorn A., van der Marel K., Dijkhuizen R.M. (2008) Longitudinal in vivo MRI of alterations in perilesional tissue after transient ischemic stroke in rats. *Experimental Neurology,* Vol. 212, pp. (207-212).

van der Zijden J.P., Wu O., van der Toorn A., Roeling T.P., Bleys R.L., Dijkhuizen R.M. (2007) Changes in neuronal connectivity after stroke in rats as studied by serial manganese-enhanced MRI. *Neuroimage,* Vol. 34, pp. (1650-1657).

Vila, Nicolás, Castillo, J., Dávalos, A., Esteve, A., Planas, A. M., & Chamorro, A. (2003). Levels of anti-inflammatory cytokines and neurological worsening in acute ischemic stroke. *Stroke,* Vol. 34, No. 3, pp. (671–675).

Vila, N, Castillo, J., Dávalos, A., & Chamorro, A. (2000). Proinflammatory cytokines and early neurological worsening in ischemic stroke. *Stroke,* Vol. 31, No. 10, pp. (2325–2329).

Wang, T., Wang, J., Yin, C., Liu, R., Zhang, J. H., & Qin, X. (2010). Down-regulation of Nogo receptor promotes functional recovery by enhancing axonal connectivity after experimental stroke in rats. *Brain Research,* Vo. 1360, pp. (147–158).

Ward N.S., Brown M.M., Thompson A.J., Frackowiak R.S. (2006) Longitudinal changes in cerebral response to proprioceptive input in individual patients after stroke: An FMRI study. *Neurorehabilitation and Neural Repair,* Vol. 20, pp. (398-405).

Ward, N. S., Brown, M. M., Thompson, A. J., & Frackowiak, R. S. (2003). Neural correlates of outcome after stroke: A cross-sectional fMRI study. *Brain : A Journal of Neurology,* Vol. 126, No. 6, pp. (1430-1448).

Weber R., Ramos-Cabrer P., Justicia C., Wiedermann D., Strecker C., Sprenger C., Hoehn M. (2008) Early prediction of functional recovery after experimental stroke: Functional magnetic resonance imaging, electrophysiology, and behavioral testing in rats. *Journal of Neuroscience,* Vol. 28, pp. (1022-1029).

Wei L., Erinjeri J.P., Rovainen C.M., Woolsey T.A. (2001) Collateral growth and angiogenesis around cortical stroke. *Stroke,* Vol. 32, pp. (2179-2184).

Weiller C., Ramsay S.C., Wise R.J., Friston K.J., Frackowiak R.S. (1993) Individual patterns of functional reorganization in the human cerebral cortex after capsular infarction. *Annals of Neurology,* Vol. 33, pp. (181-189).

Weishaupt, N., Silasi, G., Colbourne, F., Fouad, K. (2010). Secondary damage in the spinal cord after motor cortex injury in rats. *Journal of Neurotrauma,* Vol. 27, pp. (1387-1397).

Werring, D. J., Toosy, A. T., Clark, C. A., Parker, G. J., Barker, G. J., Miller, D. H., et al. (2000). Diffusion tensor imaging can detect and quantify corticospinal tract degeneration after stroke. *Journal of Neurology, Neurosurgery, and Psychiatry,* Vol. 69, No. 2, pp. (269-272).

Wiessner, C., Bareyre, F. M., Allegrini, P. R., Mir, A. K., Frentzel, S., Zurini, M., et al. (2003). Anti-nogo-A antibody infusion 24 hours after experimental stroke improved behavioral outcome and corticospinal plasticity in normotensive and spontaneously hypertensive rats. *Journal of Cerebral Blood Flow and Metabolism : Official Journal of the International Society of Cerebral Blood Flow and Metabolism,* Vol. 23, No. 2, pp. (154-165).

Winship, I. R., & Murphy, T H. (2009). Remapping the Somatosensory Cortex after Stroke: Insight from Imaging the Synapse to Network. *The Neuroscientist*, Vol. 15, No. 5, pp. (507–524).

Winship I.R. & Murphy T.H. (2008) In vivo calcium imaging reveals functional rewiring of single somatosensory neurons after stroke. *Journal of Neuroscience,* Vol. 28, pp. (6592-6606).

Witte, O. W., Bidmon, H. J., Schiene, K., Redecker, C., & Hagemann, G. (2000). Functional differentiation of multiple perilesional zones after focal cerebral ischemia. *Journal of Cerebral Blood Flow and Metabolism : Official Journal of the International Society of Cerebral Blood Flow and Metabolism,* Vol. 20, No. 8, pp. (1149-1165).

Wolf, T., Lindauer, U., Reuter, U., Back, T., Villringer, A., Einhaupl, K., et al. (1997). Noninvasive near infrared spectroscopy monitoring of regional cerebral blood oxygenation changes during peri-infarct depolarizations in focal cerebral ischemia in the rat. *Journal of Cerebral Blood Flow and Metabolism : Official Journal of the International Society of Cerebral Blood Flow and Metabolism,* Vol. 17, No. 9, pp. (950-954).

Yu, C., Zhu, C., Zhang, Y., Chen, H., Qin, W., Wang, M., & Li, K. (2009). A longitudinal diffusion tensor imaging study on Wallerian degeneration of corticospinal tract after motor pathway stroke. *NeuroImage,* Vol. 47, No. 2, pp. (451–458). ISSN: 1053-8119

Zai, L., Ferrari, C., Dice, C., Subbaiah, S., Havton, L. A., Coppola, G., et al. (2011). Inosine augments the effects of a nogo receptor blocker and of environmental enrichment to restore skilled forelimb use after stroke. *The Journal of Neuroscience : The Official Journal of the Society for Neuroscience,* Vol. 31, No. 16, pp. (5977-5988).

Zhang, S., & Murphy, Timothy H. (2007). Imaging the impact of cortical microcirculation on synaptic structure and sensory-evoked hemodynamic responses in vivo. *PLoS biology,* Vol. 5, No. 5, pp. (e119).

Zhang, Y., Xiong, Y., Mahmood, A., Meng, Y., Liu, Z., Qu, C., & Chopp, M. (2010). Sprouting of corticospinal tract axons from the contralateral hemisphere into the denervated side of the spinal cord is associated with functional recovery in adult rat after traumatic brain injury and erythropoietin treatment. *Brain Research,* Vol. 1353, pp. (249–257).

Zipfel, G. J., Babcock, D. J., Lee, J. M., & Choi, D. W. (2000). Neuronal apoptosis after CNS injury: The roles of glutamate and calcium. *Journal of Neurotrauma,* Vol. 17, No. 10, pp. (857-869).

2

Excitotoxicity and Oxidative Stress in Acute Ischemic Stroke

Ramón Rama Bretón[1] and Julio César García Rodríguez[2]
[1]*Department of Physiology & Immunology, University of Barcelona*
[2]*CENPALAB*
[1]*Spain*
[2]*Cuba*

1. Introduction

The term "stroke" is applied to a heterogeneous group of diseases caused by decreased perfusion of the brain due to occlusion of the blood vessels supplying the brain or a haemorrhage originating in them. Most strokes (~ 85%) are ischemic; that is, they result from occlusion of a major cerebral artery by a thrombus or embolism. This results in reduced blood flow and a major decrease in the supply of oxygen and nutrients to the affected region. The rest of strokes are haemorrhagic: caused by the rupture of a blood vessel either in the brain or on its surface.

Strokes deprive the brain not only of oxygen but also of glucose and of all other nutrients, as well as disrupting the nutrient/waste exchange process required to support brain metabolism. The result is the development of a hypoxic-ischemic state. Ischemia is defined as a decrease in blood flow to tissues that prevents adequate delivery of oxygen, glucose and others nutrients. Ischemic stroke is the result of total or partial interruption of cerebral arterial blood supply, which leads to oxygen and glucose deprivation of the tissue (ischemia). If cerebral arterial blood flow is not restored within a short period, cerebral ischemia is the usual result, with subsequent neuron death within the perfusion territory of the vessels affected. Ischemic stroke is characterized by a complex sequence of events that evolves over hours or even days [1-3]. Acute ischemic stroke results from acute occlusion of cerebral arteries. Cerebral ischemia occurs when blood flow to the brain decreases to a level where the metabolic needs of the tissue are not met. Cerebral ischemia may be either transient (followed by reperfusion) or essentially permanent. In all cases, a stroke involves dysfunction and death of brain neurons and neurological damage that reflects the location and size of the brain area affected [1, 2].

2. Ischemic core and ischemic penumbra

Neuropathological analysis after focal brain ischemia reveals two separate areas: the ischemic core, and ischemic penumbra. Once onset of a stroke has occurred, within minutes of focal ischemia occurring, the regions of the brain that suffer the most severe degrees of blood flow reduction experience irreversible damage: these regions are the "ischemic core". This area exhibits a very low cerebral blood flow (CBF) and very low metabolic rates of oxygen and glucose [2, 3]. Thus, reduced or interrupted CBF has negative effects on brain structure and function. Neurons in the ischemic core of the infarction are killed rapidly by total bioenergetic failure and breakdown of ion homeostasis, lipolysis and proteolysis, as well as cell membrane fragmentation [4]. The result is cell death within minutes [5]. Tissue in the ischemic core is irreversibly injured even if blood flow is re-established.

The necrotic core is surrounded by a region of brain tissue which suffers moderate blood flow reduction, thus becoming functionally impaired but remaining metabolically active; this is known as the "ischemic penumbra" [6]. This metabolically active border region remains electrically silent [7]. From experiments in non-human primates, it has been shown that in this region, the ability of neurons to fire action potentials is lost. However, these neurons maintain enough energy to sustain their resting membrane potentials and when collateral blood flow improves, action potentials are restored. The ischemic penumbra may comprise as much as half the total lesion volume during the initial stages of ischemia, and represents the region in which there is an opportunity to salvage functionality via post-stroke therapy [8, 9].

Ischemic penumbra refers to the region of brain tissue that is functionally impaired but structurally intact; tissue lying between the lethally damaged core and the normal brain, where blood flow is sufficiently reduced to result in hypoxia that is severe enough to arrest physiological function, but not so complete as to cause irreversible failure of energy metabolism and cellular necrosis [8]. The ischemic penumbra has been documented in laboratory animals as severely hypoperfused, non-functional, but still viable brain tissue surrounding the irreversibly damaged ischemic core [10]. The penumbra can be identified by the biochemical and molecular mechanisms of neuron death [11, 12] and by means of clinical neuroimaging tools [10, 13].

Thus, the ischemic penumbra refers to areas of the brain that are damaged during a stroke but not killed. The concept therefore emerges that once onset of a stroke has begun, the necrotic core is surrounded by a zone of less severely reduced blood flow where the neurons have lost functional activity but remain metabolically active. Tissue injury in the ischemic penumbra is the outcome of a complex series of genetic, molecular and biochemical mechanisms, which contribute either to protecting -and then penumbral tissue is repaired and recovers functional activity- or to damaging -and then the penumbral area becomes necrotic -brain cells. Tissue damage and functional impairment after cerebral ischemia result from the interaction between endogenous neuroprotective mechanisms such as anti-excitotoxicity (GABA, adenosine and K_{ATP} activation), anti-inflammation and anti-apoptosis (IL-10, Epo, Bcl-proteins), and repair and regeneration (c-Src formation, vasculogenesis, neurogenesis, BM-derived cells) on the one hand, with neurotoxic events such as excitotoxicity, inflammation and apoptosis that ultimately lead to cell death, on the other [14]. The penumbra is the battle field where the ischemic cascade with several deleterious mechanisms is triggered, resulting in ongoing cellular injury and infarct progression. Ultimately, the ischemic penumbra is consumed by progressive damage and coalesces with the core, often within hours of the onset of the stroke. However, the penumbra can be rescued by improving the blood flow and/or interfering with the ischemic cascade. At the onset of a stroke, the evolution of the ischemic penumbra is only partially predictable from the clinical, laboratory and imaging methods currently available [3, 10].

3. Pathophysiological basis of the stroke

In the last 30 years, experimental and clinical results have led to characterizations of the pathophysiological basis of strokes [1-3]. Cerebral ischemia (ischemic stroke) triggers a complex series of physiological, biochemical, molecular and genetic mechanisms that impair neurologic functions through a breakdown of cellular integrity mediated by ionic imbalance, glutamate-mediated excitotoxicity and also such phenomena as calcium overload, oxidative stress, mitochondrial dysfunction and apoptosis [1-3, 15, 16]. These mediate injury to neurons, glia cells and vascular elements by means of disturbing the function of important cellular organelles such as mitochondria, nuclei, cell membranes, endoplasmic reticula and lysosomes. The result is cell death via mechanisms that promote rupture, lysis, phagocytosis or involution and shrinkage [11, 16]. Knowledge of the molecular mechanisms that underlie neuron death following a stroke is important if we are to devise effective neuroprotective strategies.

We will examine how ischemic injury occurs, which cell death mechanisms are activated, especially excitotoxicity and oxidative stress, and how these can be manipulated to induce neuroprotection. Unfortunately, despite their effectiveness in preclinical studies, a large number of neuroprotectants have failed to produce the desired effects in clinical trials involving stroke sufferers, which suggests that we still lack essential knowledge of the triggers and mediators of ischemic neuron death. We will discuss why, after 30 years or so of intense basic and clinical research, we still find it extremely difficult to translate experimental neuroprotective success in the laboratory to the clinical setting [17-20].

3.1 Acute ischemic injury in strokes

Acute ischemic injury is the result of a transient or permanent reduction of CBF in a restricted vascular territory. Normal CBF is between 45 and 60 ml blood/100 g/min. It is well documented that time-dependent neuronal events are triggered in response to reduced CBF [21, 22]. The brain has critical thresholds for CBF and for oxygen tension. Oxygen supply to the brain below a critical level reduces, and eventually blocks, oxidative phosphorylation, drastically decreases cellular ATP and leads to the collapse of ion gradients. Neuron activity ceases and if oxygen is not re-introduced quickly, cells die [22]. A reduction of cortical blood flow to levels of approximately 20 ml/100 g/min may be tolerated without functional consequences, but it is associated with the loss of consciousness and ECG alterations. At values of CBF below 18 ml/100 g/min, the tissue infarction is time dependent: CBF of 5 ml/100 g/min lasting about 30 minutes cause infarction; CBF of 10 ml/100 g/min needs to last for more than 3 hours to cause infarction; permanent CBF below 18 ml/100 g/min causes irreversible damage [22, 23]. In focal ischemia, complete cessation of blood flow is uncommon because collateral vessels sustain CBF at 5 to 15 ml/100 g/minute in the ischemic core and at 15 to 25 ml/100 g/minute in the outer areas of the ischemic zone [5, 21, 24]. Global ischemia results from transient CBF below 0.5 ml/100 g/min or severe hypoxia to the entire brain. When CBF falls to zero within seconds, loss of consciousness occurs after approximately 10 s, EEG activity ceases after 30–40 s, cellular damage is initiated after a few minutes, and death occurs within 10 min, at least under normothermic conditions [25].

The brain is highly vulnerable to ischemia. In part, the vulnerability of brain tissue to ischemia reflects its high metabolic demands. The brain has a relatively high energy production demand and depends almost exclusively on oxidative phosphorylation for energy production. Although the weight of the human brain is only about 2% of the total bodyweight, it has high metabolic activity and uses 20% of the oxygen and 25% of the glucose consumed by the entire body [23]. Proper functioning of brain cells depends on an abundant and continuous supply of oxygen. Even with such high metabolic demands, there is essentially no oxygen storage in cerebral tissue, and only limited reserves of high-energy phosphate compounds and carbohydrate substrates are available. More than 90% of the oxygen consumed by the brain is used by mitochondria to generate ATP. Energy in the brain is mainly formed when glucose is oxidized to CO_2 and water through mitochondrial oxidative phosphorylation. At rest, about 40% of cerebral energy is used to maintain and restore ionic gradients across cell membrane; even more energy is used during activity [23]. The brain requires large amounts of oxygen to generate sufficient ATP to maintain and restore ionic gradients.

3.2 Basic mechanisms of ischemic cell death

After the onset of a stroke, the disruptions to the blood flow in areas affected by vascular occlusion limit the delivery of oxygen and metabolic substrates to neurons causing ATP reduction and energy depletion. The glucose and oxygen deficit that occurs after severe vascular occlusion is the origin of the mechanisms that lead to cell death and consequently to cerebral injury. These mechanisms include: ionic imbalance, the release of excess glutamate in the extracellular space, a dramatic increase in intracellular calcium that in turn activates multiple intracellular death pathways such as mitochondrial dysfunction, and oxidative and nitrosative stress that finally cause neuron death.

After ischemic onset, the primary insult that ischemia causes neurons is a loss of oxygen and glucose substrate energy. While there are potentially large reserves of alternatives substrates to glucose, such as glycogen, lactate and fatty acids, for both glycolysis and respiration, oxygen is irreplaceable in mitochondrial oxidative phosphorylation, the main source of ATP in neurons. Consequently, the lack of oxygen interrupts oxidative phosphorylation by the mitochondria and drastically reduces cellular ATP production, which results in a rapid decline in cellular ATP [26, 27]. Although there are potentially large reserves of substrates such as glycogen, lactate and fatty acids that may be alternatives to glucose, anaerobic metabolism is insufficient to produce sufficient ATP. Reduced ATP stimulates the glycolytic metabolism of residual glucose and glycogen, causing an accumulation of protons and lactate, which leads to rapid intracellular acidification and increases the depletion of ATP [26]. When the lack of oxygen is severe and glucose is diminished, inhibition of oxidative phosphorylation leads to ATP-synthase functioning backwards and consuming ATP, thus contributing to an increase in the loss of ATP [27]. If ATP levels are low, the Na^+/K^+-ATPase function fails [27]. After several minutes, inhibition of the Na^+/K^+-ATPase function causes a profound loss of ionic gradients and the depolarization of neurons and astrocytes [28]. Membrane depolarization and changes in the concentration gradients of Na^+ and K^+ across the plasma membrane result in activation of voltage-gated calcium channels. This leads to excessive release of excitatory amino acids -particularly glutamate- to the extracellular compartment (Fig. 1).

Uncontrolled membrane depolarization by massive changes in the concentration gradients of Na^+ and K^+ across the plasma membrane results in a large and sustained release of glutamate and other neurotransmitters to the extracellular compartment [29]. Simultaneously, neurotransmitter re-uptake from the extracellular space is reduced [30, 31]. The rise in the extracellular glutamate concentration initiates a positive feedback loop, with further activation of glutamate receptors in neighbouring neurons and as a result, more Na^+ inflow to neurons via monovalent ion channels that decrease ionic gradients and consume ATP, both of which promote further release of glutamate [32, 33]. Simultaneously, glutamate transporters in neurons and astrocytes can function backwards, releasing glutamate into the extracellular space [31, 34] and contributing to glutamate overload there. A marked and prolonged rise in the extracellular glutamate concentration kills central neurons [2, 11, 32]. Excessive glutamate in the synapses activates the ionotropic glutamate receptors at a pathophysiological level; this type of neuronal insult is called excitotoxicity [29] and is defined as cell death resulting from the toxic actions of excitatory amino acids. Because glutamate is the most important excitatory neurotransmitter in primary perception and constitutes the basis of synaptic transmission in about 10^{14} synapses in the human brain, neuronal excitotoxicity usually refers to the injury and death of neurons arising from prolonged intense exposure to glutamate and the associated ionic imbalance in the cell. Excessive activation of glutamate receptors by excitatory amino acids leads to a number of deleterious consequences, including impairment of calcium buffering, generation of free radicals, activation of the mitochondrial permeability transition and secondary excitotoxicity.

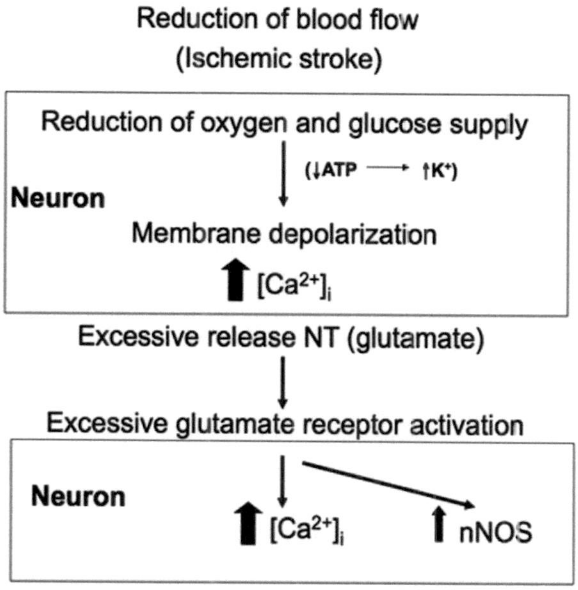

Fig. 1. Excitotoxicity in ischemic stroke. The reduction of blood flow supply to the brain during ischemic stroke results in oxygen and glucose deprivation and thus a reduction in energy available to maintain the ionic gradients. This results in excessive neuronal depolarization and deregulated glutamate release.

3.3 Excitotoxic mechanisms

Excitotoxicity is considered to be the central mechanism underlying neuron death in stroke [29, 32-35]. Excitotoxicity is considered to trigger tissue damage in both focal experimental ischemia [34, 36] and clinical ischemia [37]. Glutamate is released at high concentrations in the penumbral cortex [38], particularly if blood flow is reduced for a long period, and the amount of glutamate released correlates with early neurological deterioration in patients with acute ischemic stroke [37]. Glutamate concentrations greater than 200 mmol/l in plasma and greater than 8.2 mmol/l in CSF are associated with neurological deterioration in the acute phase of cerebral infarction.

The excitotoxic mechanisms which lead to neuron death are complex, but primarily involve the generation of free radicals [35; 39, 40], mitochondrial dysfunction [41, 42] and the participation of various transcription factors as activators of gene expression [43, 44]. All of these mechanisms acting synergistically can damage cellular proteins [45], lipids [46] and DNA [47, 48], which leads to the deterioration of cellular architecture and signalling, resulting in necrosis, apoptosis or both depending on the severity of the insult and of relative speed of each process [49-51].

3.4 The role of glutamate receptors in excitotoxicity

The excitatory effects of glutamate are mediated through two kinds of glutamate receptors – ionotropic receptors and metabotropic receptors linked to G-protein [52]– found in the pre- and post-synaptic neuron membranes of the central nervous system (CNS). Glutamate ionotropic receptors are ligand-gated cation channels permeable to Ca^{2+}. Although virtually all members of the glutamate receptor family are believed to be involved in mediating excitotoxicity [90], *N*-methyl-d-aspartate (NMDA) glutamate receptors are believed to be the key mediators of death during excitotoxic injury [53].

In recent years, the role of the structure of the NMDA glutamate receptors (NMDARs) in excitotoxicity has caused great therapeutic interest. NMDARs are complex heterotetramer combinations of three major subfamilies of subunits: the ubiquitously expressed NR1 subunit together with one of the four possible NR2 (A-D) subunits and, in some cases, two NR3 (A and B) subunits [54, 55]. Subunit NR1 contains the site where the glutamate is united to the receptor, whereas subunit NR2 contains the site where the glycine is united [56]. The NR3 subunit is present predominantly during brain development [57]. The distinct pharmacological and biophysical properties mediated by NMDARs are largely determined by the type of NR2 subunits incorporated into the heteromeric NR1/NR2 complex [58, 59]. Specific NR2 subtypes appear to play a pivotal role in strokes [60]. In a four-vessel occlusion model of transient global ischemia in rats, the blocking of NMDARs that contained NR2A enhanced neuron death and prevented the induction of ischemic tolerance, whereas inhibiting NMDARs that contained NR2B attenuated ischemic cell death and enhanced preconditioning-induced neuroprotection [61]. It has been suggested that excitotoxicity is triggered by the selective activation of NMDARs containing the NR2B subunit [61, 62] and a correlation between NR2B expression, a rise in cytosolic calcium and excitotoxicity was observed in cortical neurons [63]. Because NR2A and NR2B are the predominant NR2 subunits in the adult forebrain, where stroke most frequently occurs, NMDA receptors that contain NR2A and NR2B may play different roles in supporting neuronal survival and mediating neuron death, and hence have opposing impacts on excitotoxic brain damage after acute brain insults such as a stroke or brain trauma [60, 61].

NMDARs are found at synaptic or extrasynaptic sites [64, 65]. These different locations on cellular membrane have been considered a determining factor in excitotoxicity after a stroke [65, 66]. Depending on their location on the cell membrane, activation of NMDARs has dramatically different effects. Evidence suggests that synaptic NMDAR activity is necessary for neuronal survival while the extrasynaptic NMDARs are involved in cell death [65, 66]. Stimulation of synaptic NMDARs leads to expression of pro-survival proteins, such as BDNF (brain-derived neurotrophic factor) whereas activation of extrasynaptic NMDARs leads to expression of pro-apoptotic proteins and suppression of survival pathways [64,65, 67]. However, it has also been postulated that the apparent differences in excitotoxicity mediated by NMDARs could be due to differences in synaptic/extrasynaptic NMDAR molecular composition as opposed to the location of the receptors *per se*. In adults brain, NMDARs located in synapses predominantly contain the NR2A subtype; while extrasynaptic NMDARs predominantly contain NR2B [67-69]. Although there is little evidence that differences in subunit composition explain the differences between the synaptic and extrasynaptic effects of glutamate, a recent study showed that activation of NMDARs containing NR2B subunits tends to promote neuron death, irrespective of location, whereas activation of NMDARs containing NR2A subunits promotes survival [66]. However, have been shown that NR2A-NMDARs are capable of mediating excitotoxicity [70] and NR2B-NMDARs are capable of mediating both pro-survival and pro-death signalling, depending on the stimulation paradigm [69].

It has further been proposed that lethal Ca2+ signalling by NMDARs is determined by the molecules with which they interact [85]. At the synapse, NMDAR receptors are found localized within electron-dense structures known as the postsynaptic densities (PSDs) where they form large and dynamic multiprotein signalling complexes [71-73]. NMDARs interact with multiple intracellular synaptic and cytoskeletal proteins, mainly through the cytoplasmatic C-termini of the NR1 and NR2 subunits [74, 75]. The PSD is a multiprotein complex that includes a group of proteins called MAGUKs (membrane-associated guanylate kinases) [74-76]. These proteins contain several PDZ (post-synaptic density-95/discs large/zonula occludens-1) protein interaction domains through which they are connected to other proteins. PDZ is a common structure domain of 80-90 amino acids found in the signalling proteins. PDZ domains often function as modules in scaffolding proteins that are involved in assembling large protein complexes in the cell [73]. A prominent protein component in the PDZ complex is post-synaptic density-95 (PSD-95) [74, 75], which couples NMDARs to intracellular proteins and signalling enzymes. It also functions as a scaffolding and organizer protein of PSD [75, 76]. PSD-95 contains three PDZ domains, of the which the first two (PDZ1 and PDZ2) interact with the C termini of the NMDAR NR2B subunit. The NMDAR is linked to nNOS through the first and second PDZ domains of PSD-95 [76, 77]. Activation of the nNOS by NMDARs leads to the production of excessive levels of nitric oxide (NO) [71]. NO serves as a substrate for the production of highly reactive free radicals such as peroxynitrites, which promote cellular damage and ultimately neuron death [78-80]. Thus, during ischemia, Ca2+ influx through NMDARs promotes cell death more efficiently than through other Ca2+ channels [81], suggesting that proteins responsible for Ca2+-dependent excitotoxicity reside within the NMDAR signalling complex. Disrupting the NMDAR-PSD-95 or nNOS-PSD-95 complexes may reduce the efficiency by which Ca2+ ions activate excitotoxic signalling through molecules such as nNOS. In cortical neurons, suppression of PSD-95 selectively blocks NO production by NMDARs without affecting NOS expression [71]. In cultured neurons and in experimental animals, through the use of small peptides that disrupted the interaction of NMDARs with PSD-95, neurons were rendered resistant to focal cerebral ischemia [82]. It has been shown that inhibition of the NMDAR/PSD-95 interaction prevents ischemic brain damage, while the physiological function of the NMDAR remains intact [83]. The use of small peptides that bind to the PDZ domains of PSD-95 and block protein-protein interactions protected cultured neurons from excitotoxicity and dramatically reduced cerebral infarction in rats subjected to transient focal cerebral ischemia, and effectively improved their neurological function. The treatment was effective when applied either before, or 1 h after, the onset of excitotoxicity in vitro and cerebral ischemia in vivo [83]. Perturbing NMDAR/PSD-95 interactions with peptides that comprise the nine C-terminal residues of the NR2B subunit reduces the vulnerability of neurons to excitotoxicity and ischemia. Proteomic and biochemical analysis of all the known human PDZs with synaptic signalling proteins that include NR1 or NR2A-NR2D, shows that only neurons lacking PSD-95 or nNOS exhibited reduced excitotoxic vulnerability. Of all the PDZs examined, only PSD-p5 and nNOS participated significantly in excitotoxicity signalling. Thus, despite the ubiquity of proteins that contain the PDZ domain, the importance of the role of PSD-95 and nNOS over and above that of any other PDZ proteins in mediating NMDAR-dependent excitotoxicity was recently demonstrated [70]. Deletion of the PSD-95 dissociates NMDAR activity from NO production and suppresses excitotoxicity [84].

It remains an open question whether the death of neurons is mediated by different types of NMDAR subunits [66, 68] or only by distinct locations of the receptors [64, 65]. It is possible that Ca^{2+} toxicity is linked to the route of Ca^{2+} entry and the different second messenger pathways activated by Ca^{2+} entry [85].

Perhaps consideration of the NMDARs as the route to excitotoxicity is over-simplistic, since others mechanisms may be involved [86]. AMPA receptors are not normally calcium permeable due to their GluR2 subunit, nevertheless, after ischemia this subunit is reduced and the permeability of these receptors by calcium increases 18-fold, allowing AMPARs to contribute to increased intracellular calcium [87]. As just mentioned, injury during stroke may result from Ca^{2+}-overload due to overstimulation of AMPA receptors together with indirect Ca^{2+} entry through gated voltage-channels, Ca^{2+}-permeable acid-sensing ion channels [88], activation of metabotropic glutamate receptors via the release of Ca^{2+} from endoplasmic reticulum and via a cleavage of Na^{+}/ Ca^{2+} exchangers [89]. Consequently, it seems that in relation to the mechanisms that mediate cell death in stroke, the more important factor is the amount of cytosol Ca^{2+} free to accumulate and not the route of entry.

3.5 Ca^{2+} cytoplasmic overload, mitochondria dysfunction and oxidative stress

After a stroke, as a consequence of excessive extracellular glutamates, NMDARs are excessively activated resulting in increased Ca^{2+} influx [35, 81, 84]. Calcium plays a critical role in the excitotoxic cascade, because either removing Ca^{2+} from extracellular medium [90] or preventing Ca^{2+} from entering mitochondria by uncouplers [91] protects neurons against excitotoxic injury. There is strong evidence that perturbed cellular Ca^{2+} homeostasis is pivotal in the death of neurons following a stroke [35, 81, 84, 92]. It is now well established that a strong relationship exists between excessive Ca^{2+} influx and glutamate-triggered neuronal injury during stroke [2, 43, 93]. The earliest studies of the mechanisms resulting in neuron death as a consequence of glutamate excitotoxicity established the essential role of calcium in neuron cell death resulting from excessive NMDAR activation [93-95]. Sustained overstimulation of NMDARs leads to Ca^{2+} and Na^{+} overload in postsynaptic neurons [92, 94, 95]. After ischemia, cytoplasmic Ca^{2+} levels rise to 50-100 μM. Such excessive Ca^{2+} levels can trigger many downstream neurotoxic cascades [35, 92, 94, 95], including the activation and overstimulation of proteases, lipases, phosphatases and endonucleases (Fig. 2). The results include the activation of several signalling pathways, mainly causing an overproduction of free radicals, dysfunction of mitochondria, cell membrane disruption, and DNA fragmentation, which acting synergistically cause neuron death [1, 2, 11, 84, 96].

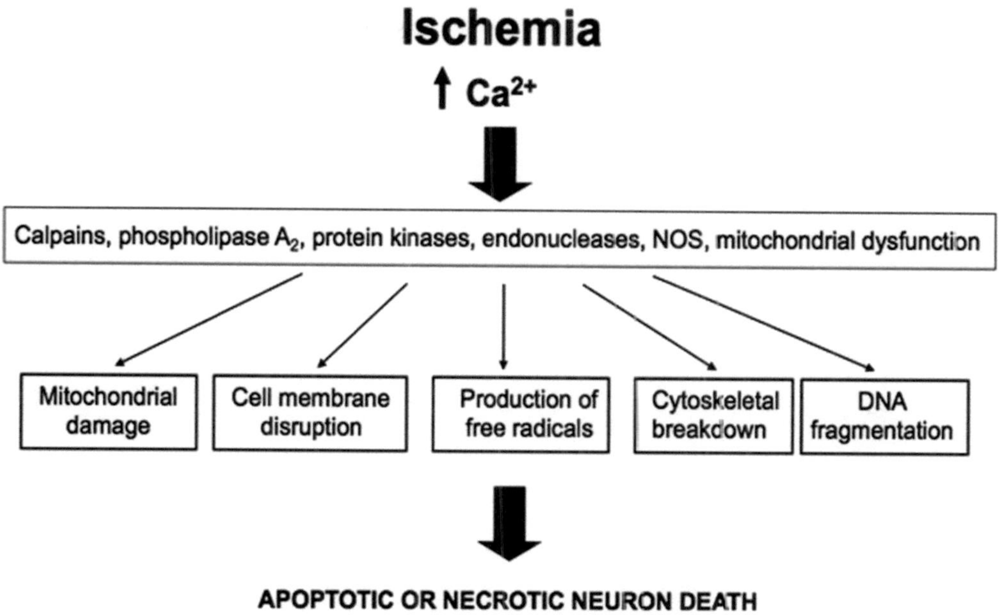

Fig. 2. Effects of very high Ca^{2+} accumulation in neurons after ischemia. Excitotoxicity causes a sudden increase in cytoplasmic Ca^{2+} concentrations in neurons after ischemia, which induces activation of several signaling pathways, leading to apoptototic or necrotic neuronal death. Activation of calpains, caspases, other proteases, kinases and endonucleases, cause mitochondrial disturbance, overproduction of free radicals and DNA fragmentation, that synergistically lead to neuronal death.

Major excitotoxic events promoted by cytoplasmic Ca^{2+} overload due to massively activated glutamate receptors include mitochondrial dysfunction, oxidative/nitrosative stress and calpain activation (Fig. 3).

The excitotoxicity can contribute to neuron death by altering the functions of mitochondria. Mitochondrial disturbance is the result of both oxidative-nitrosative stress and a direct effect of excessive Ca^{2+} intracellular levels. Mitochondrial dysfunction is caused by free radicals and the mitochondrial disturbance, in turn, increases the production of free radicals. Mitochondria play an important role in calcium homeostasis [97, 98]. Under conditions of cytoplasmic excess of Ca^{2+}, mitochondria are very important for cell survival, as they have the ability to sequester large amounts of Ca^{2+}. From *in vitro* studies [98] it can be inferred that mitochondria within intact neurons will act as temporary reversible stores of Ca^{2+}, accumulating the cation when cytoplasmic Ca^{2+} is above a set point, and releasing the cation back to the cytoplasm when the plasma membrane Ca^{2+}-ATPase succeeds in pumping down cytoplasmic Ca^{2+} to below the set point [96, 99]. For this cytoplasmic buffering to occur with no deleterious effects for the mitochondria and hence the cell, the time during which cytoplasmic $Ca^{2+}$is above the set point must be brief, thus avoiding mitochondrial Ca^{2+} overload [96]. During stroke, electron microscope analyses show that Ca^{2+} accumulates in mitochondria very soon after global ischemia and this state persists for several hours [100]. Excessive and prolonged uptake of Ca^{2+} in mitochondria causes mitochondrial dysfunction [41, 96, 101], which is considered the primary event in neuron death due to excitotoxicity [41].

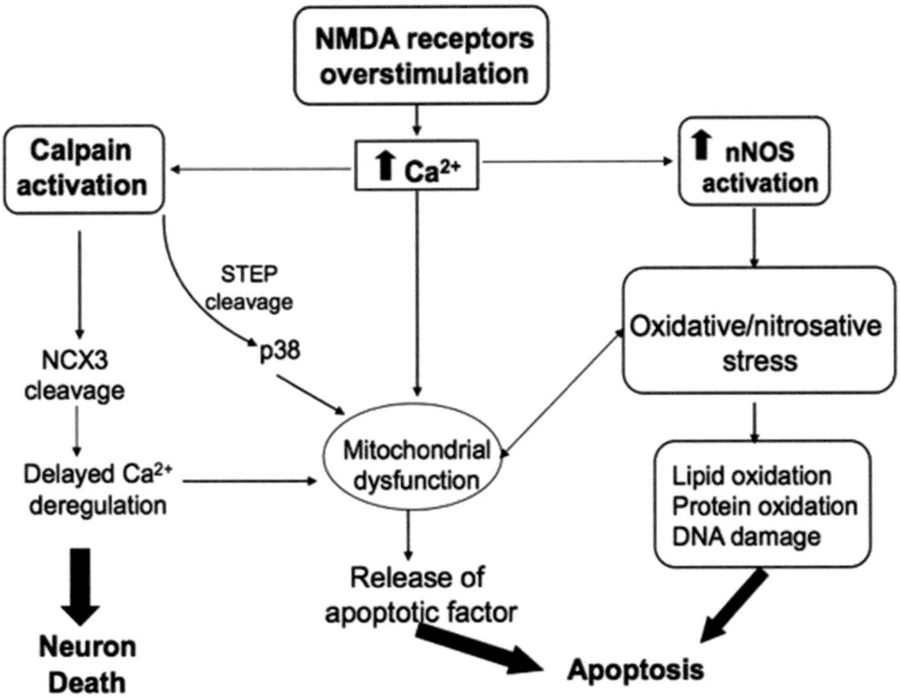

Fig. 3. Excitotoxic signaling by overstimulation of the NMDA receptors. Major excitotoxic events promoted by extrasynaptic NMDAR activation. Cerebral ischemia elevates cytosolic Ca^{2+} levels through the stimulation of NMDARs. The calcium overload: a) activates calpains that inactivate of the Na^{+}/Ca^{2+} exchanger (NCX3), b) induces mitochondrial disturbance that activate intrinsic apoptotic pathway and c) activates NOS that increases the NO production. Higher concentrations of nitric oxide can produce irreversible modifications of proteins, lipids and impairment of mitochondrial respiration. All of these processes trigger pathological mechanisms leading to neuronal death.

Mitochondrial dysfunction as a consequence of prolonged accumulation of Ca^{2+} is considered a major source of free radicals that are generated after ischemia-reperfusion [102, 103]. As a result of the mitochondrial dysfunction induced by the free Ca^{2+} cytosol accumulation, two events seem to play an important role in the death of neurons: the increase in the production of free radicals associated with a diminution of the antioxidant defences [102, 103], and the induction of the apoptotic cascade (Fig. 4) [104, 105].
Under physiological conditions, free radicals are generated at low levels and play important roles in signalling and metabolic pathways (106-108]. However, free radicals avidly interact with a large number of molecules including other small inorganic molecules as well as proteins, lipids, carbohydrates, and nucleic acids. Through such interactions, free radicals may irreversibly destroy or alter the function of the target molecule. Consequently, free radicals have been increasingly identified as major contributors to damage in biological organisms. The significance of free radicals as aggravating or primary factors in numerous pathologies is firmly established [109, 110].

Importantly, free radicals are produced continually during normal oxidative metabolism, but there are counteracted by a sophisticated system of enzymes and non-enzymatic antioxidants which maintains physiological homeostasis [111](Fig. 5). Enzymatic components mainly comprise superoxide dismutases (SOD) [112], catalases [111], glutathione [113] glutathione reductase/glutathione peroxidases (GR/GPX) [114], and peroxiredoxins [115]. Also, small molecular non-enzymatic antioxidants are important in scavenging free radicals. These include ascorbic acid, pyruvate, α-tocopherol and glutathione, which are also involved in the detoxification of free radicals, provision of antioxidant defence and prevention of tissue damage [111].

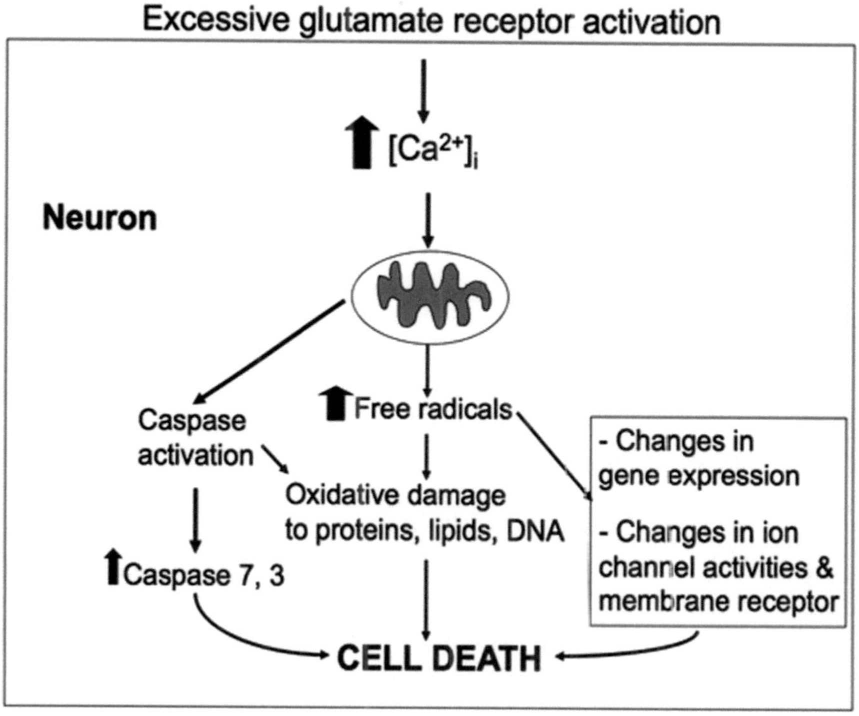

Fig. 4. Mitochondrial dysfuntion by disruption of calcium homeostasis leads to oxidative stress and apoptosis. Mitochondria are involved in both, the necrosis and the apoptotic pathways, which depend on the severity of the insult or nature of the signaling pathways. When cytosolic Ca^{2+} reaches non-physiological levels, the mitochondrial membrane may become more permeable, which causes release of cytochrome c and activation of the apoptotic pathway. Ca^{2+}-induced mitochondria disturbance involves dysfunction of ETC, increased ROS and oxidative stress.

When an imbalance occurs, either by increasing free radical formation or decreased anti-oxidant defences, and the formation of free radicals exceeds the protective capacity of antioxidant systems, the accumulation of free radicals is known as a state of "oxidative stress" [116]. Oxidative stress is generally defined as an imbalance that favours the production of free radicals over their inactivation by antioxidant defence systems [117].

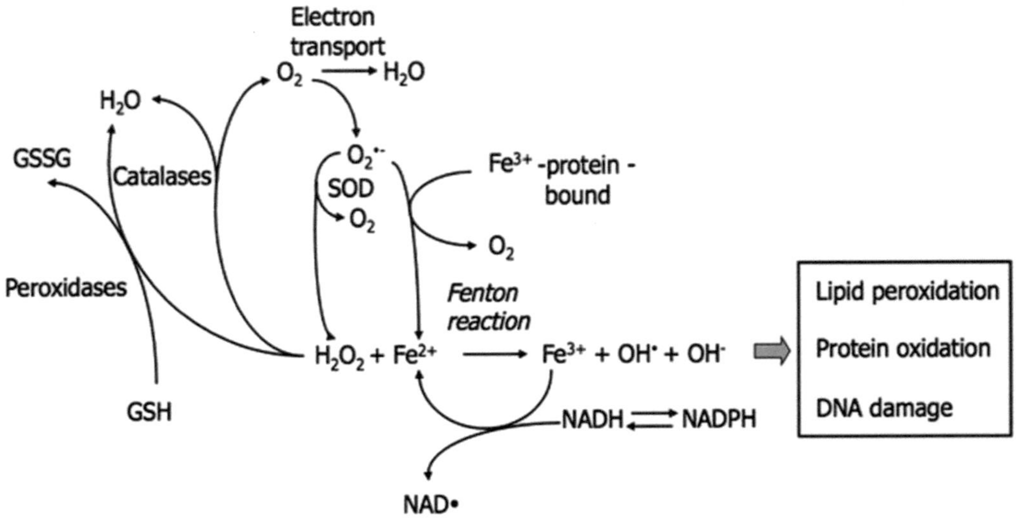

Fig. 5. Cellular reactions lead to oxidative damage of lipids, proteins and DNA via the Fenton reaction and their protection by main endogenous antioxidant enzymes (SOD, catalases and proxidaxes). The deleterious effects of ROS and RNS are controlled by antioxidant defences. Neurons are particularly vulnerable to oxidative stress owing to their high metabolic activity and oxygen consumption, which leads to high levels of ROS production, together with relatively low levels of endogenous antioxidant enzymes, particularly catalase. Moreover, the high lipid content of the brain can react with ROS to generate peroxyl radicals, leading to lipid oxidation of the neuronal membrane. The combination of these factors makes the CNS particularly vulnerable to oxidative damage.

Oxidative stress induced by excitotoxicity is considered the main event leading to brain damage after cerebral ischemia [35, 103, 109]. The most important free radicals induced by excitotoxicity are molecular derivates of oxygen and oxide nitric. Owing to their high oxidizing power, the intermediate reduction states of oxygen are called *reactive oxygen species* (ROS) and nitrogen-containing oxidants are called *reactive nitrogen species* (RNS). ROS are small oxygen-derived molecules, including the superoxide anion radical ($O_2^{\bullet-}$), hydroxyl radical ($OH^{\cdot}$), and certain non-radicals that are either oxidizing agents or easily converted into radicals, such as hydrogen peroxide (H_2O_2) and the oxygen singlet ($^1O_2$). RNS are nitrogen-derived molecules, such as nitric oxide ($NO^{\bullet}$), which has a relatively long half-life (approx. 1 s) and whose reactions with biological molecules are slow due to its very rapid diffusion into the blood and consequent inactivation by haemoglobin. $NO^{\bullet}$ is an important free radical because it combines with H_2O_2 and $O_2^{\bullet-}$ to form $OH^{\bullet}$ and peroxynitrite ($ONOO^-$), which is stable at an alkaline pH and fairly non-reactive, but it is readily protonated at cellular pH to peroxynitrous acid (ONOOH), which is very cytotoxic.

Following early suggestions [118], free radicals and other small reactive molecules have emerged as important players in the cell mechanisms involved in the pathophysiology of strokes [35, 119-121]. Several lines of research indicate that oxidative stress is a primary mediator of neurologic injury following cerebral ischemia [103, 120, 121]. After cerebral ischemia and particularly reperfusion, robust oxidants are generated including superoxide and hydroxyl radicals, which overwhelm endogenous scavenging mechanisms [122, 123] and are directly involved in the damage to cellular macromolecules, such as lipids, proteins, and nucleic acids, eventually leading to cell death [1,2] (Fig. 6). Re-oxygenation during reperfusion provides oxygen to sustain neuronal viability and also provides oxygen as a substrate for numerous enzymatic oxidation reactions that produce reactive oxidants. In addition, reflow after occlusion often causes an increase in oxygen to levels that cannot be utilized by mitochondria under normal physiological flow conditions. During reperfusion, perturbation of the antioxidative defence mechanisms is a result of the overproduction of oxygen radicals, inactivation of detoxification systems, consumption of antioxidants, and failure to adequately replenish antioxidants in the ischemic brain tissue [122-123].

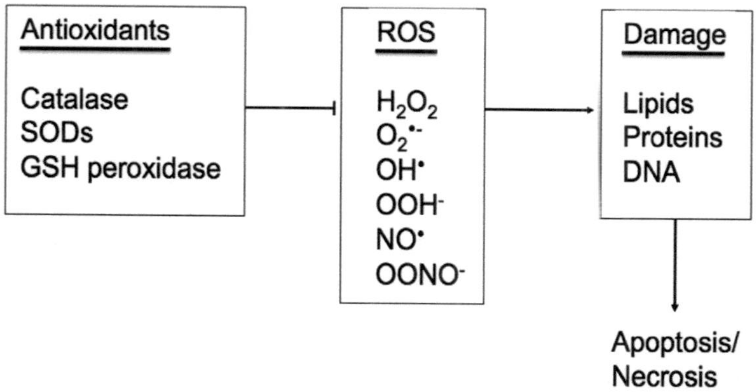

Fig. 6. ROS-mediated damage of cellular macromolecules may lead to neuron death. Excessive release of glutamate can trigger ROS increase. Antioxidant defences include several enzymes. In the healthy subjects, there is a balance between the production of antioxidants defences and of reactive species. When an imbalance occurs, either by increasing free radical formation and/or decreased anti-oxidant defences, and the formation of free radicals exceeds the protective capacity of antioxidant systems, the accumulation of free radicals leads to oxidative stress.

The important role of free radicals in cell damage during stroke is emphasized by the fact that even delayed treatment with the use of antioxidants and inhibitors of free radical producing enzymes can be effective in experimental focal cerebral ischemia [124, 125]. In addition, the overproduction of radical-scavenging enzymes protects against stroke [126] and animals that are deficient in radical-scavenging enzymes are more susceptible to cerebral ischemic damage [127]. In addition, neuroprotection is evident in animal models where genes coding for enzymes that promote oxidative stress are knocked down or out, and where genes coding for antioxidant enzymes, e.g., superoxide dismutase (SOD) are over-expressed [44, 126].

Increased levels of ROS and RNS generated extra- and intra-cellularly can, by various processes, initiate and promote neuron death during ischemic stroke. ROS and RNS can directly oxidize and damage macromolecules such as DNA, proteins, and lipids, culminating in neuron death[1, 2, 45-47]. ROS and RNS can also indirectly contribute to tissue damage by activating a number of cellular pathways resulting in the expression of stress-sensitive genes and proteins that cause oxidative injury [43].

Intracellular sources of ROS include the mitochondrial electron transport chain (ETC), xanthine oxidase, arachidonic acid, and NADPH oxidases. It is generally thought that mitochondria are the primary source of ROS involved in oxidative stress induced after cerebral ischemia. Free radicals are produced in the mitochondria as by-products of respiratory chain reactions. While passing through the mitochondrial ETC, some electrons escape from the mitochondrial ETC, especially from complexes I and III, and react with O_2 to form superoxide anion radicals ($O_2^{\bullet -}$) (Figure 7), which rapidly dismutate to H_2O_2 either spontaneously, particularly at low pH, or catalyzed by superoxide dismutase [128, 129]. Approximately 1%–2% of the molecular oxygen consumed during normal physiological respiration is converted into superoxide radicals [130].

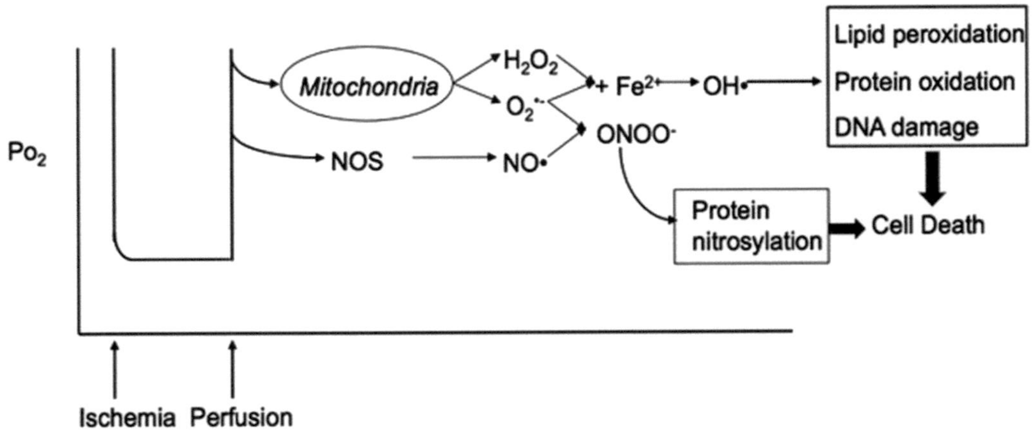

Fig. 7. Cerebral ischemia and reperfusion generated reactive oxygen species by mitochondria and reactive nitrogen species by nitric oxide synthase. The generation of peroxynitrite ($ONOO^-$), formed by the reaction of nitric oxide with superoxide anion, and subsequent hydroxil radical ($OH^{\bullet}$) production can directly damage lipids, proteins, and DNA and lead to neuron death.

4. Oxidative stress in acute ischemic stroke

Neurons are particularly vulnerable to oxidative stress owing to their high metabolic activity and oxygen consumption which lead to high levels of ROS production, together with relatively low levels of endogenous antioxidant enzymes, particularly catalase [131]. Moreover, the high lipid content of the brain can react with ROS to generate peroxyl radicals that lead to neuron membrane lipid oxidation [132]. The combination of these factors makes the CNS particularly vulnerable to oxidative damage [113].

The primary source of free radical generation in cells during cerebral ischemia has been reported to be due to a decrease in mitochondria redox potential causing ROS production from the ETC, mainly at the level of cytochrome III [102, 103, 118, 130]. After ischemia, an excess of cytosolic free Ca^{2+} due to excitotoxicity may overload the mitochondrial proton circuit, which leads to failure in oxidation together with increased ROS production [102, 109]. Overproduction of ROS by mitochondria causes the impairment of the ETC, which in turn, leads to decreased ATP production, increased formation of free radicals, altered calcium homeostasis and mitochondrial dysfunction [130]. In the rat, transient middle cerebral artery occlusion (MCAO) induces ROS production and mitochondrial dysfunction, including the inactivity of ETC enzymes. The mitochondrial dysfunction is attenuated by treatment with an antioxidant [133] or by the over-expression of mitochondrial Hsp70/Hsp75 [134], both of which decrease the ROS concentration.

Although mitochondrial dysfunction has been considered as a major source of ROS, other excitotoxic pathways may also be important in inducing oxidative stress. Recently, it has been suggested that NADPH oxidase is the primary source of superoxide production following neuronal NMDAR activation [135]. All NADPH oxidase (NOX) family members are transmembrane proteins that transport electrons across biological membranes. In general, the electron acceptor is oxygen and the product of the electron transfer reaction is $O_2^{\bullet-}$. The biological function of NOX enzymes is therefore the generation of ROS. NADPH oxidase was originally described in neutrophils, but has subsequently been identified in many other cell types including neurons [136]. While NMDAR activation induces $O_2^{\bullet-}$ production by NADPH oxidase, a near-complete absence of $O_2^{\bullet-}$ production was observed in neurons lacking functional NADPH oxidase and in neurons in which NADPH oxidase function had been inhibited. Markedly reduced NMDA neurotoxicity was also observed under these conditions [137].

During the ischemic phase, some Ca^{2+}-dependent enzymes, such as phospholipase A_2 (PLA_2) and cyclooxygenase (COX), produce oxygen free radicals. It has been shown that PLA_2 levels increase in the brain within 2-30 min of ischemia [138]. The activation of PLA_2 by Ca^{2+} results in the release of arachidonic acid from the phospholipids, which is further metabolized by cyclooxygenase to eicosanoids along with the production of free radicals [139]. Cyclooxygenase catalyzes the addition of two O_2 molecules to arachidonic acid to produce the prostaglandina PGG_2, which in turn is rapidly peroxidized to PGH_2 with a simultaneous release of $O_2^{\bullet-}$ [11, 140]. In addition, PLA_2 activation generates lysophosphatides that alter membrane structures. Activation of PLA_2 and cyclooxygenase generates free-radical species that overwhelm endogenous scavenging mechanisms, producing lipid peroxidation and membrane damage [2, 140].

During stroke, a high influx of Ca^{2+} through NMDA receptors may lead to the activation of nNOS and increase the production of NO [71, 77]. As described above, in neurons, $NO^{\bullet}$ is produced by neuronal NO synthase (nNOS), an enzyme tethered to the NMDA receptor complex by the postsynaptic density protein-95 (PSD95) [71]. During stroke NO production in the brain increases dramatically due to the activation of the neuronal and inducible isoforms of nitric oxide synthases [79]. The $NO^{\bullet}$ combines with H_2O_2 and $O_2^{\bullet-}$ to form $OH^{\bullet}$ and peroxynitrite ($ONOO^-$) [141]. which is generated at high levels and strongly contributes to ischemic brain damage [79]. After ischemia an important target of NO-induced $ONOO^-$ is mitochondria causing mitochondrial dysfunction and the consequent increased generation of oxygen free radicals leading to prompt dysfunction of cellular membranes causing necrosis. The ROS generated from the ETC can readily react with NO to form the highly reactive peroxynitrite, which can damage lipids, proteins and DNA [45-47, 79]. Mitochondrial Ca^{2+} overload, concomitant generation of free radicals, and depression of cell energy metabolism are thought to play important roles in the pathogenesis of ischemic brain damage [35, 36, 84, 101]. There is increasing evidence that NO is involved in the mechanisms of cerebral ischemia [78, 80]. After MCAO, the NO concentration in the ischemic area increases to micromolar levels. The surge in NO concentration can be inhibited by glutamate receptor antagonists, which show that increased production of NO is initiated by glutamate [78, 80]. In a clinical study in patients with acute ischemic stroke, increased NO metabolite in CSF was associated with greater brain injury and early neurological deterioration [142].

The H_2O_2 formed from $O_2^{\bullet -}$ has two possible fates: (i) conversion to hydroxyl radical ($OH^{\bullet}$), the most reactive free radical produced in biological systems, by means of the Haber-Weiss reaction ($H_2O_2 + O_2^{\bullet -} \rightarrow O_2 + OH^{\bullet} + OH^{-}$) [143] which is favoured by iron ions in Fenton reaction ($Fe^{2+} + H_2O_2 \rightarrow Fe^{3+} + OH^{\bullet} + OH^{-}$) [144] or (ii) conversion to water by oxidation of the small tripeptide glutathione (GSH) via a reaction catalyzed by the enzyme glutathione peroxidase (GPX) ($H_2O_2 + 2GSH \rightarrow GSSG + 2H_2O$) or mutated to water and oxygen ($H_2O_2 \rightarrow H_2O + ½ O_2$) by the catalase enzyme [106]. Reduction of the oxidized glutathione (GSSG) in a reaction catalyzed by glutathione reductase creates more GSH, which then converts more H_2O_2 to H_2O (Fig. 8). About 1% of the mitochondrial ROS escape elimination by antioxidant defence mechanisms. The major contribution of mitochondria to cytosolic ROS comes from H_2O_2 escaping the GPX degradation in the matrix and by residual $O_2^{\bullet -}$, which can enter the cytosol via the porin (VDAC). The greatest oxidative cellular damage produced by superoxide, however, is derived from its participation in peroxinitrite ($ONOO^{-}$) formation ($O_2^{\bullet -} + NO^{\bullet} \rightarrow ONOO^{-}$) [141].

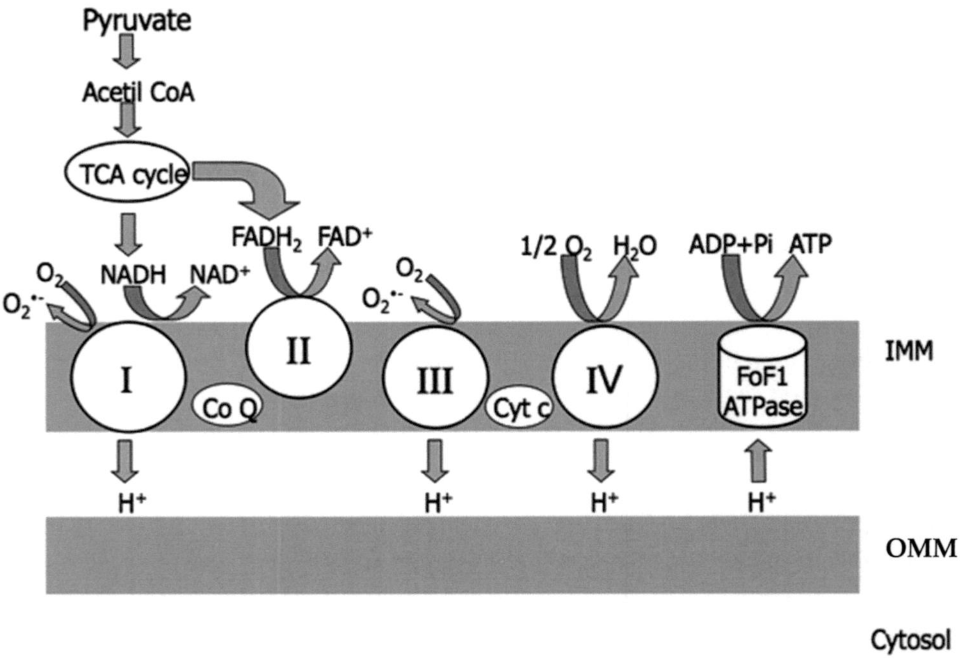

Fig. 8. The neurons, under physiological conditions, generate ATP mainly by mitochondrial phosphorylation via the electron transport chain (ETC). In this process, mainly complexes I and III carry out electrons to molecular oxygen, serving as the primary source of superoxide production. IMM: Inner mitochondrial membrane, OMM: Outer mitochondrial membrane.

Oxidative/nitrosative stress may damage different cellular components, including oxidation of membrane lipids [132], essential cell proteins [145] and DNA [48] as well as initiating cascade reactions, which lead to mitochondrial dysfunction [109] caspase activation [146] and the activation of signal transduction pathways [14], which finally lead to neuron death. On the basis of experimental models, there is ample evidence for enhanced free radical production in the brain after stroke [1-3, 35, 120, 121].

5. Apoptotic mechanisms after cerebral ischemia

After ischemia, excitotoxicity can lead to apoptotic or necrotic cell death [65-68]. The route involved depends on the time elapsed, the intensity of the stimulus and the degree to which energy production is maintained. While necrosis occurs mainly in the earliest moments after the onset of ischemia in the core [2, 49-51], programmed cell death begins hours later and lasts for several days [104]. This delayed cell death occurs mainly in the penumbra and is thus temporally and spatially different from the rapid necrotic neuron death in the core.

There are two general pathways for activation of apoptosis: the extrinsic and intrinsic pathways. Studies of tissue from patients and of animal models have shown that mitochondria-mediated apoptosis is the mode by which many neurons die after an acute stroke [105]. Oxidative stress and cytotoxic accumulation of intracellular Ca^{2+} initiate a series of cytoplasmic and cellular events, including the triggering of the intrinsic apoptotic pathway (Figure 9) [2, 105]. Increased ROS/RNS and intracellular free Ca^{2+} levels mediate induction/activation of pro-apoptotic proteins such as prostate apoptosis response 4 (Pr4), pro-apoptotic Bcl-2 members (Bax, Bad and others) and p53 [147], leading to changes in the mitochondrial membrane permeability (MMP) [148]. Proteins in the anti-apoptotic Bcl-2 family as well as anti-apoptotic kinase Akt and ERK protect the mitochondrial integrity by inhibiting pro-apoptotic Bcl-2 family members. Following cerebral ischemia, several pro-apoptotic members of the Bcl-2 family (tBid, Dp-5, Bim, Bax, Bak, and BAD) may antagonize the anti-apoptotic Bcl-2 family proteins to induce mitochondrial damage. Once the balance is shifted towards apoptosis, the mitochondria release apoptotic proteins such as cyt-*c* and AIF [104]. Alterations in expression of members of the Bcl-2 protein family, including increased expression of Bax and Bad, and reduced expression of Bcl-2 and Bcl-w, are found in the ischemic core and in the penumbra of the infarct [14]. A rapid translocation of cytosolic Bax to the mitochondria has been observed after cerebral ischemia [149]. After the opening of the mitochondrial pores, pro-apoptotic proteins are released into the cytosol; these include cytochrome *c* (cyt *c*) and Smac/DIABLO [149]. The release of cyt *c* and other pro-apoptotic proteins can trigger caspase activation and apoptosis. Once released into the cytosol from the mitochondrial intermembrane space, cyt *c* binds with apoptotic protein-activating factor-1 (Apaf-1) and procaspase-9 to form an "apoptosome", which actives caspase-9 and subsequently caspase-3. Activated caspase-3 dismantles a wide range of homeostatic, reparative and cytoskeletal proteins including nDNA repair enzymes, such as poly (ADP-ribose) polymerase (PARP), and activates caspase-activated DNase (CAD) [149] which cleaves nuclear DNA and leads to DNA damage and neuron cell death. Apoptotically damaged mitochondria also release other factors, such as AIF and EndoG, to facilitate DNA fragmentation and Smac/DIABLO to facilitate caspase activation [149]. There is a large body of evidence suggesting that cerebral ischemia can cause activation of caspases, certain types of protease that can cleave a larger number of cellular substrates [14, 105, 146]. Up regulation and activation of caspase-3 have been found to precede neuron death in focal and global cerebral ischemia [104].

Experiments involving manipulation of the molecular systems linked to the pathogenesis of apoptosis suggest that apoptosis is involved in neuron death following focal ischemic insults. Over-expression of human BCL-2 [150] reduces infarction in rodent brains subjected to focal ischemic insults. In addition, p53 knock-out transgenic mice also exhibit reduced brain vulnerability to focal ischemic insults. Interestingly, a greater protective effect was seen in heterozygous animals than in animals that were homozygous for the p53 null gene, which is consistent with some beneficial actions of p53 and some gene dose effect [151].

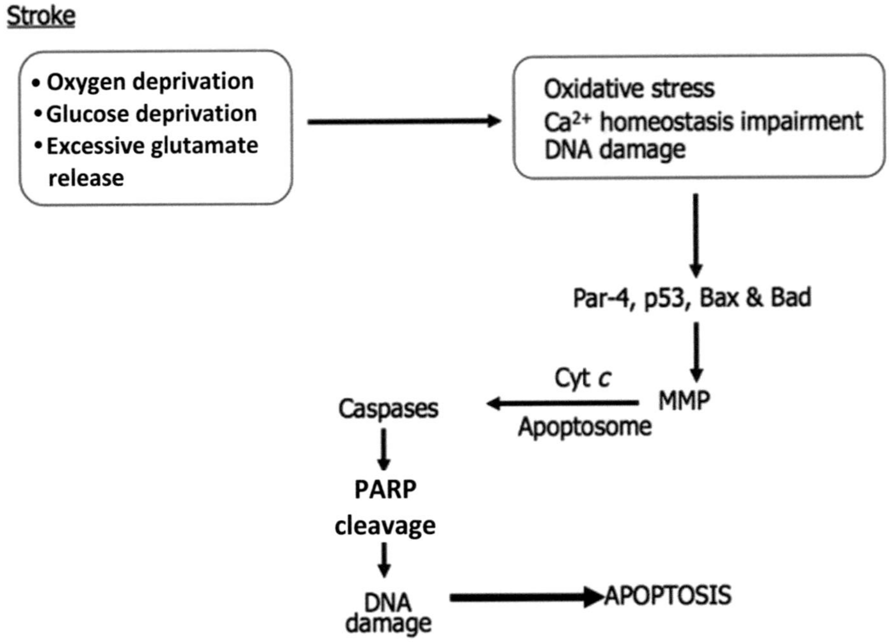

Fig. 9. The intrinsic apoptosis pathway in neurons is initiated by moderate overactivation of glutamate receptors, oxidative stress and DNA damage. The apoptotic trigger often activate transcriptions factor such as p53 that induce the expression of the pro-apoptotic Bcl-2 family members bax and bad which increased permeability of the outer mitochondrial membrane and the subsequent release of cytochrome c to the cytosol. In the cytosol, cytochrome c binds to the apoptosome which then activitates the caspase cascade that, in turn, cleaves numerous protein substrates leading to the neuronal death.

6. The role of calpains in strokes

One of the key events induced after ischemia by Ca^{2+} overload is a massive activation (either directly or indirectly) of calpains, important contributors to excitotoxic cell death [152]. The calpain family consists of about 15 members of cellular cysteine proteases that are activated by calcium in the cytosol [153]. Calpains can modulate a variety of physiological processes [153]. Regulated activation of calpains in the CNS may be critical to synaptic function and memory formation. All calpains can act in two modes: under physiological conditions they undergo controlled activation (involving only a few molecules of calpain) whereas during sustained calcium overload under pathological conditions they undergo hyperactivation (involving all the available calpain molecules) [152].

Although neurons behave very differently in acute and chronic cerebral ischemia, there is a pervasive view that Ca^{2+}-dependent calpain protease inhibitors are protective to varying degrees in animal models of stroke [154, 155]. Ample evidence documents the activation of calpains in brain ischemia and excitotoxic neuronal degeneration [152, 156]. Two mechanisms have recently been suggested which involve calpains as mediators of neuron death in strokes. In a rat model of focal ischemia, Ca^{2+}-overload activated calpain cleavage of Na^{+}/Ca^{2+} exchangers (NCX) thus precluding the possibility of restoring NCX [157], which are among the most potent regulators of Ca^{2+} concentrations in neuronal cells, and are a contribute to Ca^{2+} cytosol accumulation during ischemia [87, 89]. Cleavage of NCX leads to an irreversible increase in the intracellular Ca^{2+} concentration. The inhibition of calpain prevents cleavage of NCX and prevents the secondary Ca^{2+} overload linked to neuronal demise [89]. So, calpain activation by excessive cytoplasmic Ca^{2+} can contribute to the mediation of cleavage of NCX and increase cytoplasmic calcium deregulation [157].

7. Anti-excitotoxic mechanisms and their potential as therapeutic targets

In the treatment of acute cerebral ischemia, two primary therapeutic strategies are applied: (1) limitation of cerebral ischemia by early reperfusion after cerebral ischemia (the vascular approach), and (2) interference with the patho-biochemical cascade leading to ischemic damage (the neuroprotective approach) [158]

7.1 The vascular approach

After many years without any therapeutic treatment for strokes, and since seminal studies [6, 7] showed the existence of an ischemic penumbra where neurons maintain membrane potential for several hours or more after the onset of a stroke, recanalization therapies that aim to recover the flow of blood in the ischemic penumbra have been developed.

The results of the intravenous application the tissue plasminogen activator (tPA) to reopen occluded blood vessels [159] led the US Food and Drug Administration to approve the use of tPA for treatment of acute ischemic stroke in 1996. The early recovery of blood flow in the cerebral ischemic region is the principal factor that prevents neuronal injury. Early recanalization with thrombolytic therapy clearly improves patient outcome after an acute stroke [159]. The use of tPA therapy when administered intravenously within the first 3 h, significantly improves patient outcome by approximately 30%. In addition, tPA is the only drug licensed and available for treatment of ischemic stroke that can lead to a recanalization of occluded vessels and to an improvement in clinical outcome. However, less than 5% of potentially eligible patient are currently being treated with tPA therapy in the USA or in Europe [160] and the use of tPA therapy remains limited. The reasons for this situation are complex, but in clinical practice the main obstacle is the narrow therapeutic time window, currently limited to 3 h, together with insufficient public knowledge of the stroke warning signs, the small number of centres able to administer thrombolysis on a 24-h basis and also some physicians' excessive fear of haemorrhagic complications [161]. The use of tPA is associated with an increased risk of intracerebral haemorrhage (ICH) and mortality [162] and it requires sophisticated pre-treatment imaging [163].

7.2 The neuroprotective approach

The second major therapeutic approach, neuroprotection, aims: to rescue ischemic tissue and improve functional outcome by intervention on the ischemic cascade; and to reduce the intrinsic vulnerability of brain tissue to ischemia. Cellular neuroprotective approaches have focused mainly on blocking excitotoxicity, that is, neuron death triggered by the excitatory transmitter glutamate, and mediated by cytotoxic levels of calcium influx. Many experimental trials have demonstrated that many agents are effective in infarction volume reduction in animal models of stroke but have not been successfully translated to humans [164]. Neuroprotective strategies have failed to show clinical benefit despite promising laboratory results. Unfortunately, to date, none of tested neuroprotective agents has been shown to improve outcomes in phase III clinical trials [165]. All attempts to find effective neuroprotective drugs for the treatment of strokes have failed to demonstrate unequivocal efficacy in clinical trials [166]. Because the brain is a complex organ that is capable of many intricate functions, it has proved difficult to develop drugs for the treatment of neurodegenerative disorders that do not interfere with the normal functioning of the nervous system.

Preclinical research require rigorous attention to a variety of variables that may influence the outcome. The widely touted STAIR criteria represent constructive guidelines for preclinical testing [167] but, as experience has shown, have not increased the translational success. The failure to translate these strategies from the laboratory to clinical trials is a disappointment and many agents have been brought to clinical trial despite only modest or inconsistent preclinical evidence of neuroprotective efficacy.

These recurrent clinical failures might be due to heterogeneous populations of stroke patients, drug-associated toxicity at the doses required for efficacy. They may also be due to low dose administration, irregular study design and inadequate statistical evaluation, the limited time window required for initiating treatment, or the lack of adequate CNS penetration across the blood–brain barrier (BBB*)* [165]. The future of neuroprotection is seen to lie in concentrating on the subgroup of patients with an existing penumbra, the combination of neuroprotection and thrombolysis and in prophylactic neuroprotection. Current therapeutic targets have focused on the preservation of the ischemic penumbra in the hope of improving clinical outcomes. Neuroprotective strategies may aid in prolonging time windows, thereby potentially increasing the number of patients who could benefit from reperfusion treatments. Reperfusion therapies are rapidly evolving and have been shown to improve clinical outcomes. There has been significant progress with successful reperfusion treatments associated with improved clinical outcomes. The use of neuroprotective agents to prolong time windows prior to reperfusion or to prevent reperfusion injury may present future therapeutic targets for the treatment of ischemic stroke.

In recent years, over a thousand experimental and over four hundred clinical studies have been published. A close survey of the most extensively evaluated neuroprotection agents and their classes as well as the results of the clinical trials, have been published [164, 165, 168]. The outcome at the clinical trial phase of some compounds for the treatment of acute ischemic stroke, are shown (Table 1) [18].

These considerations have led to the possibility of a future multidrug therapeutic approach that will probably have to include peptide growth factors for early induction of survival of signal transduction and recovery of translational competence, inhibition of calpain, inhibition of radical damage, and caspase inhibition. Rigorous studies to establish such an approach will require the evaluation of neurologic and histopathologic outcomes as well as of the molecular endpoints associated with each component to establish the role of each drug. Such a multi-factorial therapeutic approach to molecular injury mechanisms now appears essential for the development of substantially improved reperfusion.

A new neuroprotective therapy opens interesting and hopeful perspectives. It is becoming increasingly clear that erythropoietin (Epo) is potentially neuroprotective in different models of brain injury [169-171]. Epo exerts its effects through the activation of the neuronal erythropoietin receptor (EpoR), part of the cytokine-receptor type I superfamily, where it acts as an anti-apoptotic, antioxidant, anti-inflammatory and neurothropic factor. Numerous preclinical findings and some clinical pilot studies [170-172] suggest that recombinant human Epo (rHuEpo) provides neuroprotection that may be beneficial in the treatment of patients suffering from ischemic stroke. Epo theoretically represents an ideal compound for neuroprotection, not only against strokes, but also against other brain disease. (See the chapter devoted to this issue in this book).

Compound	Mechanism of action	Inclusion period (h)	Outcome (Phase)	Reason[b]
Selfotel	NMDA receptor antagonist	6	Negative (III)	Adverse events
Aptiganel	NMDA receptor antagonist	6	Negative (III)	Lack of efficacy
Gavestinel	NMDA glycine-site antagonist	6	Negative (III)	Lack of efficacy
Eliprodil	NMDA, polyamine site blocker	6	Negative (II)	Adverse events
Magnesium sulphate	NMDA, channel blocker	12	Negative (III)	Lack of efficacy
Cervene	Kappa opioid receptor antagonist	6	Negative (III)	Lack of efficacy
Lubeluzole	NOS inhibitor and Na+ channel blocker	8	Negative (III)	Lack of efficacy
Fosphenytoin	Sodium channel blocker	6	Negative (III)	Lack of efficacy
BMS-204352	K+-channel blocker	6	Negative (III)	Lack of efficacy
Calcium antagonists	Ca2+ channel antagonists	6–24	Negative	
			(Meta-analysis)	Lack of efficacy
Enlimomab	Anti-ICAM antibody	6	Negative (III)	Lack of efficacy
				and adverse events
Citicoline	Cell membrane stabilizer	24	Negative (III)	Lack of efficacy
Clomethiazole	GABAA receptor mimetic	12	Negative (III)	Lack of efficacy
Tirilazad	Lipid peroxidation inhibitor	4–24	Negative (III) 6 trials	Lack of efficacy
Ebselen	Lipid peroxidation inhibitor	12–48	Negative (II)	Lack of efficacy
Repinotan	5-HT1A receptor antagonist	6	Negative (IIb)	Lack of efficacy
ONO-2506	Astrocyte modulating factor	6	Negative (II)	Lack of efficacy in
				futility analysis
Trafermin	Basic fibroblast growth factor	6	Negative (II/III)	Lack of efficacy
UK-279,276	Neutrophil inhibitory factor	6	Negative (II)	Lack of efficacy in
				Futility analysis

[a] Abbreviations: BMS-204352, [35]-[+]-[5-chloro-2-methexyphenyl]-1,3-dihydro-3-fluoro-6-[trifluoromethyl]-2H-indol-2-one; ICAM, intercellular adhesion molecule; NMDA, **N**-methyl-Daspartate;
NOS, nitric oxide synthase.
[b] Lack of efficacy means that efficacy was not demonstrated.
From Green A & Shuaib A. Drug Discovery Today 11(15/16) 681-694 (2006).

Table 1. Some compounds that have failed in clinical evaluation for the treatment of acute ischaemic stroke[a]

8. Conclusions

After the onset of a stroke, the disruptions to the blood flow in areas affected by vascular occlusion limit the delivery of oxygen and metabolic substrates to neurons causing ATP reduction and energy depletion. The glucose and oxygen deficit that occurs after severe vascular occlusion is the origin of the mechanisms that lead to cell death and consequently to cerebral injury. These mechanisms include: ionic imbalance, the release of excess glutamate in the extracellular space, a dramatic increase in intracellular calcium that in turn activates multiple intracellular death pathways such as mitochondrial dysfunction, and oxidative and nitrosative stress that finally cause neuron death.

During more than two decades, many neuroprotect drugs have emerged as potent inhibitors with different targets of the ischemic cascade in acute stroke. However, until now none of them succeeded in clinical trials. Despite the potential of Epo in animal models that enhanced resistance of the neurons to glutamate toxicity and other positive effects in different targets of ischemic cascade, Epo or its no erythropoietic variants as Neuro-EPO may be overcome by alternative non–traumatic administration methods, such as intranasal delivery.

Many questions remain unanswered yet concerning this new molecule of Epo, which will try to be answered in the next chapter as we always learn from past mistakes in developing new drugs to stroke. A more biological basis is necessary in preclinical experimental research. This is the prerequisite to design an adequate molecule and administration delivery system. Finally, we want to give the reader a novel vision of how to face the acute treatment of the stroke with the application of Neuro-EPO via nasal. This will be the fundamental objective of the following chapter, in explaining the quick clinic application of this new molecule by nasal delivery for acute stroke therapy.

9. References

[1] Lo EH, Dalkara T, Moskovitz MA. Mechanisms, challenges and opportunities in stroke. Nat Rev Neurosci 4: 399-415 (2003).

[2] Dirnagl U, Iadecola C, Moskovitz MA. Pathobiology of ischemic stroke: an integrated view. Trends Neurosci 22: 391-397 (1999).

[3] Moustafa RR, Baron J-C. Pathophysiology of ischaemic stroke: insights from imaging, and implications for therapy and drug discovery. Br J Pharmacol 153: S44-S54 (2008).

[4] Martin RL, Lloyd HG, Cowan AI. The early events of oxygen and glucose deprivation: setting the scene for neuronal death? Trends Neurosci 17: 251-257 (1994).

[5] Hossmann KA. Viability thresholds and the penumbra of focal ischemia. Ann Neurol 36: 557-565 (1994).

[6] Astrup J, Symon L, Branston NM, Lassen NA. Cortical evoked potential and extracellular K^+ and H^+ at critical levels of brain ischemia. Stroke 8: 51-57 (1977).

[7] Astrup J, Siesjo BK, Symon L. Thresholds in cerebral ischemia -the ischemic penumbra. Stroke 12: 723-725 (1981).

[8] Ginsberg MD. Adventures in the pathophysiology of brain ischemia: penumbra, gene expression, neuroprotection: the 2002 Thomas Willis lecture. Stroke 34: 214-223 (2003).

[9] Markus R, Reutens DC, Kazui S, Read S, Wright P, Pearce DC, Tochon-Danguy HJ, Sachinidis JI, Donnan GA. Hypoxic tissue in ischaemic stroke: persistence and clinical consequences of spontaneous survival. Brain 127:1427-1436 (2004).

[10] Baron JC. Mapping the ischaemic penumbra with PET: implications for acute stroke treatment. Cerebrovasc Dis 9:193-201 (1999).

[11] Lipton P. Ischemic cell death in brain neurons. Physiol Rev 79: 1431-1568 (1999).

[12] Mehta SL, Manhas N, Raghubir R. Molecular targets in cerebral ischemia for developing novel therapeutics. Brain Res Rev 54: 34-66 (2007).

[13] Heiss WD. Ischemic penumbra: evidence from functional imaging in man. J Cereb Blood Flow Metab 20:1011-1032 (2000).

[14] Ferrer I, Planas AM. Signaling of cell death and cell survival following focal cerebral ischemia: Life and death struggle in the penumbra. J Neuropathol Exper Neurol 62: 329-339 (2003).
[15] Mergenthaler P, Dirnagl U, Meisel A. Pathophysiology of the stroke: lessons from animal models. Metab Brain Dis 19: 151-167 (2004).
[16] Hossmann KA. Pathophysiology and therapy of experimental stroke. Cell Mol Neurobiol 26:1057-1083 (2006).
[17] Cheng YD, Al-Khoury L, Zivin JA. Neuroprotection for ischemic stroke: two decades of success and failure. NeuroRx 1:36-45 (2004)
[18] Green RA, Shuaib A. Therapeutic strategies for the treatment of stroke. Drug Des Today 11:681-693 (2006).
[19] Zhang ZG, Chopp M. Neurorestorative therapies for stroke: underlying mechanisms and translation to the clinic. Lancet Neurol 8: 491-500 (2009).
[20] Zaleska MM, Mercado MLT, Chavez J, Feuerstein GZ, Pangalos MN, Wood A. The development of stroke therapeutics: Promising mechanisms and translational challenges. Neuropharmacol 56: 329-341 (2010).
[21] Heiss WD. Flow threshold of functional and morphological damage of brain tissue. Stroke 14: 329-331 (1983).
[22] Erecinska M, Silver IA. Tissue oxygen tension and brain sensitivity to hypoxia. Resp Physiology 128: 263-276 (2001).
[23] Zauner A, Daugherty WP, Bullock MR, Warner DS. Brain oxygenation and energy metabolism. Neurosurgery 51: 289-301 (2002).
[24] Obrenovitch TP. The ischaemic penumbra: twenty years on. Cerebrovasc Brain Metab Rev 7: 297-323 (1995).
[25] Kulik T, Kusano Y, Aronhime S, Sandler AL, Winn HR. Regulation of cerebral vasculature in normal and ischemic brain. Neuropharmacology 55: 281-288 (2008).
[26] Martin RL, Lloyd HG, Cowan AI. The early events of oxygen and glucose deprivation: setting the scene for neuronal death? Trends Neurosci 17: 251-257 (1994).
[27] Katsura K, Kristian T, Siesjo BK. Energy metabolism, ion homeostasis, and cell damage in the brain. Biochem Soc Trans 22: 991-996 (1994).
[28] Hansen AT, Nedergaard M. Brain ion homeostasis in cerebral ischemia. Neurochem Pathol 9: 195-209 (1988).
[29] Rothman SM, Olney JW. Glutamate and the pathophysiology of hypoxic-ischemic brain damage. Ann Neurol 19: 105-111 (1986).
[30] Camacho A, Massieu L. Role of glutamate transporters in the clearance and release of glutamate during ischemia and its relation to neuronal death. Arch Med Res 37: 11-18 (2006).
[31] Rossi DJ, Oshima T, Attwell D. Glutamate release in severe brain ischaemia is mainly by reversed uptake. Nature 403: 316-321 (2000).
[32] Choi DW, Rothman SM. The role glutamate neurotoxicity in hypoxic-ischemic neuronal death. Ann Rev Neuron 13: 171-178 (1990).
[33] Hossmann KA. Glutamate-mediate injury in focal cerebral ischemia: the excitotoxin hypothesis revised. Brain Pathol 4: 23-36 (1994).
[34] Choi DW. Excitotoxic cell death. J Neurobiol 23: 1261-1276 (1992).
[35] Siesjo BK, Zhao Q, Pahlmark K, Siesjo P, Katsura K, Folbergrova J. Glutamate, calcium and free radicals as mediators of ischemic brain damage. Ann Thorac Surg 59: 1316-1320 (1995).

[36] Arundine M, Tymiansky M. Molecular mechanisms of glutamate-dependent neurodegeneration in ischemia and traumatic brain injury. Cell Mol Life Sci 61: 657-668 (2004).

[37] Castillo J, Dávalos A, Noya M. Progression of ischaemic stroke and excitotoxic aminoacids. Lancet 349: 79-83 (1997).

[38] Takagi K, Ginsberg MD, Globus MY, Dietrich WD, Martínez E, Kraydieh S, Busto R. Changes in amino acid neurotransmitters and cerebral blood flow in the ischemic penumbral region following middle cerebral artery occlusion in the rat: Correlation with histopathology. J Cereb Blood Flow Metab 13: 575-585 (1993).

[39] Pelligrini-Giampietro DE, ChericiG, Alesiani M, Carla V, Moroni F. Excitatory amino acid release and free radical formation may cooperate in the genesis of ischemia-induced neuronal damage. J Neurosci 10: 1035-1041 (1990).

[40] Oh SM, Betz L. Interaction between free radicals and excitatory amino acids in the formation of ischemic brain edema in rats. Stroke 22: 915-921 (1991).

[41] Shinder AF, Olson EC, Spitzer NC, Montal M. Mitochondrial dysfunction is a primary event in glutamate neurotoxicity. J Neurosci 16: 6125-6133 (1996).

[42] Nicholls DG, Budd SL. Mitochondria and neuronal glutamate excitotoxicity. Biochim Biophys Acta 1366: 97-112 (1998).

[43] Akins PT, Liu PK, Hsu CY. Immediate early gene expression in response to cerebral ischemia. Stroke 27: 1682-1687 (1996).

[44] Clemens JA. Cerebral ischemia: gene activation, neuronal injury, and the protective role of antioxidants. Free Radic Biol Med 28: 1526-1531 (2000).

[45] Berlett BS, Stadtman ER. Protein oxidation in aging, disease, and oxidative stress. J Biol Chem 272: 20313-20316 (1997).

[46] Sakamoto A, Ohnishi ST, Ohnishi T, Ogawa R. Relationship between free radical production and lipid peroxidation during ischemia-reperfusion injury in the rat brain. Brain Res 554: 186-192 (1991).

[47] Hayashi T, Sakurai M, Itoyama Y, Abe K. Oxidative damage and breakage of DNA in the rat brain after transient MCA occlusion. Brain Res 832: 159-163 (1999).

[48] Cui J, Holmes EH, Greene TG, Liu PK. Oxidative DNA damage precedes DNA fragmentation after experimental stroke in rat brain. FASEB J 14: 955-967 (2000).

[49] Bonfoco E, Krainc D, Ankarcrona M, Nicotera P, Lipton SA. Apoptosis and necrosis: two distinct events induced, respectively, by mild and intense insults with *N*-methyl-D-aspartate or nitric oxide/superoxide in cortical cell cultures. Proc Natl Acad Sci U S A 92:7162–7166 (1995).

[50] Nicotera P, Leist M, Manzo L. Neuronal cell dath: a demise with different shapes. Trends Pharmacol Sci 20: 46-51 (1999).

[51] Ünal-Çevik I, Kilinç M, Can A, Gürsoy-Ózdemir, Dalkara T. Apoptotic and necrotic death mechanisms are concomitantly activated in the same cell after cerebral ischemia. Stroke 35: 2189-2194 (2004).

[52] Nakanishi S. Molecular diversity of glutamate receptors and implications of brain functions. Science 258: 597-603 (1992).

[53] Waxman EA, Lynch DR. N-methyl-D-aspartic receptor subtypes: multiple role in excitoxicity and neurological disease. Neuroscientist 11: 37-49 (2005).

[54] Madden DR.: The structure and function of glutamate receptor ion channels. Nat Rev Neurosci 3: 91-101 (2002).

[55] Paoletti P, Neyton J. NMDA receptor subunits: function and pharmacology. Curr Opin Pharmacol 7: 39-47 (2007).

[56] Clements JD, Westbrook GL. Activation kinetics reveals the number of glutamate and glycine binding sites on the *N*-methyl-D-aspartic receptor. Neuron 7: 605-613 (1991).

[57] Wong H-K, Liu X-B, Matos MF, Chan SF, Pérez-Otaño I, Boysen M, Cui J, Nakanishi N, Trimmer JS, Jones EG, Lipton SA, Sucher NJ. Temporal and regional expresión of NMDA receptor subunit NR3A in the mammalian brain. J Comp Neurol 450: 303-317 (2002).

[58] Lynch DR., Guttmann RP. NMDA receptor pharmacology perspectives from molecular biology. Curr Drug Targets 2: 215-231 (2001).

[59] Furukawa, H., Singh, S. K., Mancusso, R. & Gouaux, E. Subunit arrangement and function in NMDA receptors. Nature 438: 185-192 (2005).

[60] Liu Y, Wong TP, Aarts M, Rooyakkers M, Liu L, Lai TW, Wu DC, Lu J, Tymianski M, Craig AM, Wang YT. NMDA receptor subunits have differential roles in mediating excitotoxic neuronal death both in vitro and in vivo. J Neurosci 27: 2846-2857 (2007).

[61] Chen M, Lu TJ, Chen XJ, Zhou Y, Chen Q, Feng XY, Xu L, Duan WH, Xiong ZQ. Differential roles of NMDA receptor subtypes in ischemic neuronal cell death and ischemic tolerance. Stroke 39: 3042-3048 (2008).

[62] Zhou M, Baudry M. Developmental changes in NMDA neurotoxicity reflect developmental changes in subunit composition of NMDA receptors. J Neurosci 26: 2956-2963 (2006).

[63] Cheng C, Fass DM, Reynolds IJ. Emergence of excitotoxicity in cultured forebrain neurons coincides with larger glutamate-stimulated $[Ca^{2+}]i$ increases and NMDA receptor mRNA levels. Brain Res 849: 97-108 (1999).

[64] Hardinghan GE, Fu-kunaga Y, Bading H. Extrasynaptic NMDARs oppose synaptic NMDARs by triggering CREB shut-off and cell death pathways. Nat Neurosci 5: 405-414 (2002).

[65] Sattler R, Xiong Z, Lu WY, MacDonald JF, Tymianski M. Distinct roles of synaptic and extrasynaptic NMDA receptors in excitotoxicity. J Neurosci 20: 22-23 (2000).

[66] Liu Y, Wong TP, Aarts M, Rooyakkers M, Liu L, Lai TW, Wu DC, Lu J, Tymianski M, Craig AM, Wang YT. NMDA receptor subunits have differential roles in mediating excitotoxic neuronal death both in vitro and in vivo. J Neurosci 27: 2846-2857 (2007).

[67] Léveillé F, Gaamouch F, Gouix E, Lecocq M, Lobner D, Nicole O, Buisson A. Neuronal viability is controlled by a functional relation between synaptic and extrasynaptic NMDA receptors. FASEB J 22: 4258-4271 (2008).

[68] Tu W, Xu X, Peng L, Zhong X, Zhang W, Soundarapandian MM, Balel C, Wang M, Jia N, Zhang W, Lew F, Chan SL, Chen Y, Lu Y. DAPK1 interaction with NMDA receptor NR2B subunits mediates brain damage in stroke. Cell 140: 222-234 (2010).

[69] Martel M, Wyllie DJ, Hardingham G.E. In developing hippocampal neurons, NR2B-containing NMDA receptors can mediate signalling to neuronal survival and synaptic potentiation, as well as neuronal death. Neuroscience 158: 334-343 (2009).

[70] von Engelhardt J, Coserea I, Pawlak V, Fuchs EC, Kohr G, Seeburg PH, Monyer H. Excitotoxicity *in vitro* by NR2A and NR2B-containing NMDA receptors. Neuropharmacol 53: 10-17 (2007).

[71] Sattler R, Xiong Z, Lu WY, Hafner M, MacDonald JF, Tymianski M. Specific coupling of NMDA receptor activation to nitric oxide neurotoxicity by PS-95 protein. Science 284: 1845-1848 (1999).

[72] Sheng M. Molecular organization of the postsynaptic specialization. Proc Natl Acad Sci USA 98: 7058-7061 (2001).

[73] Kim E, Sheng M. PDZ domain proteins of synapses. Nat Rev Neurosci 5: 771-781 (2004).

[74] Kornau HC, Schenker LT, Kennedy MB, Seeburg PH. Domain interaction between NMDA receptor subunits and the postsynaptic density protein PSD-95. Science 269: 1737-1740 (1995).

[75] Niethammer M, Kim E, Sheng M. Interaction between the C terminus of NMDA receptor subunits and multiple members of the PSD-95 family of membrane-associated guanylate kinases. J Neurosci 16: 2157-2163 (1996).

[76] Brenman JE, Chao DS, Gee SH, McGee AW, Craven SE, Santillano DR, Wu Z, Huang F, Xia H, Peters MF, Froehner SC, Bredt DS. Interaction of nitric oxide synthase with the postsynaptic density protein PSD-95 and R1-syntrophin mediated by PDZ domains. Cell 84: 757-767 (1996).

[77] Christopherson KS. Hillier J, Lim W A, Bredt D S. PSD-95 assembles a ternary complex with the *N*-methyl-D-aspartic acid receptor and a bivalent neuronal NO synthase PDZ domain. J Biol Chem 274: 27467-27473 (1999).

[78] Iadecola C. Bright and dark sides of nitric oxide in ischemic brain injury. Trends Neurosci 20: 132-139 (1997).

[79] Bolaños JP, Almeida A. Roles of nitric acid in brain hypoxia-ischemia. Biochim Biophys Acta-Bioenerg 1411: 415-436 (1999).

[80] Moro MA, Cárdenas A, Hurtado O, Leza JC, Lizasoain I. Role of nitric oxide after brain ischaemia. Cell Calcium 36: 265-275 (2004).

[81] Arundine M, Tymianski M. Molecular mechanisms of calcium-dependent neurodegeneration in excitotoxicity. Cell Calcium 34: 325–337 (2003).

[82] Aarts M, Liu Y, Liu L, Besshoh S, Arundine M, Gurd JW, Wang YT, Salter MW, Tymiansky M. Treatment of ischemic brain damage by perturbing NMDA receptor-PSD-95 protein interactions. Science 298: 846-850 (2002).

[83] Sun H-S, Doucette TA, Liu Y, Fang Y, Teves L, Aarts M, Ryan CL, Bernard PB, Lau A, Forder JP, Salter MW, Wang YT, Tasker A, Tymianski M. Effectiveness of PSD95 inhibitors in permanente and transient focal ischemia in the rat. Stroke 39: 2544-2553 (2008).

[84] Szydlowska K, Tymiansky M. Calcium, ischemia and excitotoxicity. Cell Calcium 47: 122-129 (2010).

[85] Sattler R, Charlton MP, Hafner M, Tymianski M. Distinct influx pathways, not calcium load, determine neuronal vulnerability to calcium neurotoxicity. J Neurochem 71: 2349-2364 (1998).

[86] Besancon E, Guo S, Lok J, Tymiansky M, Lo EH. Beyond NMDA and AMPA glutamate receptors: emerging mechanisms for ionic imbalance and cell death in stroke. Trends Pharmacol 29: 268-275 (2008).

[87] Pignarato G, Gala R, Cuomo O, Tortiglione A, Giaccio L, Castaldo P, Sirabella R, Matrone C, Canitano A, Amoroso S, Di Renzo G, Annunziato L. Two sodium/calcium exchanger gene products, NCX1 and NCX3, play a major role in the development of permanent focal cerebral ischemia. Stroke 35: 2566-2570 (2004).

[88] Xiong ZG. Neuroprotection in ischemia: blocking calcium-permeable acid-sensing ion channels. Cell 118: 687-698 (2004).

[89] Bano D, Young KW, Guerin CJ, Lefeuvre R, Rothwell NJ, Naldini L, Rizzuto R, Carasfoli E, Nicotera P. Cleavage of the plasma membrane Na^{+}/Ca^{2+} exchager in excitotoxicity. Cell 120: 275-278 (2005).

[90] Choi DW. Ionic dependence of glutamate neurotoxicity. J Neurosci 7: 369-379 (1987).
[91] Stout AK, Raphael HM, Kanterewicz BI, Klann E, Reynolds IJ. Glutamate-induced neuron death requires mitochondrial calcium uptake. Nat Neurosci 1: 366-373 (1998).
[92] Sattler R, Tymianski M. Molecular mechanisms of calcium-dependent excototoxicity. J Mol Med 78: 3-13 (2000).
[93] Tymianski M, Tator CH. Normal and abnormal calcium homeostasis in neurons: a basis for the pathophysiology of traumatic and ischemic cental nervous system injury. Neurosurgery 38: 1176-1195 (1996).
[94] Choi DW. Calcium- mediated neurotoxicity: relationship to specific channel types and role in ischemic damage. Trends Neurosci 11: 465-467 (1988).
[95] Orrenius S, Zhivotovsky B, Nicotera P. Regulation of cell death: the calcium apoptosis link. Nat Rev Mol Cell Biol 4: 552-565 (2003).
[96] Nicholls DG. Mitochondrial calcium function and dysfunction in the central nervous system. Biochim Biophys Acta 1787: 1416-1424 (2009).
[97] Berridge MJ, Bootman MD, Roderick HL. Calcium signaling: Dinamics, homeostasis and remodelling. Nat Rev Mol Cell Biol 4: 517-529 (2005).
[98] Nicholls DG. Mitochondria and calcium signalling. Cell Calcium 38: 311-317 (2005).
[99] Gunter TE, Pfeiffer DR. Mechanisms by which mitochondria transport calcium. Am J Physiol 258: C755-C786 (1990).
[100] Zaidan E., Sims NR. The calcium content of mitochondria from brain subregions following short-term forebrain ischemia and recirculation in the rat. J Neurochem 63:1282-1289 (1994).
[101] Duchen M. Mitochondria and calcium. From cell signalling to cell death. J Physiol 529: 57-68 (2000).
[102] Piantadosi CA, Zhang J. Mitochondrial generation of reactive oxygen species after brain ischemia in the rat. Stroke 27: 327-331 (1996).
[103] Niizuma K, Endo H, Chan PH. Oxidative stress and mitochondrial dysfunction as determinants of ischemic neuronal death and survival. J Neurosci 109 (Suppl. 1): 133-138 (2009)
[104] Broughton BRS, Reutens D, Sobey CG. Apoptotic mechanisms after cerebral ischemia. Stroke 40: e331-e339 (2009).
[105] Niizuma K, Yoshioka H, Chen H, KimGS, Jung JE, Katsu M, Okami N, Chan PH.: Mitochondrial and apoptotic neuronal death signaling pathways in cerebral ischemia. Biochim Biophys Acta 1802: 92-99 (2010).
[106] Dröge W. Free radicals in the physiological control of cell function. Physiol Rev 82: 47-95 (2002).
[107] Nathan C. Specificity of a third kind: reactive oxygen and nitrogen intermediates in cell signaling. J Clin Invest 111: 769-778 (2003).
[108] D' Autréaux B, Toledano MB. ROS as signalling molecules: mechanisms that generate specificity in ROS homeostasis. Nat Rev Mol Cell Biol 8: 813-824 (2007).
[109] Lin MT, Beal MF. Mitochondrial dysfunction and oxidative stress in neurodegenerative diseases. Nature 443: 787-795 (2006).
[110] Valko M, Leibfritz D, Moncol J, Cronin MTD, Mazur M, Telser J. Free radicals and antioxidants in normal physiological functions and human disease. Int J Biochem Cell Biol 39: 44-84 (2007).
[111] Yu BP. Cellular defenses against damage from reactive oxygen species. Physiol Rev 74:139-162 (1994).

[112] Fridovich I. Superoxide radical and superoxide dismutases. Annu Rev Biochem 64: 97-112 (1995).
[113] Dringen R.: Metabolism and functions of glutathione in brain. Prog Neurobiol 62: 649-671 (2000).
[114] Zimmermann C, Winnefeld K, Streck S, Roskos M, Haberl RL. Antioxidant status in acute stroke patients and patients at stroke risk. Eur Neurol 51:157-161 (2004).
[115] Rhee SG, Kang SW, Jeong W, Chang TS, Yang KS, Woo HA. Intracellular messenger function of hydrogen peroxide and its regulation by peroxiredoxins. Curr Opin Cell Biol 17: 183-189 (2005).
[116] Sies H. Oxidative stress: introductory remarks. In: *Oxidative Stress*. New York: Academic Press, pp. 1–8 (1985).
[117] Halliwell B. Antioxidant defence mechanisms: from the beginning to the end (of the be beginning). Free Radical Res 31: 261-272 (1999).
[118] Orrenius S, Gogvadze V, Zhivotovsky B.: Mitochondrial oxidative stress: implications for cell death. Annu Rev Pharmacol Toxicol 47: 143-183 (2007).
[119] Olanow CW. A radical hypothesis for neurodegeneration. Trends Neurosci 16: 439-444 (1993).
[120] Chan PH: Reactive oxygen radicals in signaling and damage in the ischemic brain. J Cereb Blood Flow Metab 21: 2-14 (2001).
[121] Sugawara T, Chan PH. Reactive oxygen radicals and patogenesis of neuronal death after cerebral ischemia. Antioxid Redox Signal 5: 597-607 (2003).
[122] Nakashima M, Niwa M, Iwai T, Uematsu T. Involvement of free radicals in cerebral vascular reperfusion injury evaluated in a transient focal cerebral ischemia model in rat. Free Radic Biol Med 26: 722-729 (1999).
[123] Schaller B, Graf R. Cerebral ischemia and reperfusion: the pathophysiologic concept as a basis for clinical therapy. J Cereb Blood Flow Metab 24: 351-371 (2004).
[124] Zhao Q, Pahlmark K, Smith ML, Siesjö BK. Delayed treatment with the spin trap alpha-phenyl-N-tert-butyl nitrone (PBN) reduces infart size following transient middle cerebral artery occlusion in rats. Acta Physiol Scand 152: 349-350 (1994).
[125] Imai H, Graham DI, Masayasu H, Macrae IM. Antioxidant ebselen reduces oxidative damage in focal cerebral ischemia. Free Radic Biol Med 34: 56-63 (2003).
[126] Weisbrot-Lefkowitz M, Reuhl K, Perry B, Chan PH, Inouye M, Mirochnitchenko O. Overexpresion of human glutatión peroxidase protects transgenic mice against focal cerebral ischemia/reperfusion damage. Mol Brain Res 53: 333-338 (1998).
[127] Murakami K, Kondo T, Kawase M, Li Y, Sato S, Chen SF, Chan PH. Mitochondrial susceptibility to oxidative stress exacerbated cerebral infarction that follows permanet focal cerebral ischemia in mutant mice with manganese superoxide dismutase deficiency. J Neurosci 18: 205-213 (1998).
[128] Loschen G, Azzi A, Richter C, Flohe L. Superoxide radicals as precursors of mitochondrial hydrogen-peroxide. FEBS Lett 42: 68-72 (1974).
[129] Turrens JF. Superoxide production by the mitocondrial respiratory chain. Biosci Rep 17: 3-8 (1997).
[130] Andreyev AY, Kushnareva YE, Starkov AA. Mitochondrial metabolism of reactive oxygen species. Biochemistry 70: 200-214 (2005).
[131] Cooper AJL, Kristal BS.: Multiple roles of glutathione in the central nervous system. Biol Chem 378:793-802 (1997).
[132] Kinuta Y, Kikuchi H, Ishikawa M, Kimura M, Itokawa Y. Lipid peroxidation in focal cerebral ischemia. J Neurosurg 71: 421-429 (1989).

[133] Kuroda S, Katsura K, Hillered L, Bates TE, Siesjo BK. Delayed treatment with alpha-phenyl-N-tert-butyl nitrote (PBN) attenuates secondary mitochondrial dysfunction after transient focal cerebral ischemia in the rat. Neurobiol Dis 3:149-57 (1996).
[134] Xu L, Voloboueva LA, Ouyang Y, Emery JF, Giffard RG. Overexpression of mitochondrial Hsp70/Hsp75 in rat brain protects mitochondria, reduces oxidative stress, and protects from focal ischemia. J Cereb Blood Flow Metab 29: 365-374 (2009).
[135] Suh SW, Shin BS, Ma H, Van Hoecke M, Brennan AM, Yenari MA, Swanson RA. Glucose and NADPH oxidase drive neuronal superoxide formation in stroke. Ann Neurol 64: 654-663 (2008).
[136] Bedard K, Krause KH. The NOX family of ROS-generating NADPH oxidases: physiology and pathophysiology. Physiol Rev 87: 245-313 (2007).
[137] Chen H, Song YS, Chan P. Inhibition of NADPH oxidase is neuroprotective after ischaemia-reperfusion. J Cereb Blood Flow Metab 29: 1262-1272 (2009).
[138] Umemura A, Mabe H, Nagai H, Supino F. Action of phospholipases A2 and C on free ftty acid release during complete ischemia in rat neocrtex. Effect of phospholipase C inhibitor and *N*-methyl-D-aspartate antagonist. J Neurosurg 76: 648-651 (1992).
[139] Muralikrishna Adidhatla R, Hatcher JF. Phospholipase A2, reactive oxygen specis, and lipid peroxidation in cerebral ischemia. Free Rad Biol Med 40: 376-387 (2006).
[140] Dumuis M, Sebben H, Haynes JP, Pin J, Bockaert A. NMDA receptors activate the arachidonic acid cascade system in striatal neurons. Nature 336: 68-70 (1988).
[141] Beckman JS. Peroxynitrite versus hydroxyl radical: the role of nitric oxide in superoxide-dependent cerebral injury. Ann N Y Acad Sci 738: 69-75 (1994).
[142] Castillo J, Rama R, Dávalos A. Nitric oxide-related brain damage in acute ischemic stroke. Stroke 31: 852-857 (2000).
[143] Liochev SI, Fridovich I. The Haber-Weiss cycle-70 years later: An alternative view. Redox Rep 7: 55–57 (2002).
[144] Winterbourn CC. Toxicity of iron and hydrogen peroxide: The Fenton reaction. Toxicol Lett 969: 82-83 (1995).
[145] Grune T, Reinheckel T, Davies KJA. Degradation of oxidized proteins in mammalian cells. FASEB J 11: 526-534 (1997).
[146] Krupinski J, Lopez E, Marti E, Ferrer I. Expression of caspases and their substrates in the rat model of focal cerebral ischemia. Neurobiol Dis 7 332–342 (2000).
[147] Culmsee C, Mattson MP. p53 in neuronal apoptosis. Biochem Biophys Res Commun 331: 761-777 (2005).
[148] Green DR, Kroemer G. The pathophysiology of mitochondrial cell death. Science 305: 626-629 (2004).
[149] Elmore S.: Apoptosis: a review of programmed cell death. Toxicol Pathol 35: 495-516 (2007).
[150] Frankowski H, Missotten M, Albertini P, Talabot D, Catsicas S, Pietra C, Huarte J. Overexpression of BCL-2 in transgenic mice protects neurons from naturally occurring cell death and experimental ischemia. Neuron 13: 1017-1030 (1994).
[151] Crumrine RC, Thomas AL, Morgan PF. Attenuation of p53 expression protects against focal ischemic damage in transgenic mice. J Cereb Blood Flow Metab 14:887-891 (1994).
[152] Liu J, Liu MC, Wang KK. Calpain in the CNS: from synaptic function to neurotoxicity. Sci Signal 1: re 1 (2008).

[153] Goll DE, Thompson VF, Li HQ, Wei W, Cong JY. The calpain system. Physiol Rev 83: 731-801 (2003).
[154] Rami A, Ferger D, Krieglstein J. Blockage of calpain proteolytic activity rescues neurons from glutamate excitotoxicity. Neurosci Res 27: 93-97 (1997).
[155] Ray SK. Currently evaluated calpain and caspase inhibitors for neuroprotection in experimental brain ischemia. Curr Med Chem13: 3425-3440 (2006).
[156] Bevers MB, Neumar RW. Mechanistic role of calpains in postischemic neuro-degeneration. J Cereb Blood Flow Metab 28: 655-673 (2008).
[157] Bano D, Nicotera P. Ca^{2+} signals and neuronal death in brain. Stroke 38 [part 2]: 674-676 (2007).
[158] Heiss WD, Thiel A, Grond M, Graf R. Which targets are relevant for therapy of acute ischemic stroke? Stroke 30:1486–1489 (1999).
[159] Tissue plasminogen activator for acute ischemic stroke. The National Institute of Neurological Disorders and Stroke rt-PA Stroke Study Group. N Engl J Med 333: 1581-87 (1995).
[160] Reeves MJ, Arora S, Broderick JP, *et al.* Acute stroke care in the US: results from the 4 pilot prototypes of the Paul Coverdell National Acute Stroke Registry. Stroke 36: 1232-1240 (2005).
[161] Caplan LR. Stroke thrombolysis: slow progress. Circulation 114: 187-190 (2006).
[162] Derex L, Nighoghossian N. Intracerebral haemorrhage after thrombolysis for acute ischaemic stroke: an update. J Neurol Neurosurg Psychiatry 79: 1093-1099 (2008).
[163] Molina CA, Saver JL. Extending reperfusion therapy for acute ischemic stroke: emerging pharmacological, mechanical, and imaging strategies. Stroke 36: 2311-2320 (2005).
[164] O´Collins VE, McLeod MR, Donnan GA, HorkyLL, van der Worp BH, Howells DW. 1026 experimental treatments in acute stroke. Ann Neurol 50: 447-448 (2006).
[165] Ginsberg MD. Neurprotection for ischemic stroke: past, present and future. Neuropharmacol 55: 363-389 (2008).
[166] Fisher M. New approaches to neuroprotective grug development. Stroke 42 [suppl 1]: S24-S27 (2011).
[167] Fisher M, Feuerstein GZ, Howells DW, Hurn PD, Kent TA, Savitz SI, Lo EH (for the STAIR group). Update for the Stroke Therapie Academic Industry Roundtable preclinical recommendations. Stroke 40: 2244-2250 (2009).
[168] Stankowski JN, Gupta R. Therapeutic targets for neuroprotecion in acute ischemic stroke: lost in translation?. Antioxid Redox Signal 14: 1841-1851 (2011).
[169] Bernaudin M, Marti HH, Roussel S, Divoux D, Nouvelot A, MacKenzie ET, Petit E. A potential role for erythropoietin in focal permanent cerebral ischemia in mice. J Cereb Blood Flow Metab 19: 643-651 (1999).
[170] Siren AL, Fratelli M, Brines M, Goemans C, Casagrande S, Lewczuk P, Keenan S, Gleiter C, Pasquali C, Capobianco A Mennini T, Heumann R, Cerami A, Ehrenreich H, Ghezzi P. Erythropoietin prevents neuronal apoptosis after cerebral ischemia and metabolic stress. Proc. Natl Acad Sci USA 98: 4044–4049 (2001).
[171] Kilic E, Kilic U, Soliz J, Bassetti CL, Gassmann M, Hermann DM. Brain-derived erythropoietin protects from focal cerebral ischemia by dual activation of ERK-1/-2 and Akt pathways. FASEB J 19: 2026-2028 (2005).
[172] Reitmer R, Kilic E, Kilic Ü, Bacigaluppi M, ElAli A, Salani G, Pluchino S, Gassmann M, Hermann DM. Post-acute delivery of erythropoietin induces stroke recovery by promoting perilesional tissue remodelling and contralesional pyramidal tract plasticity. Brain 134: 84-99 (2011).

3

Neuro-EPO by Nasal Route as a Neuroprotective Therapy in Brain Ischemia

Julio César García Rodríguez[1] and Ramón Rama Bretón[2]
[1]Life Science and Nanosecurity, Scientific Advisor's Office, State Council,
[2]Department of Physiology & Immunology, University of Barcelona, Barcelona
[1]Cuba
[2]Spain

1. Introduction

Cerebral vascular diseases (CVD) are the third leading cause of death in industrialized countries and in Cuba affect the 50% of the population above 60 years old [1-2]. The mortality is exponentially increased with age and doubles every five years. A total of 22,000 annual cases are estimated in Cuba, a country where life expectance should increase to 80 years in the near future [1].

CVD are often followed by a high social and individual cost as a consequence of disability and family affectation.

The most problematic among such diseases is ischemic cerebral vascular disease, characterized by the reduction of cerebral blood flow (CBF) below a critical level. From this initial event several processes take place to induce the clinical symptoms of cerebral ischemia [3].

Prioritized attention has been granted to CVD prevention in Cuba for reduction of mortality and morbidity indexes associated with these diseases. Risk factors and patients suffering from transient ischemic attacks (TIA) have received special consideration [4].

While most strategies, such as thrombolysis, are aimed at CBF recovery, neuroprotection intents to increment cell survival through the modification of the ischemic cascade [4, 5]. The most important therapeutic strategy in patients with ischemic stroke is directed to improve CBF and to reduce or block sub cellular and cellular metabolic consequences [6].

Some proposals point to more than just a partial solution to the problem of ischemic cascade and call for combined therapies and the use of molecules involved in endogenous neuroprotection. [5-7]. A good candidate could be human recombinant erythropoietin (rHu-EPO), which has been employed in the treatment of renal insufficiency associated anemia, and in cancer patients suffering anemia as a consequence of chemo and radiotherapy. The effect of rHu-EPO in the protection of brain cells from ischemic injury has been investigated during the last decade [8-14].

Given the systematic failures in clinical trials using proven neuroprotection ability molecules in animal models [16], it seems logical to reevaluate the therapeutic strategy for therapeutic treatment in the acute phase of stroke.

Searching within selected biological mechanisms for endogenous neuroprotection appears to be the most promising. Today this is possible by the advances science and technology have achieved through biotechnology, which allows us to obtain proteins similar to Erythropoietin to autologously use our brain to maintain homeostasis at a stroke.
Helping this process may be the way to a successful therapeutic strategy for neuroprotection against stroke and general neurological diseases and inherited degenerative diseases too.
EPO had been reported as a neuroprotective molecule in animal models with perspectives for its clinical use. However, systemic administration has shown potential side effects. For that reason, recently researchers have demonstrated neuroprotective effects in different animal models of stroke using EPO as a neuroprotector or other different types of EPO without erythropoiesis-stimulating activity. These new molecules retain their ability to protect neural tissue against injury and they include Asialoerythropoietin (asialoEPO) carbamylated EPO (CEPO), and rHu-EPO with low sialic acid content (Neuro-EPO). [15, 16]
On the other hand, some of these derivatives of EPO or rHu-EPO have been shown to have no neuroprotective effect during *in vivo* studies. [17, 18]
Indeed, nasal administration presents advantages treating the brain compared with intravenous and intraventricular routes, especially for treatments utilizing Neuro-EPO. [16]
In this chapter, the authors focus on the neuroprotective effect from treatment of nasal Neuro-EPO in the acute stroke animals' models and the security and efficacy of this treatment from the perspective of the stroke therapies.

2. Neuroprotection and endogenous erythropoietin

A drug sufficiently effective and with safe access to the central nervous system (CNS) has not been developed yet for neuroprotective treatment of neurological diseases in either chronic or acute stages.
Besides, most of neuroprotective therapeutic agents, effective in ischemia biomodels, have failed to be clinically tolerated [19]. A strategy to circumvent this problem can be the use of the same molecules expressed in the brain after different lesions, [9, 20,] helping in the maintenance of homeostasis.
The use of endogenous biomolecules with therapeutic activity is a recent proposal in neuroscience research [20]. An example of this type of molecule is erythropoietin, a glycoprotein produced in the kidney and involved in the proliferation, differentiation, and maturation of erythrocyte progenitors, increasing oxygen supply to the tissues [21]. Indeed, EPO is one of the molecules more conserved evolutionarily [22]. This can be interpreted, as the EPO molecule is affective and safe in their biological activity.
The observation that EPO and its receptor (EPO-R) are expressed in the brain has stimulated the development of studies related to the neuroprotective effect of this molecule in different models of stroke [23, 24]. EPO expression increases during cerebral ischemia, suggesting its role in the endogenous neuroprotector system of the mammalian brain [25].
rHu-EPO is one of the ten best selling products of world biotechnology. The study of the neuroprotective effect of erythropoietin has been stimulated by the fact that this drug is normally expressed within the brain and is regulated by hypoxia inducible factor 1 (HIF-1) **(Figure 1),** which is in turn activated by a wide variety of stress factors.
Indeed, in the last 5 years several reports of applications of rHu-EPO in cytoprotection were done **(Table 1)**

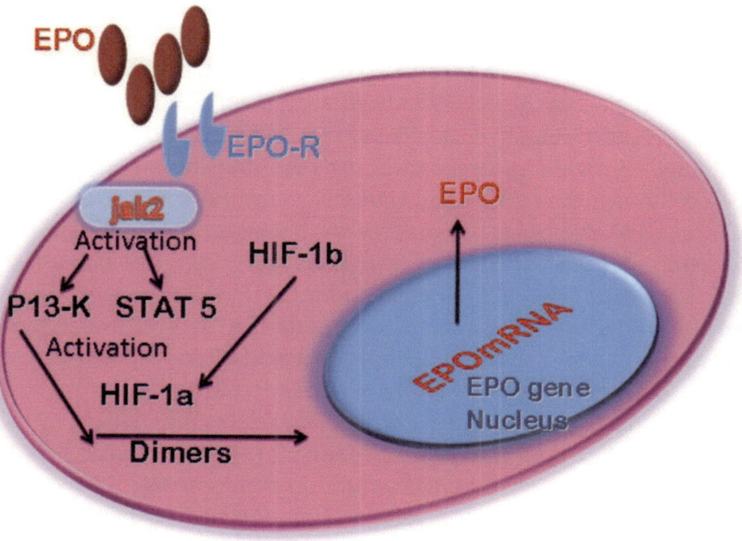

Fig. 1. Simplified diagram showing the main actors associated with neuronal protective response mediated by HIF-1. Where participating EPO, EPOR, HIF1a dimerizes with HIF-1b is the signal for transcription in the nucleus and results in EPO mRNA and finally to the synthesis of erythropoietin (EPO).

Assay	*in vivo* or *in vitro* Models	Route/dose	Reference
In vitro Primary Culture of Astrocytes	Rat	5-20 U/mL	Diaz Z, (2005)
Focal and global cerebral ischemia	Mouse	IP 25-100U	Marti HH (2004)
Focal Ischemia MCA	Rat	IN 4.8, 12, 24 U/kg	Yu YP, et al (2005)
Focal Ischemia MCA	Rat	IP 100, 1000, 5000 U/kg	Belayev L et al (2005)
Retinal Ischemia	Mouse and rat	IP 5000 U	Grimm C, et al 2006
Neonatal brain hypoxia	Rat	IP 1000 U/kg	Yamada M, et al (2011)
Spinal cord injury	Mouse and rat	IP 5000 U	Mofidi A et al (2011)
Focal cerebral ischemia	Gerbils	IN 249.4 U	Rodríguez Y et al (2010)

Table 1. Some reports of applications of rHu-EPO in cytoprotection.
U=Unit; IP= Intraperitoneal Injection; MCA=Middle Cerebral Artery; IN= Intra Nasal

3. Brain protection by erythropoietin

It has been demonstrated that EPO and its receptor are expressed in brain tissue and their expression increases during ischemia, suggesting that they are involved in an endogenous neuroprotective system in mammalian brain [25].

The neuroprotective efficacy of rHu-EPO has been tested in several animal models of nervous system injury in mouse, rat, gerbil, and rabbit, including focal and global cerebral ischemia **(Table 1),** showing a reduction of neuronal death.
Although the neuroprotective mechanism of rHu-EPO is still being investigated, it is known that this effect is mediated by receptors located at the walls of the vascular endothelia and astrocytes [26]. The neuroprotective mechanism of rHu-EPO seems to be multifactor. rHu-EPO may indirectly mediate neuroprotection by restoring the blood supply to the injured tissue or acts directly over the neurons by activating multiple molecular signaling pathways. The rHu-EPO molecule positively modulates the expression of antioxidant enzymes and reduces nitric oxide mediated formation of free radicals; by a mechanism involving JAK2 [27] and the nuclear factor NFkB [28]. Its antioxidant action is also sustained by restoring the cytosolic catalase and glutathione peroxidase activities in erythrocytes, which protects against the oxidative stress by reducing lipid peroxidation [29] and also EPO plays an important role in protecting against brain ischemia/reperfusion through inhibiting lipid peroxidation and decreasing blood brain barrier (BBB) disruption [30].
It has been demonstrated that rHu-EPO also displays neurotrophic activity [31], which implies an effect of larger latency than the inhibition of apoptosis [32] and reduces neuronal exitotoxicity, involved in many forms of cerebral injury. rHu-EPO has been also identified as a potent mediator of tolerance to ischemia [33].
Like other HIF-1 induced cytokines, this glycoprotein promotes angiogenesis as a response to hypoxia and neuronal injury [34] by stimulating the generation of microvessels through the interaction with its receptor in the blood vessels [35, 36].
Its antiapoptotic action is given through the EPOR mediated activation of JAK2, which in turns leads to the activation of NF-kB and to the overexpression of the apoptosis inhibiting genes XIAP and c-IAP2 [34]. rHu-EPO protects neurons from ischemic injury by overexpression of Bcl-x in the hippocampus of gerbils [29].
At the same time it stimulates cell survival by inhibiting the MAPK and PI3K/Akt complex which promotes apoptosis [29]. These data suggest that rHu-EPO acts by controlling the balance of the expression of either pro apoptotic or antiapoptotic molecules [37].
The neuroprotective effect attributed to rHu-EPO can be also derived from its anti-inflammatory effect signaling in neurons, glial and cerebrovascular endothelial cells and stimulates angiogenesis and neurogenesis. These mechanisms underlie its potent tissue protective effects in experimental models of stroke [38.]
A summary of the different biological activities on cells of the nervous system to explain the cytoprotective capacity of EPO is shown in **Table 2**

Activity/ Cells	**Immature Neurons**	**Neurons**	**Astrocytes**	**Microglia**	**Ependimal**	**Oligodendrocyte**
Neurogenesis	**YES**	?	?	?	?	?
Anti oxidative	?	**YES**	**YES**	**YES**	?	?
Tropic	**YES**	**YES**	?	?	?	?
Anti apoptotic	**YES**	**YES**	**YES**	?	**YES**	**YES**
Anti Inflammatory	**YES**	?	**YES**	**YES**	?	**YES**
Anti-Glutamate	?	**YES**	?	?	?	?

Table 2. Differents neuroprotective profile for rH-EPO on cells of the nervous system.
(?)= Not yet demonstrated activity; (YES) = Demonstrated Activity.

4. Delivery of drugs to CNS and BBB

The deficiency in this first decade of the century to have efficient and safe drugs to counter neurodegenerative diseases and cerebrovascular accidents are, without a doubt a pressing need for the development of pharmacology and neuroscience in general.

Some molecules have been developed with proven ability in different biomodels of neuroprotective stroke; however, none of them managed to overcome the barrier of Phase III clinical trials [35]. In this respect, several negative factors are limiting the success. At this point, we refer to the strong obstacles that represent the BBB.

We focus our commentary on the possibilities for EPO to be one of the safest and most effective drugs that has developed global biotechnology. EPO has been used in millions of peoples for over 20 years with very few adverse effects reported.

The application of EPO and its non-erythropoetic variants like Neuro-EPO through nasal delivery to the central nervous system target an area of great interest right now [39-41]. In *cynomolgus monkeys,* intra nasal route is relatively well known anatomically, physiologically as well as the transport mechanism of low molecular weight molecules and proteins to the brain [42].

In a simplified form the nasal cavity can be divided into three parts. They are: 1) Nasal vestibule, 2) Olfactory region and 3) Respiratory region **(Figure 2).**

Of these three regions, drugs released into the nostril in contact with the nasal epithelium, which has several types of cells through the *lamina propria,* and a thin layer off loose connective tissue containing blood. Vessels, lymphatic vessels, axons and glands are involved.

For a drug to travel from the olfactory region in the nasal cavity to the CSF or brain parenchyma has to go through the olfactory epithelium, depending on the path followed, also the arachnoid membrane. In principle you can consider three paths through the olfactory epithelium:

- Via endocytic pathway, primarily through subtentaculares cells, where endocytosis processes occurring receptor-mediated endocytosis of liquid phase or by passive diffusion. This path corresponds especially to small lipophilic molecules or large molecules.
- Via extra cellular through the tight junctions or open cracks in the membrane between sustentacular cells and olfactory neurons. This pathway is particularly suited to small hydrophilic molecules.
- Via axonal: The drug can be transported through the olfactory neurons (where endocytic mechanisms enters or pinocytotic) to the olfactory bulb by axonal transport intracellular

Possible mechanisms by which macromolecules applied to the nasal cavity transport to the brain are under investigation.

These mechanisms are involved in several possible anatomical structures such as olfactory and trigeminal nerves, vasculature, cerebrospinal fluid (CSF), and the lymphatic system. Possible routes for the molecules of the nasal cavity to the brain may involve several mechanisms as bulk flow and diffusion within perineural channels, perivascular spaces, or lymphatic channels directly connected to brain tissue or CSF [40].

It is known that the trigeminal nerve innervates the nasal cavity and provides a direct connection to CNS, a description of these pathways and Genc (2011) in an excellent Expert Opinion [41] has recently reported processes.

We note that there are now enough experimental evidences and clinical practice show that the olfactory BBB level can be considered highly permeable to many molecules, including proteins of medium molecular weight such as erythropoietin.
This possibility is challenges to use this route to deliver drugs to the CNS that do not allow access the BBB. What are the advantages and disadvantages offered by the nasal route to deliver molecules to the CNS will discuss below.

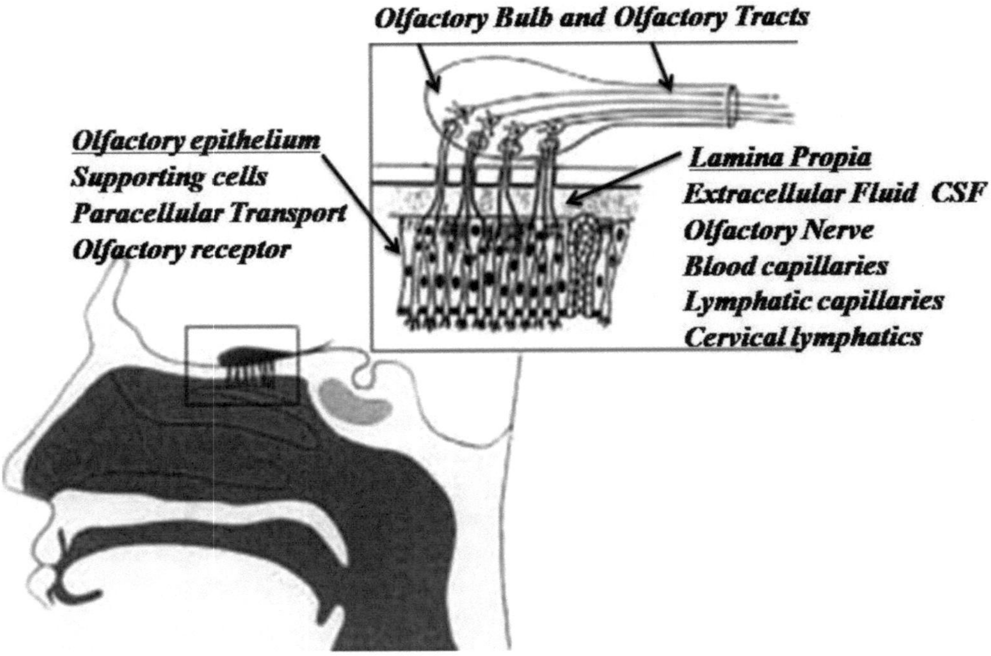

Fig. 2. Diagram of the nasal cavity. Structure of olfactory epithelium with the communication proposed for the circulation of substances by intranasal route to the CNS and possible routes to come from the Neuro-EPO to the brain when applied nasally.

5. Advantages and disadvantages of the nasal route for drug delivery to CNS

In this section, we would point out those aspects that we believe according with our experience should always be taken into account for proper projection of work with a formulation of nasal application.
It is truly remarkable to consider the anatomical differences between rodents and humans with respect to the nasal system. These become more important since most drug studies are conducted in rodents.
We must also take into account the experimental general procedure in trials where it has demonstrated the efficacy and safety of a nasal preparation. The possible influence of anesthesia methods employed (mostly placed in the supine position) and experimental factors to try to find optimal conditions, far removed from real life human beings.
Among the advantages of nasally is low cost, as opposed to systemically, this product does not require needles or syringes, which represents a negligible cost for a drug. For the same reason your application is easier and less traumatic and allows smooth, self-application.

Perhaps the biggest advantage is its rapid nasal application release to the CNS, concomitantly with a considerable less amount of drug applied and therefore a lower risk of side effects from excessive drug.
Studies carried out in nonhuman primates using rH-EPO systemically and Neuro-EPO nasally, showed that Neuro-EPO was more readily to the lumbar CSF and for more longer time and with a considerably lower dose of Neuro-EPO.
This study shows the distribution levels of Neuro-EPO content in CSF obtained by lumbar puncture at different time intervals after application intranasal (Neuro-EPO 1000 IU) or intravenously (rHu- EPO, 5000 IU).
There was a peak of 430 mIU / mL for rHu-EPO at 10 min after application, representing approximately 0.01% the total injected dose, whereas the total volume of CSF in this species is 15 mL approx. This distribution of rHuEPO from blood to the CSF is consistent with those reported by other authors in non-human primates [42] and human [43]. This finding is characteristic of those components of protein origin not permeable to the BBB, but in small amounts or traces is present in CSF, as albumin [44]. It should be noted that these small amounts physiological concentrations achieved much higher baseline levels of rHu- EPO in the CSF action ensuring already reported neuroprotective.
An analysis of the results in the model of *M. fascicular* is shows that after the first hour the behavior of both approaches (intranasally and intravenous) is very similar, suggesting rapid elimination of the molecule. This makes it possible to avoid side effects caused by an excess of circulating Neuro-EPO long time in the CNS [45].
In a study by Brines et al (2000) [46] demonstrated an application of 5000 IU / kg via intraperitoneal mouse EPO levels in CSF was highest 3.5 hours from application.
Among the disadvantages we can point to the nasal route is that we can not determine with absolute precision the dose that each nasal application is delivered to the CNS. Another aspect is the exclusion of people with allergies, deviated nasal septum, the mucus and clearings may reduce the passage of product to the CNS.
Among the side effects of intranasal application of erythropoietin, is the fact that most of the application moves into the bloodstream and therefore has the capacity to induce erythropoiesis, at least, increases the number of red blood cells. Any increase in these cells will increase the viscosity of blood, which is undesirable for patients in the acute stroke. Therefore, the development of non-erythropoietic variants from the ability to maintain protective capacity shown for erythropoietin is an emerging field within neuroscience comment below as variants not erythropoietic of erythropoietin and its neuroprotective action.

6. Non-erythropoietic variants of erythropoietin and their neuroprotective action

Recently, several different types of new EPOs without erythropoiesis-stimulating activity have been developed. These new molecules retain their ability to protect neural tissue against injury; they include Asialoerythropoietin (asialoEPO) [47,48], carbamylated EPO (CEPO)[49-,51], and rHu-EPO with low sialic acid content (Neuro-EPO)[16, 39,45].

6.1 AsialoEPO

The need for nonerythropoietic rHu-EPO derivatives that still retain neuroprotective action has led to the discovery of asialoEPO, generated by total enzymatic desialylation of rHu-

EPO. AsialoEPO has the same EPO-R affinity and neuroprotective properties as EPO, but an extremely short plasma half-life [50].

The ability to dissociate the tissue-protective actions of EPO from its erythropoietic actions may eventually be applied in the clinic to promote neurological regeneration without increasing red blood cell formation [52]. Erbayraktar and coworkers [53] have shown protective activities of the nonerythropoietic asialoEPO in models of cerebral ischemia, spinal cord compression, and sciatic nerve crush. Additionally, asialoEPO protects against neonatal hypoxia-ischemia as potently as EPO in hypoxic-ischemic brain injury in 7-day-old rats [52] and also in short-term changes in infarct volume, penumbra apoptosis and behaviors following middle cerebral artery occlusion in rats [48].

6.2 CEPO

Another modified EPO molecule that solely manifests tissue-protective action without erythropoietic activity may have a more targeted effect. As an example, transformation of lysine to homocitrulline by carbamylation gives rise to carbamylated EPO (CEPO) [50].

CEPO, similar to asialoEPO, lacks erythropoietic effect, but still shows neuroprotective effects in animal models of stroke, diabetic neuropathy, and experimental autoimmune encephalomyelitis to an extent comparable to that of EPO [54]. It is important to note that CEPO has a minimal affinity for EPO-R and that its effects are mediated via a different EPO receptor. It is thought that this receptor consists of the EPO-R monomer together with a dimer of the common β chain (CD131). Recently, an investigation carried out in a rat model of focal cerebral ischemia showed that post ischemic intravenous treatment with CEPO led to improved functional recovery [52]. In 2007, a study by Mahmood et al. [55] assessed the effect of intraperitoneally infused rHu-EPO and CEPO in a traumatic brain injury rat model, and they concluded that rHu-EPO and CEPO are equally effective in enhancing spatial learning and promoting neural plasticity, but hematocrit was significantly increased only with rHu-EPO. Similarly, a recent study by Wang et al [52], demonstrated equivalent effects of rHu-EPO and CEPO in the reduction of neurological impairment in rats subjected to embolic middle cerebral artery occlusion (MCAO). As expected, rHu-EPO, but not CEPO, produced a transient increase in hematocrit levels.

Another advantage of EPO over CEPO was demonstrated in rodents. Short-term treatment with EPO at doses optimal for neuroprotection caused significant alterations in platelet function and composition with in vivo haemostatic consequences, while CEPO treatment had no effect on these parameters [56].

6.3 Neuro-EPO

During the biotechnological production of rHu-EPO, various isoforms with different contents of sialic acid are obtained. When the sialic acid content is 4–7 mol/mol protein, it is considered a low sialic acid–containing EPO, modified to display low sialic acid content (Neuro-EPO) is very similar to the one that occurs in the mammalian brain. Low sialic acid–containing EPOs are rapidly degraded by the liver. Thus, this molecule could be administered by a no systemic route, such as the intranasal route, to prevent its hepatic degradation. The intranasal administration of Neuro-EPO has been shown to be safe; the molecule reaches the brain rapidly, does not stimulate erythropoiesis after acute treatments, and shows efficacy in some rodent models of brain ischemia and in nonhuman primates. This proposal could be considered a therapeutic option for stroke and others neurodegenerative illness. (See review García Rodriguez and Sosa Testé, 2009) [3]

There have been two strategies followed so far by different research groups. Some have postulated the safer use of erythropoietin as a neuroprotectant in cerebral ischemia. Their works have been based on existing knowledge of primary and secondary structure of the protein erythropoietin **(Figure 3)** and knowing there are differentially placed amino acid sequence with erythropoietic capacity and cytoprotective property in this cytokine.

From this knowledge has been postulated by different chemical modifications to inactivate the capacity of erythropoietic region, leaving only the resulting molecules with neuroprotective capacity. This variant has the potential disadvantage of the molecule obtained in this way; it is not similar to that naturally produced by the CNS, which may bring difficulties in recognition or neurotoxicity. These topics have not yet been fully studied in works of neurotoxicology.

The second variant, through which we get the Neuro-EPO, is characterized not by changes to chemical molecules produced by biotechnology, but selects those molecular populations with a low profile isoforms sialic acid content that make the Neuro-EPO easily degraded as it passes into the bloodstream. In addition, recent study has demonstrated in neurotoxicological study its safety and low toxicity when applied nasally [57].

Therefore, studies of effectiveness and efficiency are top priority. A synthetic form below and discussion of the work with the Neuro-nasally EPO in models of cerebral ischemia.

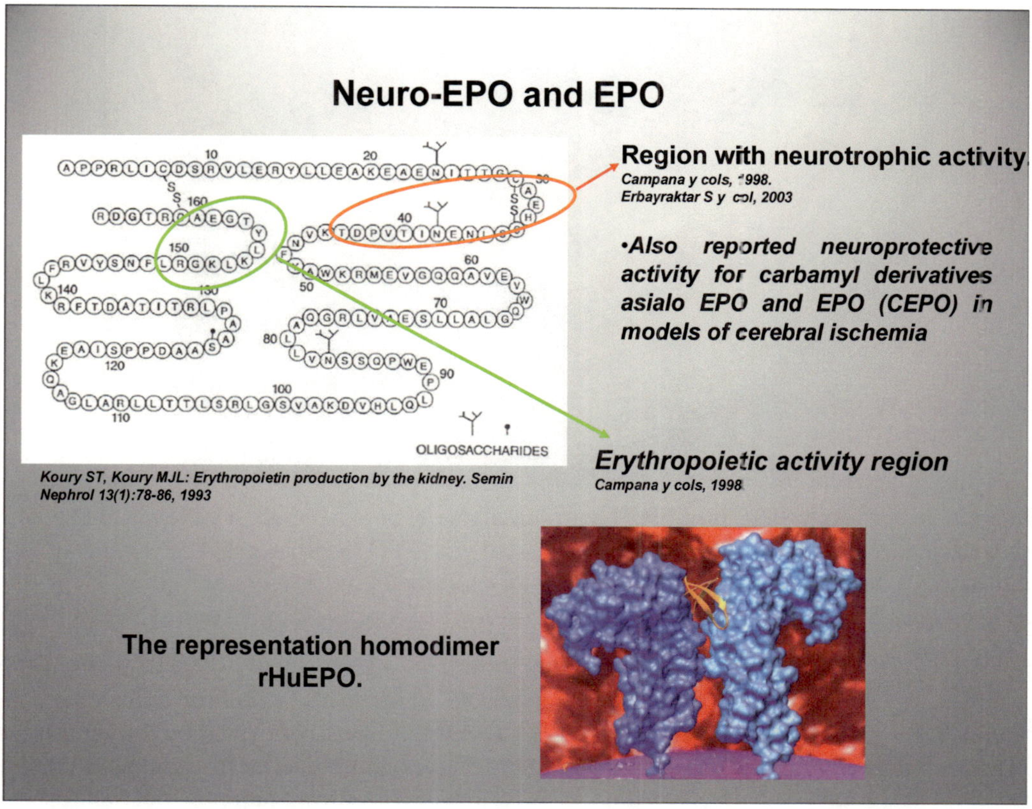

Fig. 3. *Top* Show the representation of EPO protein AA sequences and Regions with Neurotrophic and Erythropoietic activity. *Down*, Show the representation homodimer rHuEPO.

7. Security and efficacy of the nasal Neuro-EPO intra nasally preclinical studies of brain ischemia

Evaluation of whether the formulation produced allowed the arrival of the Neuro-EPO nasally applied to the CNS was one of the first tasks accomplished. The animal model was the Gerbil Mongolia. **(Figure 4)**
Activity detected molecule Neuro-EPO labeled I^{125} was detected in the olfactory bulb and cerebellum. In the CSF concentrations was in the range of physiological and therefore support an adequate therapeutic concentration.
The nasal opening is generally favored for rodents. The nasal olfactory mucosa covers approximately 50% of total nasal epithelium in the rat [58], while in human's covers only 5% [59]. Another important difference is the volume of cerebrospinal fluid (CSF) in the rat is 3.5 ml and in humans is 160 ml, therefore, the replacement time of the CSF in the rat is 1.5 hours while in humans is 5 hours, making it difficult to infer the uptake of molecules of one species to another. However studies conducted on the passage of molecules by the intranasal route in species such as nonhuman primate *Macaca fascicularis* species are recommended for pharmacokinetic studies of the nasal [45, 60].

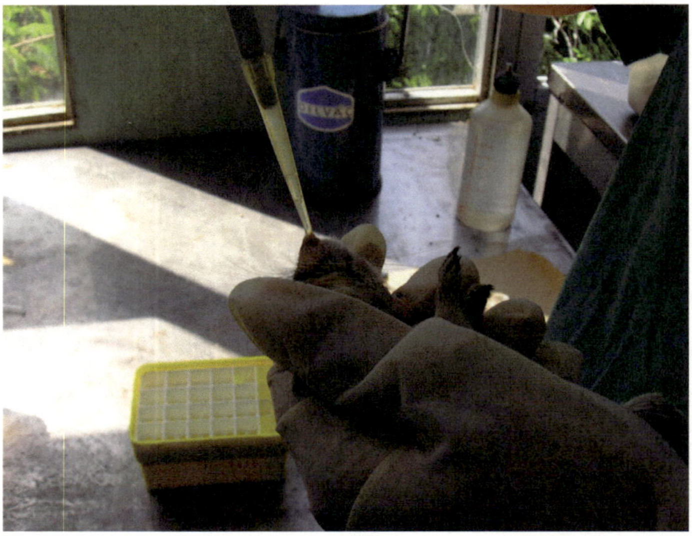

Fig. 4. Neuroprotective effects of EPO Neuro-nasal model of focal cerebral ischemia in the Mongolian Gerbils. In the group of animals treated with EPO Neuro-applied by nasal way only animals died within 24 hours. This behavior continued until 5 weeks, which demonstrates the powerful protective effect achieved by intranasal application of Neuro-EPO.

The transit of Neuro-EPO to the CNS after intranasal administration and its effect were reported by us [41]. The detection of the molecule either in the olfactory bulbs or in the cerebellum suggested its contact with the CSF. This was further confirmed by the significant increase of rHu-EPO in the CSF of *M. fascicularis* (Figure 4) 5 min after its administration by the intranasal route. In animals treated with Neuro-EPO, a preservation of the habituation behavior in spontaneous exploratory activity was observed in both models, demonstrating the conservation of the structural integrity of the brain regions related to learning, and short- and long-term memory [61].

In the model of MCAO for 2 h in rats, animals treated with Neuro-EPO by the intranasal route displayed smaller volumes of ischemic tissue and a better clinical condition at 48 h [62]. The results of this study in rodents show therapeutic efficacy in both the acute and chronic phases of ischemia, as well as in reperfusion ischemia models, suggesting neuroprotective effects in brain structure and function.

These are indirect evidences of the access of Neuro-EPO administered in the amounts equivalent to the therapeutic dose recommended for ischemia by the intranasal route.

Those results suggest additional advantages for the intranasal route, which could be safer and faster than the intravenous route, which was recently demonstrated for delivery of Neurotrophic factors BDNF, CNTF, EPO, and an NT-4 to the CNS. [63]

In correlation with these ideas, Fletcher et al. [64] demonstrated that intranasal EPO plus IGF-I penetrate into the brain more efficiently than other drug delivery methods, and could potentially provide a fast and efficient treatment to prevent chronic effects of stroke.

A general survey carried out by a group of investigators concerning the use of the intranasal route to administer drugs for the treatment of diseases affecting the CNS indicated that in the last decade, roughly 11% of the new drugs generated by the industry are administered by this route. Patients prefer intranasal administration due to the efficacy and safety of these formulations.

A recent study assessing the safety of the Neuro-EPO was carried [57] out because the use of human recombinant erythropoietin (EPO) as a neuroprotective agent is limited due to its hematological side effects. Neuro-EPO, similar to that produced in the brain during hypoxia, may be used as a neuroprotective agent without risk of thrombotic events.

The objective of this investigation was to assess the toxicological potential of a nasal formulation with Neuro-EPO in acute, subacute and nasal irritation assays in rats. Healthy Wistar rats (Cenp: Wistar) were used for the assays.

In an irritation test, animals received 15 micro liters of Neuro-EPO into the right nostril. Rats were sacrificed after 24h and slides of the nasal mucosa tissues were examined. Control and treated groups showed signs of a minimal irritation consisting of week edema and vascular congestion in all animals. In the acute toxicity test, the dose of 47,143UI/kg was administered by nasal route. Hematological patterns, body weight, relative organ weight, and organ integrity were not affected by single dosing with Neuro-EPO.

In the subacute toxicity test, Wistar rats of both sexes received 6,600 UI/kg/day for 14 days. The toxicological endpoints examined included animal body weight, food consumption, hematological and biochemical patterns, selected tissue weights, and histopathological examinations. An increase of lymphocytes was observed in males that were considered to reflect an immune response to treatment. Histopathological examination of organs and tissues did not reveal treatment-induced changes.

The administration of Neuro-EPO at daily doses of 6,600 UI/kg during 14 days did not produce hematological side effects.

In conclusion, these results suggest that Neuro-EPO could offer the same neuroprotection as EPO, without hematological side effects.

In fact the great advantage of having a formulation of erythropoietin with neuroprotective capacity but non-erythropoietic enables its possible implementation, not only in the acute phase of stroke but in its later stage, where its behavior will give us useful information, possible for the treatment of chronic neurodegenerative diseases of the CNS.

Therefore, a discussion to determine the effectiveness of the Neuro-EPO treatment in chronic phase of stroke model using Gerbils follows.

8. Nasal delivery of Neuro-EPO. Effect in acute and sub chronic phase post stroke in animal model

We are relatively poorly acquainted with the effects of erythropoietin in the central nervous system. Therefore, our bank of knowledge with the novel nasal formulation of Neuro-EPO is correspondingly miniscule.

Therefore, it is logical to want to know the effect on the CNS by administration of Neuro-EPO by the nasal route, not just over days, but when it is applied for weeks.

Of practical interest, it has been postulated that EPO activates mechanisms of neuroplasticity [65]. The mechanism through which the Neuro-EPO does this neuroprotective effect in the short and medium term is an issue that requires more basic research. In this direction a recently paper from Reitmer et al., (2011) (66) showed that EPO administered intra-cerebroventricularly at 10 IU/day; starting 3 days after 30 min of middle cerebral artery occlusion. The neurological recovery was associated with structural remodeling of ischaemic brain tissue, reflected by enhanced neuronal survival, increased angiogenesis and decreased reactive astrogliosis with expression changes of plasticity-related molecules that facilitated contralesional axonal growth, and establishes a plasticity-promoting effect of EPO after stroke. [66]. In this excellent work, unfortunately the route used to delivery EPO to the brain is not applicable to stroke patients.

If this were verified, it would be invaluable for the treatment of patients, not only in the acute phase, but also for the recovery period of mental and motor activities affected by Stroke, using pathways and molecules safer, such as nasal delivery of Neuro-EPO.

The protective effect of Neuro-EPO was also evaluated at short and medium term [24]. Not evident, at the 24-hr post ischemia time point, when the percentage of deaths in both groups was similar **(Figure 5).** However, the mortality at 48 hr after brain ischemia was greater in the Nasal-Vehicle group than that in the Nasal-Neuro-EPO group ($p=0.02$). Indeed, 50% more of the animals in the Nasal-Vehicle group were dead at 48 hr after ischemia, whereas no animals from the Nasal-Neuro-EPO group died before 48 hr post ischemia. No further mortality was recorded during the five weeks of the study. Among other tests, this result confirms the well-known phrase "*Time is Brain*". This expression is also valid for the nasal application of Neuro-EPO.

In this study, the animals treated with Nasal-Neuro-EPO showed better general states. The gerbils with higher neurological scores not only showed deterioration in the extremities corresponding to the damaged hemisphere but also showed defects on the opposite side, including bilateral palpebral ptosis. The open field-testing to evaluate the exploratory activity of the animals showed significant differences ($p<0.05$) when comparing activity before surgery to after surgery in all groups of ischemic animals, except in the groups treated with Nasal-Neuro-EPO, which showed no difference. A marked behavioral difference existed at 24 hr between the ischemic animals in both treatment groups [24]

These results taken together speak for the effectiveness and safety of nasally administered Neuro-EPO in one of the strongest models of stroke.

The concept of achieving a significantly higher survival in animals treated with Neuro-EPO nasally during the 5 weeks of the study gives clear evidence of its neuroprotective properties. If we attach to this value the protection, which it confirms to the neurological status of animals, and histological protection displayed [24] we can ensure that this molecule has strong neuroprotective effects in the short and medium terms. However, we [24] recently reported its relationship with the EPOR and the expression of another important protein in the CNS, neuroglobin.

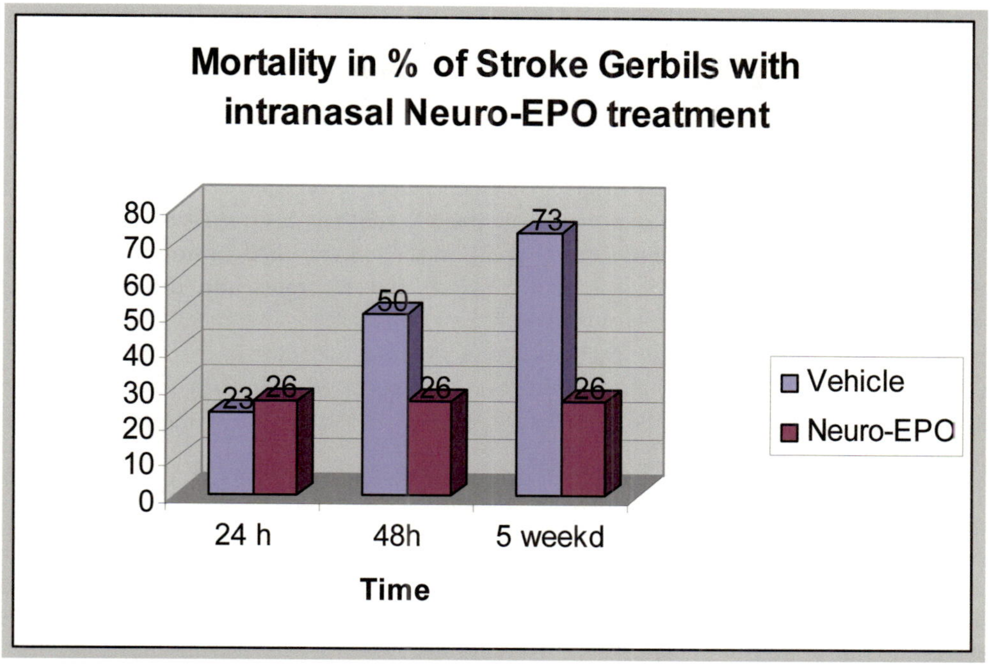

Fig. 5. The protective effect of Neuro-EPO was also evaluated at short and medium term. Not evident at 24-hr post ischemia time point; when the percentage of deaths in both groups was similar. However, no further mortality was recorded during the five weeks of the study. Among other tests, this result confirms establishes a survival-promoting effect of Neuro-EPO in the treatment of acute stroke.

In the next and final section of this chapter, we discuss the effect of Neuro-EPO application by nasal route in Gerbils Stroke model, and the effect on the expression of EPO receptor and Neuroglobin in this animal model.

9. Neuro-EPO, EPO receptor and Neuroglobin in acute phase of stroke animal model

As yet the molecular events, through which EPO makes its neuroprotective effect in the CNS have not been fully described. There are reports where it has been shown that the presence of its receptor in the hypoxic tissue is necessary for expression, which has been interpreted as the over-expression is necessary to trigger the molecular mechanisms of cytoprotection. That is, there have to be over expressed receptors for EPO and EPO existing in the region where these receptors are expressed.

The foregoing, that is the theoretical basis of EPO supplementation to hypoxic tissue as the tissue damage, mainly in the so-called ischemic penumbra region, within the mechanisms of endogen neuroprotection is the expression of new receptors to cells.

In addition, EPO has been shown to have the ability to induce the formation of new receptors. The latter should be a possible tipping point for the analysis of Neuro- EPO optimal dose, to avoid unwanted effects on the CNS in long-term treatment.

This apparent paradox of the EPO receptor should be carefully studied in the future and if in real terms for the stress neurons as a penumbra, on the limited availability to generate energy by synthesis of new receptors to the EPO. It is a challenge to the classical concept of *cellular economy*. Therefore, obviously there must exist important new functions, the EPOR, which we have not been able to elucidate to the present. Among them may be the establishment of the new homeostasis, given the change of surroundings and intrinsically in those neuron-specific functions in the new contact of damaged tissue.

As complicated and not well-recognized biochemical processes of brain endogenous neuroprotection has emerged a relatively new protein that has been investigated by several research groups, we refer to neuroglobin (NGB). In the well-studied evolutionary branch of globins, hemoglobin has played a critical role in all vertebrates and their evolutionary adaptation to the oxygen atmosphere.

At this point, we must not forget that oxygen is the final acceptor in the respiratory chain and the key atom of the vital energy production in mitochondria in the cells. We have long conceived that this step has been free of oxygen and is therefore a thermodynamically favored process.

But what happens in critical conditions where there really is not enough oxygen? A few possibilities can be unwanted interaction with the simple entry of oxygen into a cell under stress or normal. These and many more are questions that motivated us to study the expression patterns of NGB and EPOR in the Cerebral Cortex and Hippocampus revealed distinctive intranasal delivery of therapeutic effects of EPO for neuro-ischemic insults to the gerbil brain. Later, we discuss results of this work [24].

Indeed, our results [24] not only showed that the intranasal delivery of Neuro-EPO is a valuable neuroprotective approach for the treatment of ischemia but also suggested that Ngb and the EPO/EPOR system have a close relationship with ischemic insults and Neuro-EPO treatment.

Ngb may act as a positive neuroprotective biomarker for brain ischemic insults or brain protection in vertebrates, including humans [68]. Thus, the overall expression patterns of Ngb at different time points after ischemic insults suggested that it might be an indicator of the neuroprotective action of Neuro-EPO in the brain (**Table 3).**

Actually, recent studies have also reported that treatment with EPO after brain ischemia could up-regulate Ngb expression in the brain [67-70], concurring with our work. Furthermore, the neuroprotective effects of EPO have various complementary actions, including antagonism of the effects of glutamate, increased expression of antioxidant enzymes, changes in the production of neurotransmitters, and induction of Ngb [70].

In addition, we have recently demonstrated that Ngb has antioxidant and free-radical scavenging activities, providing fundamental evidence for the neuroprotective function of this protein [70]. Therefore, the neuroprotective functions of Ngb and EPO/EPOR in the brain are probably closely related [24].

The dramatic expression pattern of endogenous Ngb and EPOR is possibly important for improving gerbil survival with intranasal Neuro-EPO treatment. EPO played a neuroprotective role mediated by EPOR accompanied with Ngb up regulation.

In addition, the distinctive biphasic expression patterns of Ngb in the gerbil brain are largely associated with ischemic tolerance in the cerebral cortex and ischemic sensitivity in the hippocampus. These data are important for understanding the different reaction properties of different brain regions, which are subjected to ischemic insults at specific time points and also important for improving the therapeutic effects of intranasal Neuro-EPO administration.

Time post ischemic Insults		10min	1hr	12hr	24hr	48r	72hr	1Week	5 Weeks
Protein	Brain Region								
Ngb	CC	-	+	+	+	-	+	+	+
	HP	+	-	-	-	+	ND	+	+
EPOR	CC	ND	-	-	-	+	ND	ND	ND
	HP	+	-	-	-	+	-	-	+
		Golden Hour			Silver days			Late recovery Phase	

CC= Cerebral Cortex; HP= Hippocampus; EPOR= EPO receptor; ND= not determined;
(+) = Upregulation; (-) = Down regulation. All cases $p<0.05$. Gold Hours is the practical more important time "Time is Brain". The Silver day it is critical period of time. The 10 min and 48 hr seemed to be two time points for the brain to switch the expression of both Ngb and EPOR to early and late recovery phase, respectively. In addition, there were two phases, 10 min to 1 hr and 24 hr to 72 hr, respectively, closing to the "golden hour" of about 60 min and the "silver day" of 1 to 3 days, for the brain to recover from stroke onset with intranasal Neuro-EPO treatment.

Table 3. Expression Pattern of Ngb and EPOR in the Cerebral Cortex and Hippocampus of Gerbils in the Nasal-Neuro-EPO Group Compared to Nasal-Vehicle group. Data Represent of 3 independent experiments.

10. Conclusions

There is a significant amount of histologic findings, behavioral, biochemical and pharmacological to support Neuro-EPO by nasal route as a neuroprotective therapy in brain ischemia. Unlike other molecules of EPO, which have no capability for erythropoiesis yet retain their neuroprotective capacity, the Neuro-EPO is not a carrier of chemical alterations that may cause unwanted effects, when in contact with the CNS.

Various studies have not identified adverse effects and it has been shown to be safe and effective in protecting cortical regions and sub cortical hypoxic brain 18 hours after the occurrence of hypoxia in models where the effect has been studied.

Evaluation of its safety and effectiveness in the clinic is the new challenge is to address Neuro-EPO nasally as a new neuroprotective drug to combat ischemic acute stroke.

11. References

[1] Anuario Estadístico de Salud en Cuba. [Ref Type: Electronic Citation]. http://www.infomed.sld.cu/servicios/estadisticas/; 2009.

[2] AHA. Heart and stroke uptake. 2010

[3] Guevara GM, Rodríguez R, Álvarez LA, Riaño MA, Rodríguez P. Mecanismos celulares y moleculares de la enfermedad cerebrovascular isquémica. Rev Cubana. Med 2004;43(4). Disponible en: http:// scielo.sld.cu/scielo.php?script=sci_arttext&pid=S0034-75232004000400-008&lng=es&nrm=iso.

[4] Rodríguez ML, Galvizu SR, Álvarez GE. Neuromodulación farmacológica en la Enfermedad cerebrovascular. Temas actualizados. Rev Cubana Med 2002;41: 34-9.

[5] Krieglstein J, Klump S. Pharmacology of cerebral ischemia. Rev Mex 2002; 3(3):179.

[6] Hacke W. Neuroprotective strategies for early intervention in acute ischemic stroke. Cerebrovascular disease 1997; Suppl 4. 201-220.

[7] Buergo Zuaznábar MA, Fernández-Concepción O, Pérez Nellar J, Pando Cabrera A. Guías de práctica clínica para las enfermedades cerebrovasculares. Medisur 2007 (Número Especial):1-25 In: http://medisur.sld.cu/index.php/medisur/article/view/246/730.

[8] García Salman JD. Protección neuronal endógena: un enfoque alternativo. Rev Neurol 2004;38:150-5.

[9] Dirnagl U, Simon RP, Hallenbeck JM. Ischemic tolerance and endogenous neuroprotection. Trends Neurosci 2003;26:248-54.

[10] Villa P, Bigini P, Mennini T, Agnello D, Laragione T, Cagnotto A, *et al.* Erythropoietin selectively attenuates cytokine production and inflammation in cerebral ischemia by targeting neuronal apoptosis. J Exp Med 2003;198:971-5.

[11] Weiss MJ. New insights into erythropoietin and epoetin alfa: mechanisms of action, target tissues, and clinical applications. Oncologist 2003;8(3):18-29.

[12] Sakanaka M, Wen T-C, Matsuda S, Seiji Masuda S, Morishita E, Nagao M, *et al. In vivo* evidence that erythropoietin protects neurons from ischemic damage. Proc Natl Acad Sci PNAS 1998;95:4635-40.

[13] Marti HH, Gassmann M, Wenger RH, Kvietikova I, Morganti-Kossmann MC, Kossmann T, *et al.* Detection of erythropoietin in human liquor: intrinsic erythropoietin production in the brain. Kidney Int 1997;51:416-8.

[14] Van der Meer P, Voors A, Lipsic E, Van Meer G, Dirk J, Van Veldhuisen D. Erythropoietin in cardiovascular diseases. Eur Heart J 2004;25:285-91.

[15] Sirén A L, Faßhauer T, Bartels C and Ehrenreich H. Therapeutic potential of erythropoietin and its structural or functional variants in the nervous system Neurotherapeutics Vol 6 (1), 2009, 108-127.

[16] Rodríguez Cruz Y, Mengana Támos Y , Muñoz Cernuda A, Subirós Martines N, González-Quevedo A, Sosa Testé I, and García Rodríguez J C. Treatment with Nasal Neuro-EPO Improves the Neurological, Cognitive, and Histological State in a Gerbil Model of Focal Ischemia. TheScientificWorldJOURNAL (2010) 10, 2288–2300

[17] MAC Gil J, Leist M, Popovic N, Brundin P and Petersén A. Asialoerythropoetin is not effective in the R6/2 line of Huntington's disease mice. *BMC Neuroscience* 2004, 5:17

[18] Na'ama A. Shein,Nikolaos Grigoriadis, Alexander G. Alexandrovich, Constantina Simeodinou, Evangelia Spandou, Jeanna Tsenter, Ido Yyatsiv, Michal Horwitz, and Esthe Shohami. Differential Neuroprotective Properties of Endogenous and Exogenous Erythropoietin in a Mouse Model of Traumatic Brain Injury. Journal of Neurotrauma 25:112–123 (February 2008)

[19] Fisher M. The ischemic penumbra identification, evolution and treatment concepts. Cerebrovasc Dis 2004;17 (1):1-6.

[20] García Salman, J.D. (2004) Protección neuronal endógena: un enfoque alternativo. *Rev. Neurol.* 38(2), 150–155.

[21] Jelkmann, W. (2004) Molecular biology of erythropoietin. Intern. Med. 43, 649–659.

[22] Rahat O, Yitzhaky A, Schreiber G. Cluster conservation as a novel tool for studying protein-protein interactions evolution. Proteins. 2008 May 1;71(2):621-30.

[23] Marti, H.H., Bernaudin, M., Petit, E., and Bauer, C. (2000) Neuroprotection and angiogenesis: dual role of erythropoietin in brain ischemia. News Physiol. Sci. 15(5), 225–229.

[24] Gao Y, Mengana Y, Rodríguez Cruz Y, Muñoz A, Sosa Testé I, García J D, Wu Y, García Rodríguez J C, and Zhang C. (2011) Journal of Histochemistry & Cytochemistry 59(2) 214–227

[25] Siren, A.L., Fratelli, M., Brines, M., et al. (2001) Erythropoietin prevents neuronal apoptosis after cerebral ischemia and metabolic stress. Proc. Natl. Acad. Sci. U. S. A. 98(7), 4044–4049.

[26] Juul SE, Yachnis AT, Rojiani AM, Christensen RD. Immunohistochemical localization of erythropoietin and its receptor in the developing human brain. Pediatr Dev Pathol. 1999 Mar-Apr;2(2):148-58.

[27] Garcia-Ramírez M, Hernández C, Ruiz-Meana M, Villarroel M, Corraliza L, García-Dorado D, Simó R. Erythropoietin protects retinal pigment epithelial cells against the increase of permeability induced by diabetic conditions: Essential role of JAK2/ PI3K signaling. Cell Signal. 2011 May 19.

[28] Toth C, Martinez JA, Liu WQ, Diggle J, Guo GF, Ramji N, Mi R, Hoke A, Zochodne DW. Local erythropoietin signaling enhances regeneration in peripheral axons. Neuroscience. 2008 Jun 23;154(2):767-83.

[29] Chattopadhyay A, Choudhury TD, Bandyopadhyay D, Datta AG. Protective effect of erythropoietin on the oxidative damage of erythrocyte membrane by hydroxyl radical. Biochem Pharmacol 2000;59:419-25.

[30] Bahcekapili N, Uzüm G, Gökkusu C, Kuru A, Ziylan YZ. The relationship between erythropoietin pretreatment with blood-brain barrier and lipid peroxidation after ischemia/reperfusion in rats. Life Sci. 2007 Mar 13;80(14):1245-51.

[31] Leconte C, Bihel E, Lepelletier FX, Bouët V, Saulnier R, Petit E, Boulouard M, Bernaudin M, Schumann-Bard P. Comparison of the effects of erythropoietin and its carbamylated derivative on behaviour and hippocampal neurogenesis in mice. Neuropharmacology. 2011 Feb-Mar;60(2-3):354-64.

[32] Deng H, Zhang J, Yoon T, Song D, Li D, Lin A. Phosphorylation of Bcl-associated death protein (Bad) by erythropoietin-activated c-Jun N-terminal protein kinase 1 contributes to survival of erythropoietin-dependent cells. Int J Biochem Cell Biol. 2011 Mar;43(3):409-15.

[33] Zhu H, Sun S, Li H, Xu Y. Cerebral ischemic tolerance induced by 3-itropropionic acid is associated with increased expression of erythropoietin in rats.J Huazhong Univ Sci Technolog Med Sci. 2006;26(4):440-3.

[34] Juul S. Erythropoietin in the central nervous system, and its use to prevent hypoxicischemic brain damage. Acta Paediatr Suppl 2002;91:36-42.

[35] Buemi M, Donato V, Bolignano D. [Erythropoietin: pleiotropic actions. Recenti Prog Med. 2010 Jun;101(6):253-67.

[36] Siren AL, Knerlich F, Schilling L, Kamrowski-Kruck H, Hahn A, Ehrenreich H. Differential glial and vascular expression of endothelins and their receptors in rat brain after neurotrauma. Neurochem Res 2000; 25:957-69.

[37] Gassmann M, Heinicke K, Soliz J, Ogunshola O. Non-erythroid functions of erythropoietin. In: Roach RC, ed. Hypoxia: Through the lifecycle. Kluwer Academic/ Plenum Publishers, New York, 2003:1-8.

[38] Byts N, Sirén AL. Erythropoietin: a multimodal neuroprotective agent. Exp Transl Stroke Med. 2009 Oct 21;1:4.

[39] García Rodríguez JC and Sosa Teste I: Intranasal Delivery of Erythropoietin in Stroke TheScientificWorldJOURNAL (2009) 9, 970–981

[40] Dhuria SV, Hanson LR, Frey WH II. Intranasal delivery to the central nervous system: mechanisms and experimental considerations. J Pharm Sci 2010;99:1654-73

[41] Genc S, Zadeoglulari Z, Oner M G, Genc K & Digicaylioglu M. Intranasal erythropoietin therapy in nervous system disorders. Expert Opin. Drug Deliv. (2011) 8(1):19-32

[42] Coscarella, A. ; Liddi, R. ; Bach, S. ; Zappitelli, S. ; Urso, R.; Mele, A. ; De Santis, R. (1998) :Pharmacokinetic and immunogenic behavior of three recombinant human GM-CSF-EPO hybrid proteins in cynomolgus monkeys. Mol. Biotechnol. Oct; 10(2): 115-22.

[43] Olsen, N.V. (2003): Central nervous system frontiers for the use of erythropoietin. Clin Infect Dis. 37 (Suppl 4), S323.

[44] Fantacci M; Bianciardi P; Caretti A; Coleman T.R.; Cerami, A.; Brines M L, .; Samaja M (2006) Carbamylated erythropoietin ameliorates the metabolic stress induced in vivo by severe chronic hypoxia. PNAS, November 14, 103(46): 17531-17536.

[45] Sosa I, Cruz J, Santana J, Mengana Y, García-Salman J.D, Muñoz A, Ozuna y García Rodriguez J.C.. Paso De La Molécula De Eritropoyetina Humana Recombinante Con Bajo Contenido De Ácido Siálico Al Sistema Nervioso Central Por La Vía Intranasal En Los Modelos Del *Meriones unguiculatus* Y EL PRIMATE NO HUMANO Macaca fascicularis. Rev. Salud Anim. Vol. 30 No. 1 (2008): 39-44

[46] Brines, M.L.; Ghezzi, P.; Keenan, S. (2000): Erythropoietin crosses the blood brain barrier to protect against experimental brain injury. Proc. Natl. Acad. Sci. U.S.A. 97: 10526-31

[47] Yamashita, T; Nonoguchi, N,; Ikemoto, T., Miyatake,S., and Kuroiwa,T. (2010) Asialoerythropoietin attenuates neural cell death in the hippocampal CA1 region after transient forebrain ischemia in a gerbil model. Neurol.\res.32(9),957-962.

[48] Price, C.D.; Yang, Z., Karinoski, R., Kumar, D., Chaparro, R, & Camporesi, E.M. (2010) Effect of continous infusion of asialo erythropoietin on hort-term changes in infarct volume, penumbra apoptosis and behavior following middle cerebral artery occlusion in rats. Clin Exp Pharmacol Physio 37, 185-192.

[49] Kirkeby, A., Torup, L., Bochsen, L., et al. (2008) High-dose erythropoietin alters platelet reactivity and bleeding time in rodents in contrast to the neuroprotective variant carbamyl-erythropoietin (CEPO). *Thromb. Haemost.* 99(4), 720–728.

[50] Lundbeck, H. (2009) Safety Study of Carbamylated Erythropoietin (CEPO) to Treat Patients With Acute Ischemic Stroke. Report No. NCT00756249. ClinicalTrials.gov

[51] Villa, P., van Beek, J., Larsen, A.K., et al. (2006) Reduced functional deficits, neuroinflammation, and secondary tissue damage after treatment of stroke by nonerythropoietic erythropoietin derivatives. J. Cereb. Blood Flow Metab. 27(3), 552–563.

[52] Wang, X., Zhu, C., Wang, X., et al. (2004) The nonerythropoietic asialoerythropoietin protects against neonatal hypoxia-ischemia as potently as erythropoietin. J. Neurochem. 91(4), 900–910.

[53] Erbayraktar, S., Grasso, G., Sfacteria, A, Xie, Q; W. Coleman, T; Kreilgaard, M., et al. (2003) Asialoerytropoietin is a nonerythropoietic cytokine with broad neuro– protective activity in vivo. Proc Natt Acad Sci USA 100, 6741-6746.
[54] Velly l, Pellegrini, Guillet B, Bruder, N, Pisano. P. Erythropoietin 2nd cerebral protection after acute injuries: A double-egged sword? Pharmacology & Therapeutics 128 (2010) 445-459
[55] Mahmood A, Lu D, Qu C, Goussev A, Zhang ZG, Lu C, Chopp M.T reatment of traumatic brain injury in rats with erythropoietin and Carbamylated erythropoietin. J Neurosurg. 2007 Aug;107(2):392-7.
[56] Kirkeby A, Torup L, Bochsen L, Kjalke M, Abel K, Theilgaard-Monch K, Johansson PI, Bjørn SE, Gerwien J, Leist M. High-dose erythropoietin alters platelet reactivity and bleeding time in rodents in contrast to the neuroprotective variant carbamyl-erythropoietin (CEPO). Thromb Haemost. 2008 Apr;99(4):720-8.
[57] Lagarto A, Bueno V, Guerra I, Valdés O, Couret M, López R, Vega Y. Absence of hematological side effects in acute and subacute nasal dosing of erythropoietin with a low content of sialic acid. Exp Toxicol Pathol. 2010 May 18.
[58] Hilger PA. Applied anatomy and physiology of the nose. In: Boies Fundamentals of Otolaryngology, edited byAdams GL, Boies LR, Hilger PA. Philadelphia: W. B. Saunders, 1989.
[59] Illum L. Transport of drugs from the nasal cavity to the central nervous system. Eur J Pharm Sci 2000;11:1-18
[60] Jansson B. Models for the transfer of drugs from the nasal cavity to the central nervous system. Acta Universitatis Upsaliensis Comprnsive Summaries of Uppala Dissertations from the Faculty fo Farmacy 305: 46, 2004.
[61] Sosa Testé I., García Rodríguez J.C., García Salman J.D., Santana J., Subirós Martínez N.2, González Triana C.1, Rodríguez Cruz Y.4, Cruz Rodríguez J. Intranasal Administration Of Recombinant Human Erythropoietin Exerts Neuroprotective Effects On Post-Ischemic Brain Injury In Mongolian Gerbils. Pharmacologyonline (2006)1: 100-112.
[62] Estudio Del Efecto Neuroprotector De La Eritropoyetina Humana Recombinante Con Bajo Contenido De Ácido Sialico Aplicada Por Vía Intranasal En Biomodelos Experimentales De Isquemia Cerebral. Trabajo para optar por el Grado de Doctor en Ciencias Veterinarias . Dra. MV. MSc. Iliana María Sosa Testé, Tutor. Profesor PhD.. Julio César García Rodríguez, Havana, 2007.
[63] Alcalá-Barraza SR, Lee MS, Hanson LR, McDonald AA, Frey WH 2nd, McLoon LK: Intranasal delivery of neurotrophic factors BDNF, CNTF, EPO, and NT-4 to the CNS. J Drug Target; 2010 Apr;18(3):179-90
[64] Fletcher L, Kohli S, Sprague SM, Scranton RA, Lipton SA, Parra A, Jimenez DF, Digicaylioglu M. Intranasal delivery of erythropoietin plus insulin-like growth factor-I for acute neuroprotection in stroke. Laboratory investigation. J Neurosurg. 2009 Jul;111(1):164-70.
[65] Sargin D, El-Kordi A, Agarwal A, Müller M, Wojcik SM, Hassouna I, Sperling S, Nave KA, Ehrenreich H. Expression of constitutively active erythropoietin receptor in pyramidal neurons of cortex and hippocampus boosts higher cognitive functions in mice. BMC Biol. 2011 Apr 28;9:27.

[66] Reitmeir R, Kilic E, Kilic U, Bacigaluppi M, El Ali A, Salani G, Pluchino S, Gassmann M and Hermann D M.. Post-acute delivery of erythropoietin induces stroke recovery by perilesional tissue remodelling and contralesional piramidal tract plasticity. Barin, 2011: 134; 84-99

[67] González, F.F., Mc Guillen, P., Mu, D., Chang,Y., Wendland, M., Vexler, Z., M; et al (2007) Erythropoietin enhances long-term neuroprotection and neurogenesis in neonatal stroke. Dev Neurosci 29, 321-330.

[68] Jink K, Mao X, Xie L, Greenerg DA. (2010). Neuroglobin expression in ischemic stroke. Stroke.41. 557-559.

[69] Ye S, Tang Y, Li Y. (2009) Protective effect of erythropoietin agains cerebral ischemia-reperfusion injury. J. Int Neurol Neurosurg 36: 391-394.

[70] Li RC, Guo SZ, Lee SK, Gozal D. Neuroglobin protects neurons against oxidative stress in global ischemia. J Cereb Blood Flow Metab. 2010 Nov;30(11):1874-82.

4

Dysphagia and Respiratory Infections in Acute Ischemic Stroke

Claire Langdon
Sir Charles Gairdner Hospital & Curtin University of Technology, Australia

1. Introduction

Eating and swallowing are activities that are normally performed without conscious thought. This complex behaviour - involving 5 pairs of cranial nerves and 26 pairs of muscles - can be interrupted by a stroke, leading to dysphagia. Dysphagia is associated with aspiration (where material passes into the respiratory tract) and aspiration carries a risk of pneumonia seven times greater than that of the normal population. Around 15% - 20% of all stroke patients will develop respiratory tract infections during the acute phase of their stroke. Pneumonia is one of the leading causes of mortality in the acute stroke patient. Respiratory infections add to hospital length of stay and are associated with significant increases in the cost of patient care, as well as being associated with poorer outcomes for the patient. This chapter will outline the association of dysphagia and other risk factors in the development of respiratory infections in acute ischemic stroke patients.

2. High early incidence of dysphagia, its causes, presentation and implications

Swallowing is a vital motor activity that serves alimentary purposes and protects the upper airway (Jean, 2001). Dysphagia (difficulty eating and swallowing) is very common after an ischemic stroke, affecting between 13% and 94% of all ischemic stroke patients, with the incidence depending on the size and location of the lesion (Barer, 1989; DePippo, Holas, Reding, Mandel & Lesser, 1994; Daniels, 2000; Ding & Logemann, 2000; Aydogdu, Ertekin, Tarlaci, Turman & Klyliogly, 2001; Marik, 2001). Dysphagia can lead to malnutrition, dehydration, aspiration pneumonia and increased length of hospital stay.

In a recent review of the costs to the US health system, dysphagia was found to be associated with significantly increased costs due to increased length of stay and infections. The median hospitalization days for patients with dysphagia was 4.04 compared with 2.40 days for those patients without dysphagia. Mortality was substantially increased in patients with dysphagia associated with rehabilitation, intervertebral disk disorders, and heart diseases (Altmann, Yu & Schaefer, 2010). A cohort study of 330 stroke survivors found that those who developed infections during their hospital admission had a median length of stay of 26 days, significantly longer than the median length of stay of 11 days of those who did not require antibiotic treatment (Langdon, Lee and Binns, 2010).

Best practice management of dysphagia in acute stroke encompasses the need to consider the patient holistically. The impact of various eating difficulties on nutritional status has not received great attention in research (Westergren, 2006). Impaired arm movement, lip closure and swallowing have all been found to be significant predictors of decreased energy intake over 24-hours in patients with stroke (McLaren & Dickerson 2000).

Dysphagia that occurs due to a stroke is associated with an increased risk of material being aspirated during swallowing. This is due to the disruption to motor and sensory input and to protective reflexes (Holas, DePippo & Reding, 1994; Aviv, Martin, Sacco, Zager, Diamond, Keen & Blitzer, 1996; Daniels, Brailey, Priestly, Herrington, Weisberg & Foundas, 1998; Addington, Stephens, Gilliland, Rodriguez, 1999; Nakajoh, Nakagawa, Sekizawa, Matsui, Arai & Sasaki, 2000). 'Aspiration' occurs when matter (food, fluid, saliva or secretions), enters the airway and passes below the level of the true vocal folds. Pneumonia is up to seven times more likely to occur in patients who are known to aspirate (DePippo, Holas & Redding, 1994; Kidd, Lawson, Nesbitt & MacMahon, 1995; Smithard, O'Neill, England, Park, Wyatt, Martin & Morris, 1997). Dysphagia has been found to be associated with an increased risk of chest infections, dehydration and death (Gordon, Hewer & Wade, 1987). In stroke patients, pneumonia has been associated with an increased cost to the health system of US$14,836 per patient (Katzan, Dawson, Thomas, Votruba & Cebul, 2007) and is strongly associated with poorer outcomes (Smithard, O'Neill, Park, Morris, 1996; Wang, Lim, Levi, Heller & Fischer, 2001; Wang, Lim, Heller, Fisher & Levi, 2003).

2.1 Infection in acute stroke

Infection in acute stroke has been, and remains, a significant problem, with pneumonia and urinary tract infections occurring the most frequently. In the GAIN study, a multicentre, multinational study of 1455 patients with strokes, 142 died during the first week following hospital admission. Thirty four (23.9%) of these died from pneumonia (Aslanyan, Weir, Diener, Kaste & Lees, 2004).

A study of 124 stroke patients who were admitted to Neurological Intensive Care Units in Cologne reported an incidence of pneumonia of 21%, occurring an average 1.8 days (±1.9 days), post stroke, although these figures did not distinguish between patients who required ventilator support for respiration and those who did not (Hilker, Poetter, Findeisen, Sobesky, Jacobs, Neveling & Heiss, 2003). Ventilator-associated pneumonia is common in patients who require mechanical respiratory support and is discussed in greater detail later in the chapter.

A Scandanavian study of 1,156 patients reported 19.4% developed infections within 3 days of hospital admission, with 49% of the infections diagnosed males and 27% of infections in females being respiratory tract infections. Early infection added 9.3 days on average to the patient's hospital admission (Kammersgaard, Jorgensen, Reith, Nakayama, Houth, Weber, Pederse, & Olsen, 2001).

Using videofluoroscopy to examine swallowing, Kidd et. al., (1995) found 25 (42%) of a cohort of 60 stroke patients were aspirating at 72 hours post stroke. In the first 14 days after their stroke, 19 patients developed lower respiratory tract infections. Of these 19 patients, 17 (89%) were known to be aspirating. Of the 25 aspirators, 22 had returned to normal swallowing function when followed up at 3 months post stroke (Kidd, Lawson, Nesbitt & MacMahon, 1995).

Mann, Hankey and Cameron followed 128 acute stroke patients for six months and reported an incidence of dysphagia in 82 patients (64%) when examined using videofluoroscopy. In the six months of follow up, 26 patients (20%) experienced a chest infection (Mann, Hankey & Cameron, 1999). A limitation of this study was the exclusion of stroke patients who were unable to tolerate the videofluoroscopy procedure, which excludes those patients with impaired conscious state. Often these patients with poor conscious level are the ones who are at greatest risk of aspiration due to the impairment in their ability to protect their airway.

A study of 88 patients admitted to hospital with ischemic strokes found infection occurred in 25 of 80 survivors during the first month post stroke. Respiratory infection was significantly more likely to occur in patients with dysphagia (Langdon, Lee & Binns, 2007).

In a cohort of 330 acute ischemic stroke patients followed up for the first month after their stroke, there were 51 respiratory infections, with dysphagia again a significant predictor of patients who developed infections (Langdon, Lee & Binns, 2009).

2.2 Normal swallowing

Swallowing is something that is often taken for granted, yet is a complex and tightly controlled event that coordinates breathing and deglutition, with an average of 2,400 swallows occurring daily. The frequency of swallowing changes depending on the activity. It occurs on the average at 6 swallows an hour during sleep to 10 per hour during normal activity to around 300 per hour while eating (Miller, 1982). The body produces 1500ml - 2000ml saliva daily (Witt, 2005), which is swallowed without conscious thought.

Successful swallowing is an extremely complex and dynamic process, involving 5 pairs of cranial nerves and coordination of some 26 pairs of striated muscles (Dodds, Stewart & Logemann, 1990; Bass & Morrell, 1992; Matsuo & Palmer, 2008) involved in the act of moving food or fluid from the oral cavity to the stomach. There is an extremely elaborate reflex mechanism that provides a close functional relationship between the pharynx (throat), larynx and oesophagus during swallowing, belching and reflux to help prevent aspiration or food/fluids going 'the wrong way' (Shaker, 2006). Studies have provided evidence that the process of swallowing is governed by specialised neural networks in a finely-tuned partnership with respiration and speech (Zald & Pardoe, 1999). Neural control of swallowing is multidimensional. The brainstem contains the swallowing central pattern generator – the first level of control. The second level of control incorporates the sub cortical structures; basal ganglia, hypothalamus, amygdala and midbrain. The third level of control is represented by suprabulbar cortical swallowing centres (Mistry & Hamdy, 2008).

Normal swallowing is generally arbitrarily divided into four stages for convenience of description, however, the normal swallow is a complex, fast, continuous sequence of coordinated muscle movements and there is some overlap between the phases. An efficient swallow involves an anticipatory phase, an oral phase, a pharyngeal phase and an oesophageal phase. These are illustrated in Figure 1 and described in greater detail below. The oral phase of swallowing is initiated voluntarily while the pharyngeal and oesophageal phases occur via intraphase reflexes (Lang, 2009). Control of the phases represent a coordination among the brain stem and central cortical pathways (Miller, 2008).

2.2.1 Oral preparatory phase (voluntary control)

The oral preparatory stage of swallow incorporates prior knowledge of feeding and swallowing, environmental, visual and olfactory cues. Once food enters the oral cavity, the lips seal, the tongue accepts and cradles the food and it is tasted. Information about the food is transmitted from the taste buds to the cortex and brainstem. The preparatory stage allows prior knowledge to impact on eating and swallowing: for example, if a stroke patient has had recent choking events due to dysphagia, they may be reluctant to accept a particular texture or type of food.

2.2.2 Oral phase (voluntary and reflexive control)

Food is chewed and mixed with saliva using movement of the jaw, tightly coordinated with movements of the tongue, cheeks, soft palate, and hyoid bone (Matsuo & Palmer, 2008). When the prepared food has been formed into a 'bolus' suitable for swallowing, it is centred on the tongue and propelled backwards by the tongue to the pharynx. Difficulties with the oral stage of the swallow may occur because of muscle weakness or nerve dysfunction. These will often lead to an extension in the time taken for oral transit and/or retention of material in the oral cavity as residue, or may cause premature spillage of the bolus into the pharynx (Dodds, Stewart & Logemann, 1990; Matsuo & Palmer, 2008) which can impact on airway protection.

Disruption to the oral phase can occur due to poor dentition or poorly fitting dentrues. Absent molar teeth can significantly impair bolus preparation, as these teeth grind food into smaller, more digestible particles. Gum disease and teeth in poor condition may cause pain when eating, which is associated with decreased intake of food. A weak tongue or jaw will also contribute to impairment of the oral phase of the swallow.

2.2.3 Pharyngeal phase (reflexive control)

The pharynx consists of the nasopharynx (superior and anterior to the soft palate) and oropharynx (from the nasopharynx to the larynx). It serves two purposes, acting as a conduit for air to and from the lungs and also moving food and liquids from the mouth to the esophagus (Miller, 2002). The pharyngeal stage of the swallow is an important and complex activity that coordinates: (1) food or liquids passing through the pharynx and upper esophageal sphincter (UES) to the osophagus and (2) airway protection - isolating the larynx and trachea from the pharynx during swallowing to prevent the bolus from entering the airway (Matsuo & Palmer, 2008). The pharynx is made up of the pharyngeal constrictor muscles (superior, middle and inferior) that overlap to form a sheath that extends from the base of skull to the esophagus. The pharyngeal swallow also involves muscles of the soft palate, the tongue, pharynx, larynx and hyoid bone. The pharyngeal swallowing muscles are innervated by the trigeminal (V), facial (VII) glossopharyngeal (IX), vagal (X), spinal accessory (XI) and hypoglossal (XII) nerves (Miller, 2002).

Breathing and swallowing are tightly coordinated by the brainstem. During swallowing, there is a brief cessation of breathing known as 'deglutition apnea'. Studies of normal subjects have found that there is a small exhalation prior to the swallow being initiated, followed by the swallow, and finally a larger exhalation once the bolus has entered the esophagus (Martin, Logemann, Shaker & Dodds, 1994). Swallowing normally finishes with an exhalation of air. This serves to assist clearance of any material that may have entered the laryngeal vestibule during the swallow. This normal breathing/swallowing rhythm has been shown to break down in stroke patients (Leslie, Drinnan, Ford & Wilson, 2002), while the apnea associated with swallowing increases with age (Leslie, Drinnan, Ford & Wilson, 2005).

Stroke can impact on the timing of the pharyngeal swallow, or weaken the muscles of one side of the pharynx, resulting in a weak or incoordinated swallow, often associated with material being aspirated before, during or after the swallow is initiated.

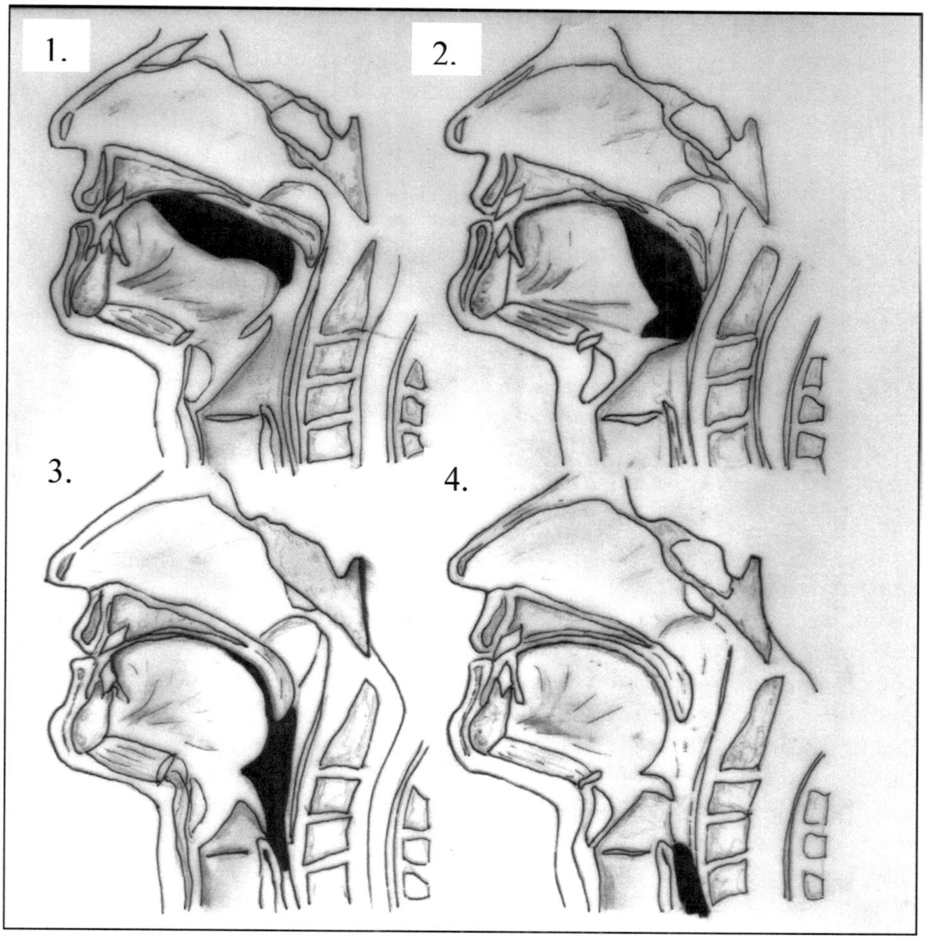

Fig. 1. Stages of Normal Swallowing:
1. Food is chewed and mixed with saliva. This is shaped into a bolus by the tongue, and centred on the tongue prior to initiation of the swallow. The soft palate elevates to form a seal with the nasopharyx.
2. The tongue tip is pressed against the alveolar ridge, then the tongue base drops and the bolus is pushed into the pharynx. The vocal folds adduct and breathing is ceased momentarily.
3. The epiglottis deflects downward and the bolus enters the esophagus due to (a) tonic relaxation of the upper esophageal sphincter (b) hyolaryngeal traction opening the sphincter (c) pharyngeal squeeze.
4. The bolus is cleared into the esophagus by pharyngeal muscles exerting a stripping action.

2.2.4 Oesophageal phase (reflexive control)

After the bolus enters the oesophagus through the UES, peristalsis moves it down to the stomach and through the lower esophageal sphincter to the stomach. The peristaltic wave consists of an initial wave of relaxation to accommodate the bolus followed by a wave of contraction that propels it onward (Matsuo & Palmer, 2008). This phase of the swallow is considered the least complex, although it can still be subject to impairment leading to decreased safety and poor oral intake.

2.3 Causes of dysphagia in ischemic stroke

Stroke is a brain injury, and may impact on swallowing, either by damage to cranial nerves or nuclei, or by interrupting the interconnecting neural networks that regulate normal deglutition. A stroke patient may be drowsy in the acute phase, which impacts on their ability to remain conscious long enough to eat or drink sufficient amounts to ensure that their nutrition and hydration needs are being met. Poor conscious level may mean that the stroke patient's ability to protect his or her airway is compromised. Difficulty in maintaining sitting balance and hemiparesis affecting the dominant hand may contribute to the person's difficulties in self-feeding. Loss of facial tone may cause dentures to become ill-fitting, making chewing difficult for the patient. Loss of facial tone may also mean that the patient has difficulty containing the bolus in the oral cavity, forming a seal with the lips to drink easily, or prevent saliva spilling from the mouth (drooling). Loss of sensation from damage to the trigeminal nerve may mean that the patient is unaware that they are drooling, or that food may be pocketed in a flaccid cheek following mealtimes. The impact of different types of stroke on feeding and swallowing is more fully discussed below.

2.3.1 Cortical lesions

Swallowing has been shown using fMRI studies to involve the precentral and postcentral gyri, the anterior cingulated gyrus and the insula (Miller, 2008). By using Transcranial Magnetic Stimulation, Hamdy and his colleagues showed that swallowing is bilaterally but asymmetrically represented in the cortical hemispheres, and that this representation is unrelated to handedness. If a stroke involves the dominant swallowing centre, dysphagia is highly likely, though this has been seen to resolve if the non-affected side subsumes the functions of the dominant centre (Hamdy, Aziz, Rothwell, Singh, Barlow, Hughes, Tallis & Thompson, 1996).

A cortical stroke may interfere with motor planning of the swallow. Large lesions may involve association or projection tracts of the brain, penetrating into the internal capsule. Significant dysphagia is commonly associated with a TACI stroke (Langdon, 2007; Sundar, Pahuja, Dwivedi, Yeolekar, 2008; Langdon, 2010). Stroke that occurs in the right hemisphere has been shown to impact on the pharyngeal phase of the swallow, with impairment to initiation and duration and increased frequency of penetration and aspiration seen (Robbins, Levine, Maser, Rosenbek & Kampster, 1993), while strokes affecting the left hemisphere result in impairement in pharyngeal transit and longer oral transit (Miller, 2008).

For many patients with unilateral cortical strokes that affect the dominant swallowing centre, dysphagia is transient, with a large percentage recovering their ability to eat and swallow very quickly. Around 50% of patients admitted with strokes demonstrate dysphagia (Gordon, Hewer & Wade, 1987; Smithard, O'Neill, England, Park, Wyatt, Martin & Morris, 1997; Broadley, Croser, Cottrell, Creevy, Teo, Yiu, Pathi, Taylor & Thompson, 2003). This incidence tends to resolve by the end of the 5-7 days post stroke once acute edema and 'cerebral shock' start to resolve (Broadley et. al., 2003). Patients who have bilateral cortical strokes tend to have more severe and prolonged dysphagia; possibly due to the impairment affecting both hemispheres and precluding the subsumption of swallowing function by an unimpaired swallowing representation.

A cortical stroke patient who presents with dysphagia may demonstrate some or all of the following:

- Facial droop
- Difficulty controlling saliva/secretions
- Slurred speech (dysarthria)
- Dysphasia/aphasia
- Weak or impaired cough
- Dysphonia
- Impaired conscious level

Any of these, or a combination of these, can impact adversely on the voluntary and reflexive aspects of the normal swallow and should be investigated and treated. This assessment is usually performed by a Speech and Language Pathologist. Formal dysphagia screening programmes for acute stroke patients are associated with a significant decrease in the risk of pneumonia and should be offered to all stroke patients (Hinchey, Shepherd, Furey, Smith, Wang & Tonn, 2005). There has been consideration in the past that patients who present with an impaired gag reflex are at high risk of swallowing problems or aspiration. The gag reflex should not be considered to be predictive of dysphagia: published evidence clearly shows that there is little or no relationship between the gag reflex and the ability to swallow safely (Smithard & Spriggs, 2003).

2.3.2 Brainstem lesions

In the brainstem, there are motor nuclei that are responsible for acting as swallowing Central Pattern Generators (CPG). The main motor nuclei involved in swallowing are the hypoglossal motor nucleus and the nucleus ambiguus. These contain motoneurons, which innervate the intrinsic and extrinsic muscles of the tongue, such as the genioglossus, geniohyoid, styloglossus and hyoglossus, and the pharynx, larynx, and esophagus (Jean, 2001). Swallowing neurons are located in two main brain stem areas:

1. In the dorsal medulla (within the nucleus tractus solitarius) (NTS) and the adjacent reticular formation, where they form the dorsal swallowing group (DSG)
2. In the ventrolateral medulla, just superior to the nucleus ambiguus, where they form the ventral swallowing group (VSG)

Anatomically, swallowing neurons are located in the same sites as neurons that belong to CPGs involved in respiration and cardiovascular regulation (Jean, 2001). Both breathing and swallowing share some interneurons. This may help to explain the close relationship between breathing and swallowing. This close relationship may be affected by an ischemic stroke in the brainstem, predisposing the person to aspiration and dysphagia.

Brainstem strokes may account for up to 15% of all strokes (Kruger, Teasell, Salter & Hellings 2007). They have been associated with severe and persisting dysphagia, although this is by no means seen in every patient who has a stroke involving the brainstem. A patient who has experienced a brainstem stroke usually presents quite differently to one who has had a cortical stroke. Commonly seen dysfunction includes hemi- or quadriplegia, ataxia, dysphagia, dysarthria, gaze abnormalities and visual disturbances. In contrast to hemispheric lesions, new onset of cortical deficits, such as aphasia and cognitive impairments, are absent. Brainstem stroke patients may demonstrate some other characteristic clinical features, including

- Dysarthria
- Vertigo, nystagmus, nausea and vomiting, due to involvement of the vestibular system
- Visual field loss or visuospatial deficits if there is occipital lobe involvement

Common findings observed in patients with vertebrobasilar stroke include an abnormal level of consciousness, as well as hemiparesis or quadriparesis. Pupillary abnormalities and oculomotor signs are common, and bulbar manifestations, such as facial weakness, dysphonia, dysarthria, and dysphagia, occur in more than 40% of patients (Kaye & Brandstarter, 2009).

Patients with brainstem lesions tend to demonstrate the most prolonged course of recovery or poorest outcomes. In an early study of dysphagia which reported on four patients with strokes involving the brainstem, two patients subsequently died, while the other two had resolution of their swallowing impairment by 25 days post onset and were discharged home (Gordon, Hewer & Wade, 1987). In a case series over a six year period, Chua & Kong (1996) reported 21 of 53 patients (40%) demonstrated dysphagia on admission, but did make some progress during their stay at a rehabilitaton facility.

3. The time course of dysphagia

While dysphagia incidence is very high in stroke patients who are admitted to hospital, there tends to be a sharp decrease in prevalence over a short period, usually in the first few days to a week.

3.1 Studies of dysphagia in acute stroke patients

In an early study of dysphagia in stroke, (Gordon, Hewer & Wade, 1987) reported on a cohort of 91 stroke patients. Forty one patients in their study (45%) had swallowing problems on admission to hospital. This study used a water swallow test; bedside swallowing examinations have been found to be less sensitive than instrumental evaluation in determining the true incidence of dysphagia and aspiration, although instrumental evaluation tends to select only those patients with conscious level good enough to tolerate testing. The reported duration of dysphagia in survivors was

8 days or less	15
9 - 14 days	3
14 – 40 days	3

Kidd examined a cohort of 60 acute stroke patients using videofluoroscopy and found 25 (42%) were aspirating at 72 hours post stroke, with resolution of aspiration in 22 of 25 patients by 3 months post stroke (Kidd, Lawson, Nesbitt & McMahon, 1995). Another study which followed 121 acute stroke patients found 61 (51%) had dysphagia on admission to hospital. When reviewed at 7 days post stroke, dysphagia had resolved in a significant number of patients, with only 28 still demonstrating swallowing impairment. By six-months post stroke, this had decreased further and dysphagia persisted in only 6 of the original 61 patients with swallowing impairment on admission (Smithard, O'Neill, England, Park, Wyatt, Martin & Morris, 1997).

Table 1 below clearly shows the decreasing prevalence of dysphagia during the first week post stroke, with a reduction from 51% to 27%, although it should be noted that this reported prevalence included cases of dysphagia that began during the first week post stroke, presumably from an extension of the original stroke, or a new event.

Day	*N*	Dysphagic (%)	New	Persistent
0	121	61 (51)	-	-
1	113	33 (39)	4	29
2	111	35 (32)	6	28
3	105	43 (39)	6	35
7	110	28 (27)	1	27
28	105	18 (17)	5	13
180	73	8 (11)	2	6

Table 1. Number of dysphagic patients at different time points in the study by Smithard et. al., (1997).

Using a combination of videofluoroscopy and bedside swallowing examination, Mann, Hankey & Cameron (2000) reported that aspiration was present in 49% of a cohort of 128 acute stroke patients. By six months post stroke, 97 of 112 survivors had returned to their pre-stroke diet (Mann, Hankey & Cameron, 1999).

Daniels, Ballo, Mahoney and Foundas (2000) reported on a cohort of 56 ischemic stroke survivors and noted that, although initially 38 (68%) presented with moderate to severe dysphagia, at the time of their discharge from hospital 52 of 54 survivors consumed a regular diet, one required food to be diced and one remained on enteral feeding.

Steinhagen, Grossman, Benecke and Walter (2008) reported on a cohort of 60 patients with ischemic strokes. This cohort demonstrated an incidence of pneumonia of 39 patients: median time to infection was 3 days (1-16 days).

In a large cohort study of 369 stroke patients, 125 of 330 survivors (38%) demonstrated some degree of dysphagia on bedside examination at 7 days post stroke. Between 48 hours post stroke and seven days post stroke, dysphagia prevalence in acute ischemic stroke patients decreased from 153 (46.4%) to 125 (37.9%). Even among the patients with the most seriously impaired swallowing function, those who were 'Nil by Mouth', there was a significant amount of swallow improvement, with the initial 63 patients who were 'Nil by Mouth' decreasing to 41 by 7 days post stroke (Langdon, Lee & Binns, 2010).

As the studies above show, dysphagia is extremely common following a stroke, but tends to resolve quite quickly in the majority of patients. It has been recommended that percutaneous endoscopic gastrostomy (PEG) tubes be considered for those patients with severe dysphagia that persists beyond 7 to 10 days post stroke if the treating medical team feels the patient is likely to survive (Broadley et. al., 2003). Previous studies have demonstrated a relatively consistent mortality rate of around 15% of all acute stroke patients (Gordon, Hewer & Wade, 1987; Aslanyan et. al., 2004; Mann, Hankey & Cameron, 1999; Langdon, Lee & Binns, 2010).

4. How good management of dysphagia prevents respiratory infections

In the early acute phase of a stroke, quality management of dysphagia is focused upon ensuring that patients' nutrition and hydration requirements are appropriately met, and that they receive medications. This needs to be done in such a way that aspiration is prevented or minimised. Stroke unit care using a multidisciplinary team with expertise in management of this population has been shown to be responsible for improved outcomes for patients.

There have been few randomized control trials of dysphagia management: this is because having a control group where treatment or management of dysphagia is withheld is unethical. In a review of the literature, Doggett, Tappe, Mitchell, Chapell, Coates and Turkelson (2001) reported an estimated incidence of 43% - 54% of stroke patients with dysphagia leading to aspiration, with approximately 37% of these patients going on to develop pneumonia. Acute-care stroke patients with dysphagia were estimated to experience malnutrition at a rate of 48%. The authors also reported that introduction of a dysphagia management program dramatically reduces pneumonia rates: one study reported frequency decreased from 6.7% (95% confidence interval 3.1% - 14%) to 4.1% (95%CI 1.8% - 9.3%) in the first year, and reduced to zero (95%CI 0% - 3%) in the second year.

4.1 Assessment of dysphagia

Optimal stroke care involves early dysphagia assessment: this often takes the form of an initial screening by medical or nursing personnel, with patients who fail the screen undergoing more thorough clinical assessment from a Speech-Language Pathologist, with the option of patients undergoing instrumental assessment. It has been argued that a reliable bedside assessment is useful in identifying patients at risk of nutritional compromise, aspiration and poorer outcomes (Smithard, et. al., 1996). The current gold standard of dysphagia assessment is the videofluoroscopic swallow study (also known as the Modified Barium Swallow Study), where patients are assessed using a moving x-ray, which is recorded to allow detailed analysis. Another alternative is a fibreoptic endoscopic evaluation of swallowing (FEES). Both assessments have been shown to have excellent reliability in detecting and assessing dysphagia.

The choice of instrumental examination should be made based upon the information that the clinician seeks to obtain from the test. Videofluoroscopy is the superior study for obtaining information about the oral phase of the swallow, and to quantify aspiration. It also provides clear visualisation of the opening of the upper oesophageal sphincter, and is very useful if a cricopharyngeal dysfunction or Zenker's pharyngoesophageal diverticulum is suspected. Negative aspects of videofluoroscopy include

- the need for patients to sit upright during the examination, which makes it a difficult procedure for patients with impaired conscious level or poor sitting balance
- the exposure to radiation, albeit a small amount of less than 0.2 mSv per procedure
- the taste and density of barium that is added to the materials to be swallowed changes the properties of the food or liquid
- the captured image is a two-dimensional representation of a three-dimensional act

The FEES examination allows excellent visualisation of the structures of the pharynx and of the larynx. It can be carried out in patients with poorer conscious state, and is comparatively portable compared to the videofluoroscopy equipment, allowing a clinician to conduct the examination in the ICU or at bedside. FEES allows the clinician to determine whether there are pooled secretions in the pharynx, and whether these are being aspirated. Due to the nature of the equipment, during the actual moment of swallowing, the view is obscured due to the action of pharyngeal squeeze against the fibreoptic camera. This phenomenon is called 'whiteout'. Judgements regarding the oral phase of the swallow are not possible, and it is not possible to quantify the amount of material that is aspirated. FEES does allow for a much longer examination, as there is no radiation exposure associated with the procedure, so it is a much better instrument to identify the effects of fatigue over the course of a meal.

Once a diagnosis of dysphagia has been made, there is liaison between members of the multidisciplinary team in how best to manage the patient's swallowing impairment. This involves communication between

- Nursing
- Speech language Pathology
- Pharmacist
- Dietitian
- Medical
- Occupational therapist
- Physiotherapist
- Family members
- Social workers

The roles of each of these are briefly discussed below.

4.1.1 Nursing

Nursing are responsible for the minute-to-minute management of the acute stroke patient. They are the eyes and ears of the ward. Nurses will be able to assist the patient with feeding and with drinking, if assistance is required. This is a skill, as careful assistance helps in preventing aspiration. Langmore et. al., (1998) showed that being dependent for feeding was associated with an increased risk of developing aspiration pneumonia of nearly 20 times greater than those subjects who were able to feed themselves.

Other important tasks that are the responsibility of the stroke patient's nurse are monitoring the performance during the meal. In acute stroke, fatigue is often a problem for the patient, and their ability to protect their airway may decline as they get increasingly tired. The patient may have demonstrated excellent control and airway protection during their swallowing assessment with the Speech Language Pathologist: this may change rapidly. A proactive nurse who is aware of the variability of the patient's swallow may decide that a reassessment is needed and act to ensure that an aspiration event is avoided. The nurse may assist the patient with finishing a meal if they are becoming too fatigued to feed themselves, or she may monitor the patient's ability to maintain sitting balance throughout the duration of the meal, and re-position them into optimal sitting position if this is required.

Nurses are responsible for one of the most important factors that contribute to the stroke patient's wellbeing - oral hygiene and care. A patient's nutritional status and immune function are closely linked. Poor oral health is associated with poor nutrition in the elderly (Mojon, Budtz-Jorgensen & Rapin, 1999). The association between poor oral hygiene and development of pneumonia is discussed in greater detail later in this chapter.

4.1.2 Speech language pathologist

The Speech Language Pathologist is well placed to assess, manage and treat the stroke patient's dysphagia. They may also determine the presence of communication difficulties and assess and treat these.

Communication impairment is common in acute stroke. This may be as a result of the stroke affecting the language areas of the brain, with the person presenting with aphasia. The person may demonstrate impairment to the motor planning of speech, with verbal dyspraxia resulting. Cranial nerve lesions may cause dysarthria, with the patient presenting with difficulty with execution of the smooth, controlled muscular movements required for precise articulation. These communication difficulties may further impact on an acute stroke patient's eating and drinking: for example, an aphasic patient who is unable to read the hospital menu may require special assistance in completing their meal requests.

It is a recommendation that stroke patients be screened for dysphagia upon admission to hospital, due to the very high initial incidence of dysphagia. If dysphagia is suspected, a more comprehensive examination by the Speech Language Pathologist should be requested. As well as assessing the patient's swallowing impairment, the Speech Language Pathologist may begin to treat the dysphagia. For some acute stroke patients, a fairly normal diet can be followed utilising strategies that overcome the impairments caused by the stroke. For example, for some patients a postural modification of tucking the chin slightly when swallowing helps to compensate for a slight delay in the triggering of the swallow.
Studies have shown that early intervention for dysphagia in acute stroke is efficacious. In a randomized control trial of 306 acute stroke patients assigned to 'usual care', 'low level intervention' or 'high level intervention', Carnaby, Hankey and Pizzi (2006) showed a significantly greater proportion of dysphagic patients who received the high level intervention had returned to their pre-morbid level of swallowing function by six months post stroke.

4.1.3 Pharmacist

A thoughtful review of a stroke patient's medications by a Clinical Pharmacist will be of benefit, particularly for the dysphagic patient. If the Speech Language Pathologist has determined that the patient has difficulty swallowing medications, the Pharmacist may be able to suggest alternative methods of delivering pharmacology. This may include transdermal, liquid form, intravenous or intra muscular or medications may be administered via suppository.
Another reason that the Pharmacist is an important member of the multidisciplinary team is to review medications to determine which may be ceased, or if a medication interaction is likely. Potential for an adverse drug reaction occurring has been estimated at 6% if two medications are taken, rising to 50% for five different medications and 100% if eight or more different medications are taken (Larsen & Martin, 1999). Polypharmacy is a problem in elderly patients. Langmore, et.al. (1998) studied a cohort of 189 elderly male subjects and demonstrated that those who were taking 6 or more different medications per day were more likely to develop aspiration pneumonia. One study in 1998 found that a typical 65-year old patient will be taking two to three medications daily, while those that are in high-level residential care take an average of eight medications each day (Barczi, Sullivan & Robbins, 2000).
In a cohort study of 330 acute stroke survivors, 109 patients were found to be taking 8 or more different medications per day, with the majority of these 109 patients aged between 65 and 84 years (n=75). Langdon, (2007) noted that of the patients taking 6 or more different medications daily, 30 (27.5%) were later diagnosed with a respiratory infection. Chi-square test indicated a significant association between taking 6 or more medications daily and developing respiratory infections, $\chi^2(1)=18.143$, $p<.0001$, with an associated Odds Ratio of 2.08 (95% CI 1.54, 2.79).

	Number of Medications per Day				
Pneumonia?	**0-2**	**3-5**	**6-8**	**9 or more**	**Totals**
Yes	13	8	16	14	**51**
No	96	104	58	21	**279**
Total	**109**	**112**	**74**	**35**	**330**

Table 2. Association between multiple medications and subsequent development of respiratory infections in acute stroke patients.

4.1.4 Dietitian

Dehydration and malnutrition are common in stroke patients, due to dysphagia, immobility and communication difficulties. These are worst in the first week after a stroke and are associated with poorer outcomes (NSF Clinical Guidelines, 2010). The dietitian's role in managing the acute stroke patient is to ensure that their nutrition and hydration are being optimally maintained. This may take the form of an enteral feeding regime, an oral feeding regime that takes into account special dietary needs (diabetic, renal, low sodium etc.) or a transitional feeding regime, where the patient is moving from enteral to full oral feeding. Speech Language Pathologists and Dietitians work closely to achieve optimal outcomes for the acute stroke patient. Patients who are re-commencing oral nutrition will require a transitional feeding regime to ensure that they continue to receive adequate hydration and calories: this may mean partial oral diet; with the Dietitian re-adjusting enteral feeding regimes based on how much is consumed orally.

4.1.5 Medical

The medical team's role includes liaising with the patient's GP or the rehabilitation facility to ensure seamless transition of care. In an acute stroke unit, the medical team is led by a Consultant Neurologist, who supervises the management of patients with support from more junior medical colleagues.

The medical team is responsible for the overall coordination of the acute stroke patient's care. They will monitor the person's recovery, and ensure that they lead and coordinate the multidisciplinary team (SIGN, 2002). Their day to day responsibilities include ordering tests and medications and reviewing these to ensure that the patient's physiological homeostasis is maintained.

4.1.6 Occupational therapist

The role of the Occupational Therapist in managing dysphagia in acute stroke patients is to assist with the promotion of self-feeding. Adaptive equipment may be needed to maximise functional independence. This includes angled cutlery, built up plates and equipment that will assist the patient overcome hemiplegia in preparing meals. Occupational Therapists will also work to provide equipment that optimises the patient's positioning, such as customising wheelchairs to compensate for poor trunk control.

4.1.7 Physiotherapist

The Physiotherapist will work towards the patient regaining movement on the hemiplegic side, and will also contribute to respiratory health. If a patient has a weak cough or has developed a chest infection, the Physiotherapist will assist with clearance of purulent secretions.

Improving movement and control allows stroke patients to sit upright and eat or drink independently and also to perform their own oral care. Being dependent for feeding and/or oral care are factors that have been shown to contribute to patients developing aspiration pneumonias (Langmore, et. al., 1998).

Physiotherapists will assist the patient to regain mobility; early mobilisation is a feature of stroke unit care which is associated with benefits to the patient (SIGN, 2002). In a cohort of 330 stroke survivors, severely impaired mobility on admission to hospital was strongly associated with subsequent development of infections, with an Odds Ratio of 2.56 (95% CI 2.01, 3.34) (Langdon, Lee and Binns, 2010).

4.1.8 Family members

In an acute ischemic stroke, stress and anxiety are frequently experienced by family members. Stroke patients and their families and carers should be offered information about stroke, its treatment and rehabilitation (SIGN, 2002). Good quality information provided to stroke survivors and family members on an ongoing basis has been shown to be beneficial in minimising stress and depression caused by the complex adjustments that need to be made by the patient and their family (NSF Clinical Guidelines, 2010).

4.1.9 Social worker

Stroke may cause additional anxiety and depression among patients and their families and carers as it may mean unexpected absence from work, with the financial implications associated with this. There may be a complicated array of government departments to negotiate. In addition, the stroke patient may require high-level care due to ongoing disability. Social workers will bring their expertise to assist patients and their families in accessing benefits and services. They also bring expertise in counselling, and may be able to assist with families and patients' adjustment to the changes that a stroke has necessitated.

5. Additional risk factors for respiratory infections in acute ischemic stroke patients

There may be other factors that the multidisciplinary team need to consider in order to provide the acute stroke patient with optimal care. These are factors other than dysphagia that may contribute to patients' developing respiratory infections during the acute stroke period.

They include

- Ventilators
- Tracheostomy
- Oral Hygiene
- Nasogastric tubes
- Gastroesophageal Reflux

These risk factors are briefly discussed below.

5.1 Ventilators

Patients who require mechanical assistance to breathe are at an increased risk of respiratory complications. Ventilator-assisted pneumonia (VAP) is a common occurrence in Intensive Care Units (ICU), with specific organisms (*Pseudomonas aeruginosa* and *Acinectobacter baumannii*) associated with the highest incidence. VAP is associated with the duration of mechanical ventilation. Other factors associated with an increased risk of VAP developing include reintubation, tracheostomy, nasogastric tube, enteral feeding, supine positioning and use of gastric pH-altering agents (Cook & Kollef, 1998).

5.2 Tracheostomy

A tracheostomy tube may be needed for patients who are slow to wean from ventilators. Generally, a cuffed tube is inserted, as this helps prevent aspiration of saliva and secretions. However, it has been demonstrated that an inflated tracheostomy cuff is more likely to lead to patients aspirating (Davis, Bears, Barone, Corvo & Tucker, 2002). Tracheostomy is associated with a high incidence of silent aspiration (aspiration without clinical signs), and it has been argued that all patients with tracheostomy should undergo instrumental examination of their swallowing function (Matthews & Coyle, 2010).

5.3 Oral hygiene

The mouth is colonised by over 400 different species of bacteria (Brook, 2003). Normal saliva has a concentration o f 10^8 organisms per millilitre, which can increase to 10^{11} per millilitre in a person with gingivitis (Mojon, 2002). Langmore et. al., (1998) demonstrated that poor oral hygiene and being dependent for oral care are both associated with a significantly increased risk of patients developing aspiration pneumonia. One small study looked at residents of chronic care and compared them with community-dwellers. Respiratory pathogens were present in dental plaque for 25% of the care facility residents, with 4 of these 7 residents classified as 'positively colonised', compared to none of the people living independently (Russell, Boylan, Kaslick, Scannapieco, Katz, 1999).
Elderly patients and hemiplegic patients may require assistance for oral care, which may mean that this is sub-optimal. Dentures of 50 elderly patients who received help from carers to maintain their dentures were analyzed. Aerobic bacteria were isolated from all 50 patients, with 23 of 50 demonstrating dental plaque that was colonised by potential respiratory pathogens (Sumi, Sunakawa, Michiwaki, Sakagami, 2002).
Acute stroke patients with dysphagia are at risk of aspirating their saliva. If this saliva is colonised by bacteria, these bacteria will be aspirated into the lungs, where they may overwhelm respiratory defences. The patient may then proceed to develop a respiratory infection. A study of 95 patients with severe aspiration pneumonia took bronchial secretion samples and compared this to the pathogens found in dental plaque. They found that the bacteria in the respiratory samples and those found in plaque were the same (El-Solh, Pietrantoni, Okada, Bhat, Zambon, Aquilina, and Berbery, 2004).
Stringent oral care and strategies to minimize reflux in the acute stroke population has the potential to reduce respiratory infections (Langdon, Lee & Binns, 2009).

5.4 Nasogastric tubes

Colonisation by bacteria has been reported to have a high incidence in patients fed by nasogastric tubes. In one study of 103 elderly patients living in residential care facilities, those patients being fed using nasogastric tubes had a much greater incidence of colonisation with gram-negative bacteria, with 34 (64%) of tube-fed patients compared to 4 (8%) of orally fed patients showing colonisation. The pathogen most frequently recovered from the nasogastric tubes was *Pseudomonas aeruginosa* (Leibovitz, Dan, Zinger, Carmeli, Habot & Segal, 2003).
One prospective cohort study investigated 100 acute stroke patients tube fed due to dysphagia: 44% were diagnosed with pneumonia in the 2nd or 3rd day after onset. The authors concluded nasogastric tubes offered limited protection against aspiration pneumonia in dysphagic stroke patients (Dziewas, Ritter, Schilling, Konrad, Oelenberg, et. al., 2004).
Langdon, Lee and Binns (2009) studied acute ischemic stroke patients and found the incidence of overall infections (respiratory, urinary tract and other infections) in stroke patients who were tube fed was 69%, with 51 infections occurring in 74 patients. Thirty of these infections were respiratory. They reported a significant effect of time-to-event, with the majority of respiratory infections diagnosed on days 3 and 4 after stroke, and 39/51

(76%) of all infections diagnosed in tube-fed survivors occurring by day 7 after stroke. The relationship between tube feeding and subsequent development of respiratory infections is shown in Figure 2.

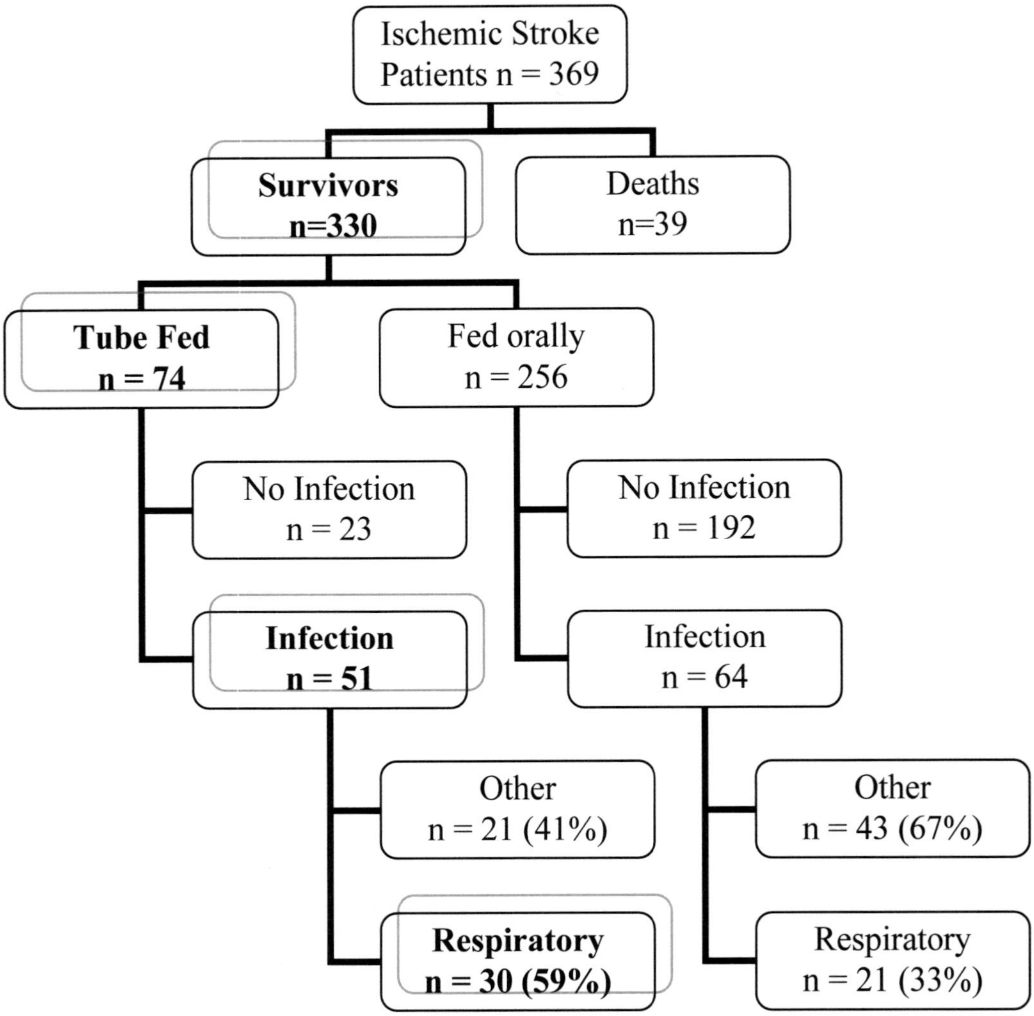

Fig. 2. Relationship Between Tube Feeding and Respiratory Infections in the First Month Following Stroke.

It has been hypothesized that nasogastric feeding tubes actually predispose patients to aspiration by

1. Loss of anatomical integrity of the upper and lower oesophageal sphincters
2. Increase in frequency of transient lower oesophageal sphincter relaxations
3. Desensitization of the pharyngoglottal adduction reflex (Gomes, Pisani, Macedo & Campos, 2003).

In addition, presence of a feeding tube may lead to formation of biofilms which become colonized by bacteria, found to have an incidence of 60% of day one and 100% on subsequent days (Leibovitz, Baumoehl, Steinberg & Segal, 2005).
Data from the FOOD trial was inconclusive on efficacy of nasogastric feeding in early stroke, however it has been suggested that enteral feeding need not begin in the first few days after a stroke (Donnan & Dewey, 2005). Langdon, Lee and Binns suggested that it may be appropriate to hold off from instituting enteral feeding in the first 3-4 days post stroke, as this appears to be a period when patients are especially susceptible to developing respiratory infections.

5.5 Gastroesophageal reflux

Patients who have gastroesophageal reflux (GOR) and also a poor conscious state are considered at very high risk of aspiration, particularly if they have a large volume of gastric content (DeLegge, 2002). Langdon, Lee and Binns (2010) found that subjects with a prior history of GOR had a significantly increased risk of developing respiratory infections in acute stroke, with 19 of 55 patients with pre-existing GOR developing respiratory infections OR 1.89 (95% CI 1.23, 2.9), p=.01.
It may be that acute stroke affects gastric motility due to the neurological insult, predisposing patients to an increased risk of reflux. Oesophageal manometry studies performed in five patients with dysphagic stroke and PEG tubes found lower oesophageal sphincter dysfunction occurred in 80% with significant gastroesophageal reflux seen in two patients. One of these two patients recovered swallow function and resumed oral feeding, while the other developed three bouts of aspiration pneumonia and died four months after PEG insertion (Elphick, Elphic, Smith, DaCosta & Riley 2006). An earlier study examined 35 acute stroke patients with severe impairment requiring tube feeding and found lower oesophageal sphincter dysfunction in 24 patients; upper oesophageal sphincter function was lower than normal in 30 patients (Lucas, Yu, Vlahos & Ledgerwood (1999).
Positioning in stroke patients can be an important prophylactic measure for GOR events. Elphick et. al., (2006) found reflux events occurred significantly more frequently when patients were in either right lateral or supine position. Supine positioning is considered a risk factor for development of reflux- related and ventilator-assisted pneumonia (Cook & Kollef, 1998; Metheny, Chang, Ye, Edwards, Defer et. al., 2002).

6. A critical period of susceptibility to infection in acute ischemic stroke

Previous studies have shown that infection commonly occurs in the acute period immediately following a stroke. Gordon, Hewer & Wade (1987) reported that all eleven chest infections developed during the first seven days post stroke in their cohort of 91 dysphagic stroke patients. Mann, Hankey and Cameron (1999) reported 26/112 patients developed chest infections during the six-month post stroke period, with 10/26 diagnosed during the first week post-onset.
In the Copenhagen study, 24.5% of female subjects and 13.6% of males developed early infections (Kammersgaard, Jorgensen, Reith, Nakayama, Houth, Weber, Pederse & Olsen, 2001). The GAIN trial noted that the majority of infections occurred in the first week of the acute stroke period (Aslanyan, 2004). In an Australian cohort of 330 ischemic stroke survivors, 115 infections were treated in the first month post stroke. Sixty (52%) of these infections were diagnosed by the third day post admission. During the first seven days post stroke, 51 infections in females, and 45 infections in males were diagnosed (Langdon, Lee &

Binns, 2010). These represent 83% of all the infections treated in the first month, and demonstrate a strong argument that the first week post stroke is associated with a greater period of susceptibility to infections.

Recent studies in animal models have suggested that stroke induces a severe depression of immune function, and predisposes patients to infections. This phenomenon, stroke induced immunodepression (SIDS) leads to lymphocytopneia and functional deactivation of monocytes and T-helper cells (Dirnafl, Klehmet, Braun, Harms, Neisel, et. al., 2007). This has been shown to be strongly related to the infarct volume and stroke severity (Hug, Dalpke, Wieczorek, Giese, Lorenz et. al., 2009).

In animal studies, stroke increases susceptibility to aspiration-induced pneumonia. In a murine model, control animals required at least a 3 order of magnitude increase in the numbers of bacteria required to induce pneumonia compared to mice with induced MCA stroke (Prass, Meisel, Hoflich, Braun, Halle, et.al., 2003).

There is evidence that overactivation of the sympathetic nervous system occurs in the first two days post stroke in humans. Within 3 days of the initial insult, up to 61% of patients will become febrile, with the most common cause being infection. Of these infections, pneumonia is most commonly reported (Mergenthaler, Dirnagl & Meiser, 2004).

In a cohort of 330 stroke survivors, 81 cases of nosocomial infection were diagnosed in the first month post stroke. Of these 81 infections, 56 (69%) were diagnosed in the first week post stroke; 28 infections in males and 28 in female subjects. Female subjects demonstrated a definite peak of infections occurring on Day 3 post stroke, while males were diagnosed on Day 3 and Day 4. Once the first 7 days post stroke were past, infection rates declined significantly for both genders (Langdon, Lee & Binns, 2010). Prass and colleagues (2006) have suggested that a stroke causes a shift from harmless aspiration to severe potentially life threatening infection.

7. Conclusions

Respiratory infections and urinary tract infections are the most common infections in acute stroke patients. Studies indicate that patients are particularly vulnerable to infection in the very acute period of their stroke: the first few days following an infarct. During this period it may be appropriate for patients to be 'Nil by Mouth' if they are at high risk of aspiration. Hydration can be maintained using either intravenous hydration or hypodermoclysis (sub cutaneous fluids), while medications can be administered transdermally, intravenously or by suppository.

Multidisciplinary care that concentrates on minimizing risk factors for infection is essential. These include minimising aspiration risk with good dysphagia management, positioning and chest care, early mobilisation, stringent oral hygiene and encouragement of self-feeding.

While dysphagia is very common in the acute stroke period, for the majority of patients it is a transitory phenomenon and they can look forward to resuming normal eating and drinking within a short period of time. For those patients with more severe and persistent dysphagia, good management will help prevent respiratory complications. Early referral to a Speech Language Pathologist with expertise in dysphagia assessment and rehabilitation will ensure that patients have their best possible chance of return to eating and drinking normally - one of life's great pleasures as well as an act essential to maintaining life.

8. References

Altman, K.W., Yu, G.P. Schaefer, S.D. (2010). Consequences of dysphagia in the hospitalized patient: impact on prognosis and hospital resources. Arch Otolaryngol Head Neck Surg. 136(9):784-789.

Addington, W.R., Stephens, R..E., Gilliland, K. (1999). Assessing the laryngeal cough reflex and the risk of developing pneumonia after stroke: An interhospital comparison. Stroke 30: 1203-1207.

Aslanyan, S., Weir, C.J., Diener, H.C., Kaste, M., Lees, D.R. (2004). Pneumonia and urinary tract infection after acute ischemic stroke: a tertiary analysis of the GAIN International trial. Eur J Neurol 11:49-53.

Aviv, J.E., Martin, J.H., Sacco, R.L., Zagar, D., Diamond, B., Keen, M.S., Blitzer, A. (1996). Supraglottic and pharyngeal sensory abnormalities in stroke patients with dysphagia. Ann Otol Rhinol Laryngol 105: 92-97.

Aydogdu, I., Ertekin, C., Tarlaci, S., Turman, B., Kiyliogly, N. (2001). Dyspahgia in lateral medullary syndrome (Wallenberg's syndrome): An acute disconnection syndrome in premotor neurons related to swallowing activity? Stroke 32:2091-2087.

Barczi, S.R., Sillivan, Pl.A., Robbins, J. (2000). How should dysphagia care of older adults differ? Establishing optimal practice patterns, Semin Speech Lang 21:347-61.

Bass, N.H., Morrell, R.M. (1992). The neurology of swallowing. *in* Dysphagia: Diagnosis and management, M.E. Groher (Ed). Butterworth-Heinemann, Boston.

Broadley, S., Croser, D., Cottrell, J., Creevy, M., Teo, E., Yiu, D., Pathi, R., Taylor, J., Thompson, P.D. (2003). Predictors of prolonged dysphagia following acute stroke. Journal of Clinical Neuroscience 10(3):300-305.

Barer, D.H. (1989). The natural history and functional consequences of dysphagia after hemispheric stroke. J Neurol Neurosurg Psychiatry 52(2):236-241.

Brook, I. (2003). Microbiology and management of periodontal infections. Gen Dent. 51(5):424-8.

Carnaby, G., Hankey, G.J., Pizzi, J. (2006). Behavioural intervention for dysphagia in acute stroke: A randomized control trial. Lancet Neurol. 5:32-7.

Chua, K.S., Kong, K.H. (1996). Functional outcome in brain stem stroke patients after rehabilitation. Arch Phys Med Rehabil. 77(2):194-7.

Cook, D.J., Kollef, M.H. (1998). Risk factors for ICU-acquired pneumonia, JAMA. 279(20):1605-06.

Daniels, S.K., Brailey, K., Priestly, D.H., Herrington, L.R., Weisberg, L.A., Foundas, A.L. (1998). Aspiration in patients with acute stroke. Arch Phys Med Rehabil 79: 14-19.

Daniels, S.K., (2000). Optimal patterns of care for dysphagic stroke patients. Seminars in Speech and Language 21:323-331.

Davis, D.G., Bears, S., Barone, J.E., Corvo, .R., Tucker, J.B. (2002). Swallowig with a treacheostomy tube in place: Does cuff inflation matter? Journal of Intensive Care Medicine. 17(3):132-135.

DeLegge, M.H. (2002). Aspiration pneumonia: Incidence, mortality and at-risk populations. Journal of parenteral and Enteral Nutrition. 26:s19-s25.

DePippo, K.L., Holas, M.A., Reding, M.J., Mandel, F.S., Lesser, M.L. (1994). Dysphagia therapy following stroke: A controlled trial. Neurology 44:1655-60.

Ding, R., Logemann, J.A. (2000). Pneumonia in stroke patients: A retrospective study. Dysphagia 15: 51-57.

Dirnagl, U., Klehmet, J., Braun, J.S., Harms, H., meisel, C., Ziemsssen, T., Prass, K., Meisel, A. (2007). Stroke-induced immunodepression: experimental evidence and clinical relevance. Stroke. 38:770-773.

Dodds, W.J., Stewart, E.T., Logemann, J.A. (1990). Physiology and radiology of the normal oral and pharyngeal phases of swallowing. Am J Roentfenol. 154(5):953-63.

Donnan, G.A., Dewey, H.M. (2005). Stroke and nutrition: FOOD for thought. Lancet. 365:729–730.

Dziewas, R., Ritter, M., Schilling, M., Konrad, C., Oelenberg, S., Nabavi, D.G., Stogbauer, F., Ringelstein, E.B., Ludemann, P: (2004). Pneumonia in acute stroke patients fed by nasogastric tube.J Neurol Neurosurg Psychiatry. 75: 852–856.

El-Solh AA, Pietrantoni C, Bhat A, Okada M, Zambon J, Aquilina A, Berbary E. (2004). Colonization of dental plaques: a reservoir of respiratory pathogens for hospital-acquired pneumonia in institutionalized elders. Chest. 2004 Nov;126(5):1575-82.

Gomes, G.F., Pisani, J.C., Macedo, E.D., Campos, A.C. (2003). The nasogastric geeding tube as a risk factor for aspiration and aspiration pneumonia. Curr Ipin Clin Nutr Metab Care. 6:327-333.

Gordon , C., Hewer, R.L., Wade, D.T. (1987). Dysphagia in acute stroke. Br Med J(Clin Res Ed). 295(6595):411-4.

Hamdy, S., Aziz, Q., Rothwell, J.C., Singh, K.D., Barlow, J., Hughes, D.G., Tallis, R.C., Thompson, D.G. (1995). The cortical topography of human swallowing musculature in health and disease. Nat Med. 2(11):1217-24.

Hinchey, J.A., Shepherd, T., Furey, K., Smith, D., Wang, D., Tonn, S. (2005). Formal dysphagia screening protocols prevent pneumonia. Stroke. 36:1972-76.

Jean, A. (2001). Brain stem control of swallowing: Neuronal network and cellular mechanisms. Physiol Rev 81(2):929-69.

Kammersgaard, L.P., Jorgensen, H.S., Reith, J., Nakayama, H., Jouth, J.G., Weber, U.J., Pederse, P.M., Olsen, T.S. Early infection and prognosis after acute stroke: The Copenhagen Stroke Study. Journal of Stroke and Cerebrovascular Diseases 10:217-221.

Katzan, I.L, Cebul, R.D., Husak, S.H., Dawson, N.V., Baker, D.W. (2003). The effect of pneumonia on mortality among patients hospitalized for acute stroke. Neurology 60: 620-625.

Kaye, V., Brandstarter, M.E. (2009). Vertebrobasilar stroke. http://emedicine.medscape.com/article/323409-overview accessed 28/03/2011.

Kidd, D., Lawson, J., Nesbitt, R., McMahon, J. (1995). The natural history and clinical consequences of aspiration in acute stroke QJM. 88(6):409-413.

Lang, I.M. (2009) Brain stem control of swallowing. Dysphagia 24(3):333-348.

Langdon, P.C. (2007). Pneumonia in acute stroke: What are the clinical and demographic factors? Doctoral Thesis, Curtin University of Technology.

Langdon, P.C., Lee, A.H., Binns, C.W. (2007). Dysphagia in acute ischaemic stroke: Severity, recovery and relationship to stroke type. J Clin Neuroscience 14(7):630-634.

Langdon, P.C., Lee, A.H., Binns, C.W. (2009). High incidence of respiratory infections in 'Nil by Mouth' acute stroke patients. Neuroepidemiology 32(2):107-13.

Langdon, P.C., Lee, A.H., Binns, C.W. (2010). Langdon PC, Lee AH, Binns CW. (2010). Pneumonia in Acute Stroke. VDM Publishers Mauritius. ISBN 978-3-639-22264-7

Langmore, S.E., Terpenning, M.S., Schork, A., Chen, Y., Murray, J.T., Lopatin, D., Loesche, W.L. (1998). Predictors of aspiration pneumonia: How important is dysphagia? Dysphagia 13:69-81.

Larsen, P.D., Martin, J.L. (1999). Polypharmacy and elderly patients. AORN J. 1999 Mar;69(3):619-22, 625, 627-8.

Leibovitz, A., Dan, M., Zinger, J., Carmeli, Y., Habot, B., Segal, R. (2003). Pseudomonas aeruginosa and the oropharyngeal ecosystem of tubefed patients. Emerg Infect Dis. 9: 956–959.

Leibovitz, A., Baumoehl, Y., Steinberg, D., Segal, R. (2005). Biodynamics of biofilms formation on nasogastric tubes in elderly patients. Isr Med Assoc J 7:428-430.

Leslie, P., Drinnan, M.J., Ford, G.A., Wilson, J.A. (2002). Swallow respiration patterns in dysphagic patients following acute stroke. Dysphagia 17:202-207.

Leslie, P., Drinnan, M.J., Ford, G.A., Wilson, J.A. (2005). Swallow respiratory patterns and aging: Presbyphagia or dysphagia? Journal of Gerontology. 60!(3):391-95.

Mann, G., Hankey, G., Cameron, D. (1999). Swallowing function after stroke: Prognosis and prognostic factors after six months. Stroke 30(4):744-748.

Mann, G., Hankey, GJ., Cameron, D. (2000). Swallowing disorders following acute stroke: prevalence and diagnostic accuracy. Cerebrovasc Dis 19(5):380-6.

Marik, P.E. (2001). Aspiration pneumonitis and aspiration pneumonia. N Engl J Med 344:665-671.

Martin, B., Logemann, J., Shaker, R., Dodds, W. (1994). Coordination between respiration and swallowing: Respiratory phase relationships and temporal integration. J App Physiol 76(2):714-23.

Matthews, C.T., Coyle, J.L. (2010). Reducting pneumoia risk factors in patients with dysphagia who have a tracheostomy: What role can SLPs play? ASHA Leader, May 18.

Matsuo, K., Palmer, J.B. (2008). Anatomy and physiology of feeding and swallowing: normal and abnormal. Phys Med Rehabil Clin N Am. 19(4):681-707,vii.

McLaren, S.M.G., Dickerson, J.W.T. (2000) Measurement of eating disability in an acute stroke population. Clinical Effectiveness in Nursing 4: 109–120.

Mergenthaler, P., Dirnagl, U., Meisel, A. (2004). Pathophysiology of stroke: lessons from animal models. Metab Brain Dis 19:151-167.

Metheny, N.A., Chang, Y.H., Ye, J.S., Edwards, S.J., Defer, J., Dahms, T.E., Stewart, B.J., Stone, K.S., Clouse, R.E.: Pepsin as a marker for pulmonary aspiration. Am J Crit Care 2002; 11: 150–154.

Miller, A.J. (1982). Deglutition. Physiol Review.62(1):129-84.

Miller, A.J., Neurobiology of swallowing. (2008). Dev Disabil Res Rev 14:77-86.

Mistry, S., Hamdy, S. (2008). Neurol control of feeding and swallowing. Phys Med Rehabil Clin N Am. 19(4):709-28.

Mojon, P. (2002). Oral health and respiratory infection. J Can Dent Assoc. 69:340-345.

Mojon, P., Budtz-Jorgensen, E., Rapin, C.H. (2002) Bronchopneumonia and oral health in hospitalized older patients. A pilot study. Gerodontology 19:66-72.

Nakajoh, K., Nakagawa, R., Sekizawa, K., Matsui, T., Arai, H., Sasaki, H. (2000). Relation between incidence of pneumonia and protective refluxes in post-stroke patients with oral or tube feeding. Journal of Internal Medicine 247: 39-42.

National Stroke Foundation. (2010). Clinical Guidelines for stroke management. http://www.strokefoundation.com.au/clinical-guidelines accessed 09.04.2011.

Prass, K., Meisel, C., Hoflich, C., Braun, J., Halle, E., Wolf, T., Ruscher, K., Victorov, I.V., Priller, J., Dirnagl, U., Vold, H.D., Meisel, A. (2003). Stroke0induced immunodeficiency promotes spontaneous bacterial infections and is medicated by sympathetic activvation reversal by poststroke T helper cell type 1-like immunostimulation. J Exp Med. 198:725-726.

Robbins, J., Levine, R.L. Maser, A., Rosenbek J.C., Kempster, G.B. (1993). Swallowing after unilateral stroke of the cerebral hemisphere. Arch Phys Med Rehabil 74:1295-1300.

Russell, S.L., Boylan, R.J., Kaslick, R.S., Scannapieco, F.A., Katz, R.V. (1999). Respitatory pathogen colonization of the dental plaque of institutionalized elders. Spec Care Dentist 19:128-134.

Scottish Intercollegiate Guidelines Network (SIGN). (2002). Management of patients with stroke: Rehabilitaiton, prevention and management of com;ications, and discharge planning. A National Clinical Guideline. http://www.sign.ac.uk/pdf/sign64.pdf accessed 09.04.2011

Smithard, D.G., O'Neill, P.A., Park, C., Morris, J. (1996). Complications and outcome after acute stroke. Does dysphagia matter? Stroke 27: 1200-1204.

Smithard, D.G., O'Neill, P.A., England, R.E., Park, C.L., Wyatt, R., Martin, D.F., Morris, J. (1997). The natural history of dysphagia following a stroke. Dysphagia 12:188-193.

Smithard, D.G., Spriggs, D. (2003). No gag, no food. Age and Ageing 32: 674–680.

Shaker, R. (2006). Reflex interaction of pharynx, esophagus and airways. GI Motility Online, 2006.

Steinhagen, V., Grossman, A., Benecke, R., Walter, U. (2009). Swallowing Disturbance Pattern Relates to Brain Lesion Location in Acute Stroke Patients. Stroke. 40:1903.

Sumi, Y., Sunakawa, M., Michiwaki, Y., Sakagami, N. (2002). Colonization of dental plawue by respiratory pathogens in dependent elderly. Gerodontology 19:25-29.

Sundar, U., Pahuja, V., Dwivedi, N., Yeolekar, M.E. (2008). Dysphagia in acute stroke: correlation with stroke subtype, vascular territory and in-hospital respiratory morbidity and mortality. Neurol India 56(4):463-70.

Wang, Y., Lim, L.L., Levi, C., Heller, R.F., Fischer ,J. (2001). A prognostic index for 30-day mortality after stroke. J Clin Epidemiol 54: 766-773.

Wang, Y., Lim, L.L, Heller, R.F., Fisher, J., Levi, C.R. (2003). A prediction model of 1-year mortality for acute ischemic stroke patients. Arch Phys Med Rehabil 84: 1006-1011.

Westergren, A. (2006). Detection of eating difficulties after stroke: a systematic review. Int Nurs Rev. 53(2):143-9.

Williams, L.S. (2006). Feeding patients after stroke: Who, when and how? Annals of Internal Medicine 144(1):59-60.

Witt, R.L. (2005). Salivary gland diseases: surgical and medical management. New York: Thieme.

Zald, D.H., Pardo, J.V. The functional neuroanatmy of voluntary swallowing. Ann Neurol. 46(3):281-6.

5

Serum Lipids and Statin Treatment During Acute Stroke

Yair Lampl
Edith Wolfson Medical Center, Holon
Sackler Faculty of Medicine, Tel Aviv University,
Israel

1. Introduction

Epidemiological studies have shown a direct correlation between total serum cholesterol level and the risk of coronary disease. The significance of lowering serum total cholesterol (TC) and low density lipoprotein (LDL-C) and increasing high density level cholesterol (HDL-C) has been shown in various kinds of these studies on stroke; even on ones concerning cardiovascular events. The relative cardiovascular risk reduction by lowering the LDL-C ranges around 20-30%. The cardiac benefit of controlling serum lipid levels is specific among patients with evidence of chronic heart disease. Among the population without previous coronary disease, the primary preventive effect is less clear.

In acute stroke, the behavior of lipids changes from day to day and even up to weeks. The exact behavior of lipids is not ultimately that clear and even though this issue is very old, the studies about it are very sparse and not up-to-date. On the other hand, it is known that the specific biological effect of lowering lipids in cardiovascular and cerebrovascular conditions by using HMG-C_oA reductase inhibitors (statins) causes a modulatory influence on the myocardial, vasculoprotective and neuroprotective areas of the brain. Some of the beneficial effects of the statins may be secondary to the "class effect" or due to the individual characteristics of each drug. An example of this is seen, when under the use of statins, there is a 1.8% reduction of body weight with a 5-7% reduction in serum LDL-C. The coronary beneficial preventive effect was shown with pravastatin in the West Scotland Coronary Prevention Study (WSCPS), with lovastatin in the Air Force coronary Atherosclerosis Prevention Study (AFCAPS), with atorvastatin in the Anglo-Scandinavian Cardiac Outcomes Study Trial (ASCOT-LLA) and with rosuvastatin in the Jupiter Study. All aspects of statin treatment during the acute stroke phases have not yet been clarified and what is known will be discussed in this chapter.

2. Lipids during acute stroke

2.1 Serum lipid levels during acute stroke

Since the end of the 60's, various articles have been published concerning the lipid level of stroke patients. Most studies of the studies analyzed the levels for weeks or months after stroke. However, none of these studies examined the lipid profile during the stroke event. In 1987, Mendez et al. [1987] studied 22 consecutive patients in three different time points, within 24 hours of stroke and 7 days and 3 months later. The mean level of total cholesterol

(225 ± 15 mg/dl) decreased to a lower level (189 ± 19 mg/dl) after 7 days and increased again to a higher level (247 mg/dl) after 3 months (significance of $p<0.05$). In transient ischemic attack patients (TIA), the profile was similar, but did not reach the level on admission at 3 months. The levels of total cholesterol were especially high among younger patients significantly. The profile of very low density lipoproteins (VLDL) was a similar one (16 ± 6 mg/dl, 13 ± 4 mg/dl, 16.5 ± 5, respectively to the time points). There was a correlation between serum levels, group of age and severity of strokes with the triglycerides (186 ± 45 mg/dl, 173 ± 36 mg/dl, 209 ± 43mg/dl., respectively), and on the low density lipoprotein (LDL) (186 ± 17 mg/dl, 149 ± 0.5 mg/dl, 202 ±19mg/dl., respectively). High density lipoprotein (HDL) showed a reciprocal profile (23 ± 3.0 mg/dl, 27 ± 4.5 mg/dl, 29 ± 4.0 mg/dl., respectively). The levels were higher in aged patients and in TIA ones. The differences in most of the tests had not reached statistical significance.

Woo et al. [1990] analyzed data of 171 patients during acute ischemic stroke (48 hours and 3 months later). They found a high level of total cholesterol in the early stage of acute stroke (221 ± 46 mg/dl vs 205 ± 50 mg/dl, $p<0.0001$) and of LDL-C (147 ± 43 mg/dl vs 135 ± 46 mg/dl, $p=0.05$). Triglycerides were lower on admission and non significant (133 ± 1.0 mg/dl vs 151 ± 89 mg/dl, $p<0.0001$).No changes were found in HDL and VLDL. There was a significant correlation toward better outcome in the higher level of total cholesterol, triglycerides, VLDL and HDL and reciprocal concerning HDL. The levels were lower in lacunar infarction patients. A significant finding was shown in lacunar infarction and was only higher in total cholesterol and LDL-C during the first 48 hours.

In 1996 Aull et al. [1996] examined the data of 37 patients with TIAs or minor strokes, during the first 24-48 hours and compared the data to the results of other patients after 49-168 hours. In spite of the severe limitations of the design of the study, they found a higher level of total cholesterol in the 24-48 hour group (231.7 ± 42.8 mg/dl vs 192.2 ± 36.0 mg/dl, $p<0.05$). There was no difference concerning the triglyceride and HDL-C levels.

A study which analyzed the post ischemic stroke cholesterol and LDL-C levels in various time points – on admission; day 2 and 3; week 1, 2 3 and 4; although in only 19 patients, was published by Kargman et al. [1998] based on the data from the Northern Manhattan study (NOMIS). They found a similar profile for cholesterol and LDL-C. The highest level was on admission, decreased to a lower level on the second day, reaching the lowest level after 1 week, and a recurrent increase on the 4th week, without reaching the original level on admission (cholesterol - 295 ± 57.6 mg/dl, 214 ± 53.2 mg/dl, 215 ± 58.2 mg/dl, 208 ± 43.5 mg/dl, 213 ± 45.3 mg/dl, 213 ± 45.3 mg/dl, 218 ± 47.9 mg/dl and 216 ± 55.8 mg/dl; LDL - 154 ± 56.0 mg/dl, 137 ± 52.1 mg/dl, 133 ± 49.4 mg/dl, 124 ± 39.2 mg/dl, 131 ± 36.6 mg/dl, 133 ± 43.3 mg/dl, 130 ± 45.6 mg/dl). The profile of triglycerides showed the lowest level on admission (181 ± 94.7 mg/dl) and a maximal level after the first week (250 ± 151.6 mg/dl). HDL-C did not show any dynamic values.

2.2 Level of lipids during acute stroke as a prognostic marker for outcome and death

Some studies analyzed the level of lipids during the acute state of stroke as a prognostic marker for the later outcome.

2.2.1 Total cholesterol

Vauthey et al. [2000] analyzed the data base of 3,273 consecutive patients with first ever stroke. They found a high mortality rate ($p=0.002$) and a poorer one month outcome ($p<0.01$) in correlation with low levels of total cholesterol. The association between low serum level of total cholesterol and worse outcome as well as with mortality rate was described also by Dyker et al. in 977 patients [1997] and by Olsen et al. [2007] when measuring the total cholesterol in 513 patients within 24 hour time window. The neurological score used for evaluation was the Scandinavian Stroke Score (SSS). Li et al. [2008] in a prospective observational study of 649 patients, including all types of stroke and intracerebral hemorrhage patients also found a high level of correlation of $p<0.005$ between low levels of total cholesterol and better 90 day outcome, using the Scandinavian Stroke Score (SSS). The correlation between high level of serum total cholesterol and better outcome was confirmed during follow-up post stroke. Simundic et al. [2008] demonstrated these findings also in their acute stroke study which included 70 patients. Pan et al. [2008] examined the functional Barthel Index Scale in 109 patients in different stages of outcome at 2 weeks and 1, 2, 4 and 6 month and confirmed this observation in each of the examination points. E. Cuadrado-Godia et al. [2009] found this association in both sexes, but also more prominently among the male. In their study, which included 591 patients, a neurological score (NIH Stroke Scale), as well as a handicap score (Modified Rankin Scale - mRS) were used. A sex dependency was found not only in the higher levels, but also in the lipid level as outcome prognostic markers. The level of total cholesterol was higher among females (187.7 ± 45.0 mg/dl vs 176.7 ± 43.8 mg/dl, $p=0.005$). The association between high level of total cholesterol and better outcome was highly significant among males and not among females ($p=0.0014$). This study included naïve and non naïve statin users, as well as patients under tPA administration. The overall lipid level was relatively low (6% total cholesterol and >250 mg/dl). Contrary to these results, von Budingen et al. [2008] in Switzerland analyzed prospectively collected data of 899 patients. Each of them neurologically scored using the NIHSS scale. The authors compared the scores on admission and day 90 and found no correlation between neurological recovery and cholesterol level.

2.2.2 High density lipoprotein (HDL) level

The HDL levels during acute stroke were analyzed as part of the lipid examination in Li et al. [2008] in 649 patients and a high correlation ($p<0.001$) was found between low HDL and severity of stroke after 90 days. Sacco et al. [2001] in a population based incident case controlled study, which included 539 patients with first ever ischemic stroke, evaluated a protective effect of high HDL-C (> 35mg/dl). The association between HDL-C level and better outcome more was significant in the serum level group of 35-39 mg/dl and as most effective in the patient group having HDL-C > 50 mg/dl. The study was designed for the elderly population (>75 years) of all ethnic groups. The previously mentioned study of Cuadrado-Godia et al. [2009] found the same tendency of higher HDL among females (52.9 ± 15.1 mg/dl vs 45.1 ± 13.4 mg/dl) and an isolated effect toward better outcome in association with higher HDL levels only among males ($p<0.001$). There was the same tendency in the total cholesterol/HDL ratio showing higher a ratio among males (3.7 ± 1.2 mg/dl vs 4.11 ± 1.4 mg/dl, $p=0.002$). A sex dependency was shown also by Russman et al. [2009]. A higher level among females (42.5 mg/dl vs 34.2 mg/dl, $p=0.05$) was demonstrated, as well as being less prone to stroke and having a better outcome (mRS $p=0.059$). It was assumed as the increase of HDL-C among females was dependent on the higher endogenous estrogen regulation APO AI [Hamalainen et al., 1986; Longcope et al., 1990].

2.2.3 Triglycerides (TG)

The association between the level of TG and outcome is more controversial. Whereas, most studies showed a correlation between high level and better outcome and recovery [Li et al.,

2008], other studies had not found a correlation or a tendency, and their results not reaching statistical significance [Simundic et al., 2008].
In summation, all studies confirmed the finding of direct, independent correlation between higher total cholesterol level, during acute stroke, and HDL-C and better outcome and recovery. This tendency was shown especially among the elderly population in different races and ethnicities. Some studies, in which the results were not absolutely clear, showed that a high triglycerol level has a tendency toward better outcome. A higher level was expected among females, and among males, the elevation of lipids in serum, and especially in total cholesterol and HDL, are of more importance as better outcome markers.

2.3 Lipid profile and outcome after thrombolysis in acute stroke

Intravenous administration of tissue plasminogen activator (tPA) is an improved tool for better outcome in a large group of acute ischemic stroke. The main severe complication of tPA is secondary bleeding after the administration of the drug. The association of lipid and tPA was examined in severe strokes and revealed controversial data. In a retrospective study, which included tPA treated patients, intraarterial thrombolysis on mechanical embolectomy found an association between secondary hemorrhagic transformation and LDL cholesterol level. Bang et al. [2007] examined 104 patients checking parameters for tPA outcome in intravenously treated patients. They found that low LDL (odds ratio (OR) 0.968 per 1 mg/dl) increases independently upon static treatment has a high risk for hemorrhagic transformation. Uyttenboogaart et al. [2008] one year later found controversial findings. They found no association between LDL, HDL and total cholesterol levels and usage of statins as predictive factors for secondary bleeding. On the other hand, they demonstrated a significant independent correlation between high levels of triglycerides and the risk of secondary bleeding, but not with unfavorable outcome in a three month analysis ($p=0.53$). Among 252 patients, they found that the mean triglyceride levels were significantly higher among secondary bleeding patients (2.5 mmol/L vs 1.8 mmol/L, $p=0.02$) and reaches statistical significance, $p=0.01$, as an independent associated factor. The difference in HDL level (1.0 mmol/L vs 1.2 mmol/L, $p=0.03$) did not reach statistical independent significance. Ribo et al. [2004] investigated low Lp(a), as an isolated marker for hemorrhagic transformation in tPA treatment, but found no association.

2.4 Lipid and hemorrhagic transformation during acute ischemic stroke

Most studies showed an association between low level of cholesterol and triglycerides and intracerebral bleeding. This assumption is controversial. Kim et al. [2009] analyzed 377 patients of different types of stroke to investigate the association between serum lipids and hemorrhagic transformation. Lipid profile was evaluated on admission (< 24 hours) and MRI done within 1 week after stroke. They found a difference between large artery artheromathosis and cardioembolic origin. In large atheromatotic patients, a low level of LDLC was significantly independently correlated with bleeding (OR 0.46/1mmol/L increase, $p=0.004$); in the lowest quartile (≤ 25 percentile) and the OR was 0.21 ($p=0.001$). The low level of cholesterol (lower quartile OR 0.63 for 1 mmol/L increase, $p=0.02$) was possibly associated with transformation into bleeding. No association at all was found in the cardioembolic group. The association between low total cholesterol and LDL-C is not yet established. Endothelial damage, blood extravasation around microvessels and the direct effect on blood brain barrier were discussed. A correlation between lipids and bleeding was shown by Ramirez-Moreno, who analyzed the data of 88 intracerebral patients. There was no correlation between low LDL-C level and death [Ramirez-Moreno et al., 2009].

2.5 Conclusion

The consensus is that total cholesterol in the LDL form decreases during acute stroke. As for VLDL and HDL, the acceptable consensus is that the serum level of lipids is irrelevant for estimation of the basic outcome of the individual, up to at least 7 days from the event. To estimate the real lipid level, it is best to wait for 30 days. It is also accepted that lower level of total cholesterol and LDL are predictor factors for a worse outcome, especially in larger cortical infarction strokes. However, the studies concerning this consensus are considered poor and include only a limited number of patients. This consensual date is also responsible for the examination of serum lipids only after a month in most of the acute stroke status studies. The very large data base of the various placebo groups of the disease of the diverse acute stroke studies, including ones on neuroprotection studies and a thrombolytic trial are not involved with lipid profile at the acute and hyperacute phases. It is also assumed that studying the subgroups of patients involving race, ethnicity, disease coexistence, various medication usage and various origins of the stroke were also neglected. A better clarification of such subgroups may be of importance for understanding the pathogenesis and clinical and therapeutic aspects in the proper care of stroke victims.

2.6 Lipoprotein and APO Lipoprotein (APO Lp) in acute stroke

Lipoprotein (a) was first described by Berg et al. in 1963. It was defined as a genetic variance of β lipoprotein and was inherited in an autosomal dominant form. The Lp(a) is a LDL-like molecule, consisting of Apo(a) which is linked by a disulphide bridge to apolipoprotein B100. Lp(a) is evaluatory being specific to humans and primates. The sequencing of Lp(a) at the protein and DNA levels has a high degree of similarity to plasminogen, leading to cross reactivity between both. A lower degree of similarity can be found with other "kringel" loop proteins, such as prothrombin, factor XII, and macrophage stimulating factor. The similarity is responsible for the endothelial cell fibrinolysis and the indication of procoagulant state.
The Apo(a) gene is highly polymorphic and more than 35 different sized alleles (ranging from 187-648 kDa) have been identified. The size of polymorphismus of Apo (a) is mostly dependent upon the genetically determined number of kringel IX type 2 repeats.
A few small studies have analyzed the quantitative profiles of Lp, APO Lp (a), and APO Lp(b) alongside the time axis after acute stroke. In the early 90s, Woo et al. [1990] discussed this topic. He examined APO Lp A_1 and APO B levels in 171 patients during the first 48 hours and 3 months later. During the acute phase, the APO Lp A_1 level was higher overall in all stroke subjects, as well as in cortical ischemic stroke and intracerebral bleeding, but not in lacunar stroke. The increase was in the range of 8-10%, but did not reach statistical significance (122.0 ± 30.9 vs 117.4 ± 26.4 mg/dl; 121.2 ± 31.8 vs 115.6 ± 26.4 mg/dl; 127.5 ± 34.7 vs 117.2 ± 29.8 mg/dl; and 119.1 ± 26.8 vs 119.1 ± 23.8 mg/dl; respectively).
The level of APO B showed a similar tendency; however, the increase of APO B level reached statistical significance among the cortical subgroup ($p<0.008$) (95.6 ± 27.9 vs 87.1 ± 23.4 mg/dl; 98.0 ± 26.5 vs 89.5 ± 27.4 mg/dl; 90.5 ± 25.3 vs 83.9 ± 22.2 mg/dl; and 98.7 ± 32.9 vs 86.9 ± 32.9 mg/dl; respectively). The Lp(a) showed reciprocal behavior. There was a decrease of Lp (a) during the acute phase (among 10-15%), significantly in cortical stroke, but not in intracerebral bleeding. The level of Lp(a) after three months of stroke was

significantly high in cortical infarct also in other studies [Yingdong & Xiuling, 1999]. These studies were contradictory with another study which involved 127 patients, having not found any difference between the acute stage level and recovery stage [Misirli, 2002].
The NMSS (North Manhattan Stroke Study) at the end of the 90s, Lp (a), APO AI and APO B were examined during the acute state of 24 hours and in the follow-up stages at 2 and 3 days and weeks 2, 3 and 4. Nineteen subjects fulfilled all the criteria, mean age was 65.0 ± 12 years and all types of ischemic infarcts were included. The Lp (a) concentration was elevated (52.0 ± 28.6 mg/dl) on admission (<24 hours) and remained (>30 mg/dl) in 15 patients after 1 month. The Lp(a) level began to decrease (46.0 ± 25.8) on day 3 and remained constant up to the 4th week (43.0 ± 29.7 mg/dl). The data did not reach statistical significance.
The APO AI level did not show any significant changes (day 1 130.0 ± 26.4 mg/dl; day 3 128.0 ± 27.1 mg/dl; 4th week128.0 ± 28.3 mg/dl). The APO B showed an increased level at the acute stage (141.0 ± 46.1 mg/dl), decreased at day 3 (131.0 ± 41.5 mg/dl) and remained stable up to the 4th week (132.0 ± 37.2 mg/dl). Another study, which analyzed the data of 31 cerebral hemorrhage patients and 10 ischemic strokes, found a decrease of APO A in the intracerebral patient group up to the 14th day. Lp(a) levels increased simultaneously up to the 7th day. In the ischemic group, APO A decreased, whereas no change was observed in the APO B and Lp(a) levels.
At the end of the 90's, Seki et al. [1997] analyzed the level of Lp(a) in association with thrombomodulin and total cholesterol levels in 28 cerebral thrombus patients during the acute phase of cerebral thromboses. The examination took place up to three days after the event. The event included large vessel thrombosis in lacunar infarction. The data was compared with 36 patients who had chronic phase cerebral thrombosis (> 1 month post event), 6 patients with chronic post intracerebral hemorrhage (> 3 months post event) and a control group of 37 volunteers. The plasma level of Lp(a) was significantly higher in the acute stage of cortical strokes (24.2 ± 20.9 mg/dl in cortical strokes; 13.4 ± 8.6 mg/dl in lacunar strokes; 24.2 ± 20.9 mg/dl in cortical strokes; and 11.6 ± 8.0 in controls; $p<0.0001$. significant higher level was found also in recurrent strokes (19.8 ± 17.6 mg/dl, $p<0.05$). Higher levels were demonstrated also in chronic post stroke phases (16.9 ± 14.7 mg/dl after 1 months), but not in bleeding ones after 3 months. The total cholesterol levels were low as expected. Van Kooten et al. [1996] in a cross sectional study which included 151 consecutive patients found a higher level of Lp(a) in 355 of stroke patients. The media values were 191 (12-1539) mg/dl in stroke and 197 (10-1255) mg/dl among transient ischemic stroke patients. In intracerebral hemorrhage, an elevation of Lp(a) to 153 (11-920) mg/dl was also found. Although the level of Lp(a) was increased in about one third of acute stroke patients, it was not characteristic of a stroke profile or outcome progress. These are contradictory to other studies having found only independent correlation between Lp (a) level and acute stroke [Misirli et al., 2007].

2.6.1 Summary

The data is inconclusive and is based on small group studies. Most of the studies indicate mild increase of APO AI and APO B in the acute stage after infarction lasting up to three days and returning to normal values after weeks or months. The data regarding Lp(a) is controversial. It seems that in cortical infarction the changes are more predominant, but in cerebral bleeding, only some of the changes may be present. The difference in results can be explained by the use of a very small patient sample, differences in laboratory techniques and homogeneity in patient populations.

2.7 Oxidized Low Density Lipoprotein ($_{ox}$LDL)

LDL particles can be modified into a form defined as oxidized LDL ($_{ox}$LDL). It is a proatherogenic and proinflammatory mediator induced by the inflammatory stimuli and the presence of oxygen enzymes (ROS), especially myeloperoxidase and nitric oxide synthase (NOS). $_{ox}$LDL looses the affinity to bind to LDL receptors and gains an affinity to bind to the protein receptor family called scavenger receptors. Their subfamily A is present on macrophages, platelets and other cells and has the affinity to bind and internalize the $_{ox}$LDL particles and other cells; plus, to gather up the cholesterol in the cells and create foam cells. This multi-functional membrane receptor shares also an effect on apoptotic cells and microbial agents.

An important scavenger type is CD 36, which has a concrete affect on $_{ox}$LDL. The signaling pathways include activation of SCR family kinase, MAP kinase, and the Vav family of quinine nucleotide exchange factors. The CD 36 deficient animal models show inhibition of thrombus formation, reduction of accumulation of microparticles and inhibition of foam cell creation. The scavenger receptor B type I (SR-R_1) plays a main role in mediating cholesterol exchange between cells and diverse lipoproteins. HDL-SR-R_1 is atheroprotective, cardioprotective and vascular protective by a direct endothelial affect on the kinase pathways. This includes plasma membrane cholesterol flux, requiring the C termination of the PDZ domain on the receptor and mediation of the membrane cholesterol binding; it includes also the upregularion of nitric oxide production.

In astrocytes surrounding the tissue of infarcts, an activity of $_{ox}$LDL was shown stimulating interleukin 6 secretion, active initiation of immunity and tissue survival [Shie et al., 2004]. The behavior of $_{ox}$LDL during acute stroke is characterized by a significant increase of its level immediately after onset of infarction, lasting up to three to seven days. Uno et al. [2003] compared the plasma level of $_{ox}$LDL in 45 patients after acute ischemic stroke and in 11 patients with intracerebral bleeding and compared it to a control group. They found a highly significant correlation ($p<0.0001$) between high level of $_{ox}$LDL and only cortical ischemic stroke. The mean values in the three groups (ischemic stroke, hemorrhagic stroke and controls) resulted in the following outcomes: 0.245 ± 0.22 vs 0.13 ± 0.007 and 0.179 ± 0.0232 ng/microg $_{ox}$LDL.

A second study of the same group [Uno et al., 2005] compared the $_{ox}$LDL of 44 patients with the imaging data DWI-PWI (diffusion perfusion weighted index) mismatched. The results showed a statistical correlation between enlargement of the ischemic phase and the serum elevation of $_{ox}$LDL. The correlation was specific for cortical infarcts and not for subcortical strokes or for huge hemispheric infarctions. The first blood sample was examined during the first 24 hours after infarction. The elevation profile showed a high level up to seven days and normalization of serum level up to 14-30 days post stroke.

Another study compared $_{ox}$LDL in 28 patients after acute atherothrombotic and lacunar infarction. There were significant ($p<0.001$) higher serum $_{ox}$LDL level in atherothrombotic strokes compared with the small vessel disease and control groups. The values were as follows: 106.85 ± 11.6 U/L; 81.0 ± 28.2 U/L; and 79.1 ± 20.4 U/L; respectively. The rationale for the elevation of the $_{ox}$LDL during acute stroke was due to the acute increase of oxidative stress and induction of the adhesion molecules.

3. Statins during acute stroke

3.1 Statins

Statins are competitive inhibitors of the enzyme HMG (3-hydroxy 2 - methylglutaryl) CoA reductase. This enzyme is considered to have the most important role for limiting cholesterol biosynthesis. The statin effect is based on the capacity of its binding to the active site of the HMG C_0A reductase. Statins reduce the intrahepatic cholestasis amount, increase the LDL receptor turnover and reduces the VDLD production by acting on the hepatic APO B secretion and reduction of the plasma triglycerides level. It also acts on the clearance of VLDL.

Six main statins are now on the market - lovastatin, pravastatin, simvastatin, fluvastatin, atorvastatin and rosuvastatine. Although all statins share the same "class effect", there are predominant differences among the various types of statin drugs. The non selective reduction of the LDL substances, especially the small, dense LDL particles, is more specific for atorvastatin and rosuvastatin. The effect of increasing HDL-C in serum and the apo lipoprotein AI is typical for simvastatin and rosuvastatin. Rosuvastatin and atorvastatin are also very effective in the dynamic changes of serum triglycerides, although the individual effect of these diverse statins and the drug's is very different from person to person, often dependent upon race and genetic ethic differences [Mangravite et al., 2008; Mangravite & Krauss; Puccetti et al., 2007].

The benefit of statins in primary and secondary prevention of coronary heart disease and the formation of atherosclerotic plaques is well established [Sandowitz et al., 2010a, 2010b]. The effect of statins on the cerebrovascular system and the brain tissue is based on their pleiotrophic effect beyond the direct lipid effect. The vasoeffective action is based on a direct upregulation of the endothelial nitric oxide synthase (eNOS), increase of the bioavialability of NO 20-22 [Ito et al., 2010; Laufs et al., 2000; Nakata et al., 2007; Yagi et al., 2010; Ye et al., 2008;] and inhibition of NADPH oxidase [Antoniades et al., 2010; Rueckschloss et al., 2001]. This vascular effect precedes the lipid one. The decrease of the asymmetric dimethylarginine (ADMA) [Nishiyama et al., 2011] stabilizes the blood barrier integrity [Sierra et al., 2011], acts on the apoptotic pathway [Carloni et al., 2006] and stimulates excitatory Neurotransmitters are other targets of the statin effects concerning its action on the vascular system and cerebrovascular event.

3.2 Statins in stroke

Statins have multiple targets of action in stroke. The main confirmed activity is in the vasculature reactivity action on the eNOS and NO and by action on the inflammatory pathways. The effect was shown in animal model studies. In human ones, it was shown that statin pretreatment has a favorable effect on outcome. The issue of initiation of statin treatment during acute stroke is not yet resolved. There are indications that the efficacy may be dependent upon type of statins and that this effect is an individual and not a "class effect". The multiple mechanisms of statins on ischemic brains are based on the different targets of action. Statins increase eNOS [Ito et al., 2010; Ye et al., 2008] and reduce activity of nicotinamide adenine dinucleotide phosphate oxidase and decrease endothelin 1 and 2 and the expression of AT_1 receptor [Yagi et al., 2010]. It also acts on the inflammatory system by decreasing the nkFB [Nakata et al., 2007; Ye et al., 2008] and the expression of interleukin (IL) 1p, IL6 and MCP. It also has an increasing effect on expression of tPA and a decreasing effect on plasminogen activator inhibitor 1. Additional targets of action are on the reactive oxygen species, the metalloproteinase 9 and blood brain barrier and on platelet activity [Sierra et al., 2011]. Also, various animal model studies demonstrated improvement in outcome by induced stroke on different types of models and administration of statins (mostly simvastatin or atorvastatin).

3.3 Acute stroke in patients under statin treatment

The issue of mortality and functional outcome after ischemic stroke in patients under statin treatment was analyzed in different prospective and retrospective studies. As inclusion criteria for all the studies, statins were defined as such without characterization of the type of statins. The results of those studies was based on the assumption of a statin "class effect" for neuroprotection and as a lipid lowering agents. The data of preclinical animal model studies [Berger et al., 2008; Bosel et al., 2005; Carloni et al., 2006; Domoki et al., 2010; Franke et al., 2007; Lee et al., 2008; Moonis et al., 2005; Sironi et al., 2003; Yrjanheikki et al., 2005] have indicated a different neuroprotective effect of the various types of statins and raises the fact that all these results must be taken into consideration.

Marti-Fabregas et al. [2004] in a prospective study, which included 167 patients, found a favorable outcome after three months post stroke and on statin pretreated patients compared with the untreated group (80% vs 51.8%, p=0.059) using handicapped mRS scores. Using functional disability Barthel Index (BI) scoring, similar results were found. Yoon et al. [2004] examined 436 patients with ischemic stroke. He found a good outcome (defined as mRS score >2) in 52% in the statin protected group, compared with 38% among controls (p=0.02). At the same time, Greisenegger et al. [2004] confirmed the findings with a cross-sectional study of 1,691 patients. They found also, that among the diabetes mellitus patients, the percentage of bad outcome (defined as mRS score of 5-6) was 16% of the untreated patient group, whereas no bad outcome was found among the statin treated group.

One year later, Moonis et al. [2005] compared 129 patients under previous statin treatment with a group of 600 untreated patients. The pretreated patient group had a significant better outcome at 12 weeks, using NIHSS (p=0.002) and mRS scoring (p=0.033).

In January 2008, Reeves et al. in Michigan analyzed the data of the Paul Coverdell National Acute Stroke Registry. They data included 1,360 ischemic stroke patients in 15 hospitals. They also confirmed the previous studies. In this study, the patients under statins were associated with lower odds of poor outcome. There was also a significant difference among race. Whereas, the odds ratio among Caucasian Americans was significantly toward better outcome from the statin treated group (OR=0.61), the odds ratio among Afro Americans was non significant (OR=1.82).

The north Dublin Population Stroke Study [Ni et al., 2011] was a population based prospective cohort one and included 448 ischemic stroke patients with 305 (134 patients) being pretreated with statins. The most common prescribed statins were atorvastatin (70.2%) and pravastatin (24.6%). NIHSS and the mRS scores were compared with 112 patients of the untreated group and 189 newly post stroke statin treated group. The odds ratio of the pretreated group in comparison to the untreated group was 0.04 (CI 0.0-0.33, p=0.003) at 7 days, 0.23 (CI 0.09-058, p=0.002) at 90 days and 0.48 (CI 0.23-1.01, p=0.05) at 1 year. The newly acute post statin group demonstrated similar results - lower OR (0.12, p=0.003) after 7 days, similar OR (0.16, p<0.001) after 90 days and better OR (0.26, p<0.001) after 1 year.

Arboix et al. [2010] collected date on 2,082 consecutive patients with first ever ischemic stroke incorporated from prospective hospital based stroke registry during 19 years. They found a better prognosis for pretreated patients concerning death (6.0% vs 11.5%, p=0.001), symptom-free (22% vs 17.5%, p=0.025) and severe bad functional outcome (6.6% vs 11.5%, p=0.002). Imaging studies confirmed the clinical data results. Stead et al. [2009] showed also that among 508 patients with ideal LDL level (≤ 100 mg/dl) the functional outcome was significantly better among statin users ($p<0.001$) [Reeves et al., 2008]. The neuroprotective pleiotrophic effect was assumed to be the reason for this phenomenon. Nicholas et al. [2008] found a smaller volume of infarcts in statin pretreated patients ($p=0.01$). Ford et al.[2011] examined the reperfusion in acute ischemic stroke using MR scan within 4.5 hours and 6 hours. Twelve of the patients were statin pretreated and 19 were not. They found a significant better reperfusion among the treated group (50% vs 13%, respectively; $p=0.014$). The findings were in association with improvement of NIHSS scores after one month.

3.3.1 Summary

All trial data indicate a significantly better for pre users of statin in ischemic stroke. This finding included mortality rate, early and late handicap and functional outcomes, as well as Neuroimaging findings.

3.4 Satin treatment withdrawal during acute stroke

The assumption that sudden discontinuation of statins may have a critical effect on the body is based on its biological characteristics and observations within in vitro studies and in vivo animal models. These studies showed dramatic down regulation of eNOS expression and reduction of eNOS protection up to 90%. This process is dependent upon changes in Rho and Rac regulation and changes in activity of Rho kinase. Platelet factor 4 and thromboglobulin change as well. This significant involvement in the vascular endothelial biology may, as usual, have a rebound effect. There are studies showing almost complete disappearance of the statin protective effect in experimental acute stroke after discontinuation of the drug for two days [Chen et al., 2005; Karki et al., 2009]. Changes of cerebral blood flow, in the posterior circulate system, was observed as well [Berger et al., 2008; Xu et al., 2008]. In humans during a randomized controlled study, Blanco et al. [2007] examined the effect of discontinuation of atorvastatin 20 mg / day in cortical stroke patients' outcomes. Of 219 patients, 89 were pretreated with statins, 43 continued the study and 43 stopped for 3 days. The data analysis showed high percentage of bad outcome ($mRS > 2$) among discontinued patients (60% vs 39%, $p=0.043$); a worse early neurological outcome (day 4-7 using NIHSS score, $p=0.002$) and a significant larger volume of stroke ($p<0.0001$). In comparison of the patient group naïve to statins, the risk of worse early neurological outcome was 19.01 and the risk of larger infarcts was 13.51 in total. However, meta analysis of 18 studies, enrolling 14,303 patients after acute coronary syndrome and initiation of statins within 14 days following event did not find reduction of stroke, similar to all cause mortality and heart attacks in a period of a four month follow-up.

3.4.1 Summary

The preclinical experimental data raise the speculation of a serious 'rebound' effect by the discontinuance of statins towards a worse outcome. There are too few clinical studies confirming this hypothesis.

3.5 Satin in tissue Plasminogen Activator (tPA) ischemic stroke patients

The association between statin treatment and intracerebral hemorrhage, especially after publication of the results of the SPARCL study [Goldstein et al., 2008; Goldstein et al., 2009; Welch, 2009], raises the very genuine issue of the adverse event after tPA treatment.

3.5.1 Intravenous tPA (IVtPA)

Uyttenboogaart et al. [2008] analyzed the data of 252 patients treated with tPA. They found that high level of triglycerides and low level of HDL were independent risk factors for bleeding (p==0.02, p=0.03, respectively). However, there was no association between statins and 90 day outcome. Makihara et al. [2010] analyzed the data of the Japanese SAMURAI rtPA Registry and confirmed the well established fact that administration of IV tPA increases the risk of intracerebral hemorrhage, but increases also the rate of favorable outcome. The usage of statins did not influence any of these findings. Miedema et al. [2010] published the results of a prospective observational cohort study of 476 patients treated with IV tPA with 20% of the patients being on statins. They did not find any favorable effect for 90 days in functional and neurological outcome (OR 1.1, P=0.87). This tendency was consistent in all five groups of stroke subtypes according to the TOAST classification. On the other hand, no increase of bleeding was observed as well.

3.5.2 Intraarterial tPA

Meier et al. [2009] in a monocenter study of 311 consecutive patients, of whom 18% were statin pretreated, found a higher rate of intracerebral bleeding among statin users (OR 3.1, P=0.004). This fact was unrelated to the 90 day functional and neurological outcome. The group of statin users included atorvastatin (36.4%), pravastatin (36.4%) and simvastatin (unknown %) users. Restrepo et al. [2009] examined the impact of statins before and after intraarterial fibrinolysis and percutaneous mechanical embolectomy. The study was a single center one in Los Angeles. Statin use was related to a better outcome with decrease of 6.5 units in the NIHSS score after discharge (P=0.016). There was no increase in the post procedure bleeding.

3.5.3 Summary

The data of the statin effect on tPA is sparse. However, it seems that intravenous administration has no beneficial effect of a better outcome, but also no higher rates of secondary bleeding adverse events.

3.6 Onset of satin treatment during acute stroke

The pleiotropic neuro- and vasculoprotection effect is already described. Simvastatin, rosuvastatin, atorvastatin and pravastatin had been shown to have a neuroprotective effect in animal models. It has been shown that simvastatin reduces stroke volume in rats up to 50% and pravastatin reduces the cerebral post stroke edema [Mariucci et al., 2011]. The usage of an intravenous statin in stroke is based on the intravenous formulation of the hydrophile types of statins - rosuvastatin and pravastatin. Rosuvastatin in intraperitoneal administration in rats improved clinical outcome and infarct volume [Prinz et al., 2008]. In humans, the studies are few. According to the latest updated cholesterol management guidelines, it is recommended that anticholesterol treatment be performed immediately after stroke. In the North Dublin Study, 134 out of 445 patients (30.1%) had begun the treatment during the first 72 hours after admission and 7% were treated with atorvastatin and 24% with pravastatin. The early and late survival and outcome were significantly better compared with the no treated group and equivalent to the previous statin treated group. In the data of the FASTER study concerning the assessment of minor stroke and transient ischemic attacks (TIAs) to prevent early recurrency, the group of patients under simvastatin within 24 hours of onset showed an increase of absolute risk of 3.3% toward bad outcome

[Kennedy et al., 2007]. Montaner et al. [2008] performed a simvastatin placebo controlled study of 60 patients having cortical stroke and receiving simvastatin 3-12 hours after onset of symptoms and found significant improvement after 3 days (44.4% vs 17.9%, p=0.022), but also a higher, non significant rate of mortality (OR 2.4 CI 1.06-5.4).

A head-to-head study was performed by Lampl et al. [2010] and included 371 patients. The administration of statin was immediate comparing three elements - simvastatin and atorvastatin at 40mg/daily and 80 mg/daily. The statistical analysis indicated that the subjects receiving simvastatin had a highly significant worser outcome as noted by neurological (NIHSS score) and functional (mRS) measurements compared with the two dose atorvastatin treated patients (p<0.001). The scores of atorvastatin 80 mg were marginally better than those of atorvastatin 40 mg (p=0.08).

3.6.1 Summary

The complete picture of statins as neuroprotectors during the acute phase of stroke is not yet resolved. Very few studies have been performed. It is plausible to assume that the pleiotropic neuroprotective effect is an individual characteristic of each drug and not a part of a "class effect". Many more studies and positive data are needed to confirm this assumption.

3.7 Satin in acute subarachnoid hemorrhage

The rationality of administration of statins in subarachnoid hemorrhage is based on the fact that statins have an effect on eNO and eNOS, as well as an anti-inflammatory mechanism. Therefore, it is assumed that statins may have an anti-vasospastic effect. These hypotheses were confirmed in animal studies using simvastatin. There have been some meta analysis studies which calculated the effect of statins on subarachnoid hemorrhage. Sillberg et al. [2008] published one meta analysis in 2008. Most of the studies used simvastatin in dosages of 20 mg/d and 80 mg/d and pravastatin at 40 mg/d. Sillberg et al.'s [2008] meta analysis consisted of three randomized controlled trials and incorporated the studies of Lynch et al. [2005], Tseng et al. [2005] and Chou al. [2008]. The overall number of included patients was only 158. The authors found that the incidence of vasospasm (RR 0.75 CI 0.54-0.99), delayed ischemic deficits (RR 0.38 CI 0.17-0.83) and mortality (RR 0.22 CI 0.06-0.82) were significantly reduced in the statin treated group.

Vergouwen et al. [2009] published another metal analysis of 4 studies and included 190 patients. Two studies were about simvastatin and one about pravastatin. No beneficial effect concerning transcranial Doppler vasospasm, delayed cerebral ischemia, poor outcome or mortality was found.

3.7.1 Summary

Although preclinical and various single center studies have been very promising, a positive conclusion about the benefit of statins in subarachnoid hemorrhage has not yet been finalized.

3.8 Satin in acute intracerebral hemorrhage

Previous studies on animals showed a significant improvement of functional outcome after use of simvastatin or atorvastatin, as well as reduction of hematoma volume at four weeks (Karki). Enhancement of neuroprotection and neuroplasticity effects in rats was assumed.

In humans, some studies analyzing the outcome of intracerebral hemorrhage patients under statin treatment. In a retrospective cohort study, Fitz-Maurice et al. [2008] compared the outcome of 149 patients pretreated with statins with 480 untreated patients. They found no difference among the groups concerning mortality, functional outcome and volume of hematoma. In a small group study, Tapia-Perez et al. [2009] examined 18 patients under ruravastatin with a control group of statin non users. The mortality rate was 5.6% among users and 15.8% in the control group. In Israel, two studies have been published. Eichel et al. [2010] found that the mortality rate among 101 statin pretreated patients was 45.5%, whereas the percentage among 298 non treated patients was 56.1%, p=0.04). The other Israeli study based on the data of the Israel Stroke Survey, compared 89 patients statin pretreated patients with a 312 untreated patient group. The patients under statin treatment had a better baseline neurological status or better outcome and a lower mortality rate [Leker et al., 2009]. In a prospective ascertained cohort study, Biffi et al. [2011] compared 238 statin pretreated intracerebral hemorrhage patients with 461 non treated patients. They extended their own results into a meta analysis of previously published data - for a total of 698 vs 1,823 patients. They found a favorable outcome for pretreated patients (OR 2.8 CI 1.37-3.17) and reduced mortality (OR 0.47 CI 0.32-0.70) at 90 days. The meta analysis results confirmed this finding concerning better outcome (OR 1.1 CI 1.38-2.65) and mortality (OR 0.55 CI 0.42-0.72).

3.8.1 Summary

Most published studies indicated a better outcome and reduced mortality among pretreated statin patients having intracerebral hemorrhage. Final decision on these issues must wait for more studies and those with a greater number of participants. No data is available concerning the issue of beginning statin treatment during the acute phase of intracerebral hemorrhage.

	Probable better outcome	Possible better outcome	Inconclusive	Probable worser outcome	Possible worser outcome
AIS under statin pretreatment	+				
AIS under statin withdrawal					+
AIS under statin and IV tpa			+		
AIS under statin and IAtpa		+			
AIS under statin as acute phase therapy		+			
SAH and statins		+			
ICH and statins		+			
Probable outcome dependent upon type of statin		+			

Abbreviations: AIS-acute ischemic stroke; tpa-tissue plasminogen activator; IV- intravenous; IA-intra-arterial; SAH-subarachnoid hemorrhage; ICH-intracerebral hemorrhage

Table 1. Statin efficacy during acute stroke

4. Conclusion

There are evidences of a favorable effect of statins in the different types of stroke. The efficacy was demonstrated in ischemic and hemorrhagic stroke. Most studies show a better recovery and decrease of mortality rate among statins pretreated patients, who did not discontinued the treatment. A newly treatment with statin during the acute phase of stroke maybe indicated. The pleiotrophic effect of statins may play a key role in the positive effect of statins. It is plausible that this effect is not a class effect of the statin group, but is an individual effect of each the drugs. Much larger well designed studies must be performed to confirm these assumptions.

5. References

Antoniades C., Bakogiannis C., Tousoulis D., Reilly S., Zhang M.H., Paschalis A., Antonopoulos A.S., Demosthenous M., Miliou A., Psarros C., Marinou K., Sfyras N., Economopoulos G., Casadei B., Channon K.M., & Stefnandis C. (2010). Preoperative atorvastatin treatment in CABG patients rapidly improves vein graft redox state by inhibition of Rac 1 and NADPH-oxidase activity. *Circulation,* 122(Suppl), (Sep 2010), pp. S66-73

Aull S., Lalouschek W., Schnider P., Sinzinger H., Uhl F., & Zeiler K. (1996). Dynamic changes of plasma lipids and lipoprotein in patients after transient ischemic attack or minor stroke. *Am J Med,* 101(3), (Sep 2010), pp. 291-298

Arboix A., Garcia-Eroles L., Oliveres M., Targa C., Balcells M., & Massons J. (2010). Pretreatment with statins improves early outcome in patients with first-ever ischaemic stroke: a pleiotropic effect of a beneficial effect of hypercholesterolemia? *BMC Neurol,* 10, (Jun 2010), pp. 47

Bang O.Y., Saver J.L., Liebeskind D.S., Starkman S., Villablanca P., Salamon N., Buck B.., Ali L., Restrepo L., Vinuela F., Duckwiler G., Janhan R., Razinia T., & Ovbiagele B. (2007). Cholesterol level and symptomatic hemorrhagic transformation after ischemic stroke thrombolysis. *Neurology,* 68(10), (Mar 2007), pp. 737-742

Berger C., Xia F., Mauer M.H., & Schwab S. (2008). Neuroprotection by pravastatin in acute ischemic stroke in rats. *Brain Res Rev* 58(1), (Jun 2008), pp. 48-56

Biffi A., Devan W.J.., Anderson C.D., Ayres A.M., Schwab K., Cortellini L., Viswanathan A., Rost N.S., Smith E.E., Goldstein J.N., Greenberg S.M., & Rosand J. (2011). Statin use and outcome after intracerebral hemorrhage: case-control study and meta-analysis. *Neurology,* 76(18), (May 2011), pp. 1581-1588

Blanco M., Nombela F., Castellanos M., Rodriguez-Yanez M., Garcia-Gil M., Leira R., Lizasoain I., Serena J., Vivancos J., Moro M.A., Davalos A., & Castillo J. (2007). Statin treatment withdrawal in ischemic stroke: a controlled randomized study. *Neuorlogy,* 69(9), (Aug 2007), pp. 904-910

Bosel J., Gandor F., Harms C., Synowitz M., Harms U., Dioufack P.C., Megow D., Dimagl U., Hortnagl H., Fink K.B., & Endres M. (2005). Neuroprotective effects of atorvastatin against glutamate-induced excitotoxicity in primary cortical neurons. *J Neurochem,* 92(6), (Mar 2005), pp. 1386-1398

Carloni S., Mazzoni E., Cimino M., DeSimoni M.G., Perego C., Scopa C., & Balduini W. (2006). Simvastatin reduces caspase-3 activation and inflammatory markers induced by hypoxia-ischemia in the newborn rat. *Neurobiol Dis*, 21(1), (Jan 2006), pp. 119-126

Chen J., Zhang C., Jiang H., Jhang H., Li Y., Zhang L., Robin A., Katakowski M., Lu M., & Chopp M. (2005). Atorvastatin induction of VEGF and BDNF promotes brain plasticity after stroke in mice. *J Cereb Blood Flow Metab*, 25(2), (Feb 2005), pp. 281-290

Chou S.H., Smith E.E., Badjatia N., Nogueira R.G., Sims JR. 2nd, Ogilvy C.S., Rordorf G.A., & Ayata C. (2008). A randomized double-blind, placebo-controlled pilot study of simvastatin in aneurysmal subarachnoid hemorrhage. *Stroke*, 39(10), (Oct 2008), pp. 2891-2893

Cuadrado-Godia E., Jimenez-Conde J., Ois A., Rodriguez-Campello A., Garcia-Ramallo E., & Roquer J. (2009). Sex differences in the prognostic value of the lipid profile after the first ischemic stroke. *J Neurol*, 256(6), (Jun 2009), pp. 989-995

Domoki F., Kis B., Gaspar T., Snipes J.A., Bari F., & Busija D.W. (2010). Rosuvastatin induces delayed preconditioning against L-glutamate excitoxicity in cultured cortical neurons. *Neurochem Int*, 56(3), (Feb 2010), pp. 404-409

Dyker A.G., Weir C.J., & Lees K.R. (1997). Influence of cholesterol on survival after stroke: retrospective study. *BMJ*, 314(7094), (May 1997), pp. 1584-1588

Eichel R., Khoury S.T., Ben-Hur T., Keidar M., Paniri R., & Leker R.R. (2010). Prior use of statins and outcome in patients with intracerebral hemorrhage. *Eur J Neurol*, 17(1), (Jan 2010), pp. 78-83

Fitz-Maurice E., Wendell L., Snider R., Schwab K., Chanderraj R., Kinnecom C., Nandigam K., Rost N.S., Viswanathan A., Rosand J., Greenberg S.M., & Smith E.E. (2008). Effect of statins on intracerebral hemorrhage outcome and recurrence. *Stroke*, 39(7), (Jul 2008), pp. 2151-2154

Ford A.L., An H., D'Angelo G., Ponisio R., Bushard P., Vo K.D., Powers W.J., Lin W., & Lee J.M. (2011). Preexisting statin use is associated with greater reperfusion in hyperacute ischemic stroke. *Stroke*, 42(5), (May 2011), pp. 1307-1313

Franke C., Noldner M., Abdel-Kader R., Johnson-Anuna L.N., Gibson-Wood W.E., Muller W.E., & Eckert G.P. (2007). Bcl-2 upregulation and neuroprotection in guinea pig brain following chronic simvastatin treatment. *Neurobiol Dis*, 25(2), (Feb 2007), pp. 438-445

Goldstein L.B., Amarenco P., Szarek M., Callahan A. 3rd, Hennerici M., Sillesen H., Zivin J.A., Welch K.M.; SPARCL Investigators. (2008). Hemorrhagic stroke in the Stroke Prevention by Aggressive Reduction in Cholesterol Levels study. *Neurology*, 70(24 Pt 2), (Jun 2008), pp. 2364-2370

Goldstein L.B., Amarenco P., Zivin J., Messig M., Altafullah I., Callahan A., Hennerici M., MacLoed M.J., Sillesen H., Zweifler R., Michael K., &Welch A. Stroke Prevention by Aggressive Reduction in Cholesterol Levels Investigators. (2009). Statin treatment and stroke outcome in the Stroke Prevention by Aggressive Reduction in Cholesterol levels (SPARCL) trial. *Stroke*, 40(11), (Nov 2009), pp. 3526-3531

Greisenegger S., Mullner M., Tentschert S., Lang W., & Lalouschek W. (2004). Effect of pretreatment with statins on the severity of acute ischemic cerebrovascular events. *J Neurol Sci*, 22(1-2), (Jun 2004), pp. 5-10

Hamalainen E., Adlercreutz H., Ehnholm C., & Puska P. (1986). Relationships of serum lipoproteins and apoproteins to sex hormones and to the binding capacity of sex hormone binding globulin in healthy Finnish men. *Metabolism*, 35(6), (Jun 1986), pp.535-541

Ito D., Ito O., Mori N., Muroya Y., Cao P.Y., Takashima K., Kanazawa M., & Kohzuki M. (2010) Atorvastatin upregulates nitric oxide synthases with Rho-kinase inhibition and Akt activation in the kidney of spontaneously hypertensive rats. *J Hypertens*, 28(11), (Nov 2010), pp. 2276-2288

Kargman D.E., Tuck C., Berglund L., Lin I.F., Mukherjee R.S., Thompson E.V., Jones J., Boden-Albata B., Paik M.C., & Sacco R.L. (1998). Lipid and lipoprotein levels remain stable in acute ischemic stroke: the Northern Manhattan Stroke Study. *Atherosclerosis*, 139(2), (Aug 1998), pp. 391-399

Karki K., Knight R.A., Han Y., Yang D., Zhang J., Ledbetter K.A., Chopp M., & Seyfried D.M. (2009). Simvastatin and atorvastatin improve neurological outcome after experimental intracerebral hemorrhage. *Stroke*, 40(10), (Oct 2006), pp. 3384-3389

Kennedy J., Hill M.D., Ryckborst K.J., Eliasziw M., Demchuk A.M., & Buchan A.M.: FASTER Investigators. (2007). Fast assessment of stroke and transient ischaemic attack to prevent early recurrence (FASTER): a randomized controlled pilot trial. *Lancet Neurol*, 6(11), (Nov 2007), pp. 961-969

Kim B.J., Lee S.H., Ryu W.S., Kang B.S., Kim C.K., & Yoon B.W. (2009). Low level of low-density lipoprotein in cholesterol increases hemorrhagic transformation in large artherothrombosis but not in cardioembolism. *Stroke*, 40(5), (May 2009), pp. 1627-1632

Lampl Y., Lorberboym M., Gilad R., Vysberg I., Tikozky A., Sadeh M., & Boaz M. (2010). Early outcome of acute ischemic stroke in hyperlipidemic patiens under atorvastatin versus simvastatin. *Clin Neuropharmacol*, 33(3), (May 2010), pp. 129-134

Laufs U., Gertz K., Huang P., Nickenig G., Bohm M., Dirnagl U., & Endres M. (2000). Atorvastatin upregulates type III nitric oxide synthase in thrombocytes, decreases platelet activation, and protects from cerebral ischemia in normcholesterolemic mice. *Stroke*, 31(10), (Oct 2000), pp. 2442-2449

Lee S.H., Kim Y.H., Kim Y.J., & Yoon B.W. Atorvastatin enhances hypothermia-induced neuroprotection after stroke. (2008). *J Neurol Sci*, 275(1-2), (Dec 2008), pp. 64-68

Leker R.R., Khoury S.T., Rafaeli G., Shwartz R., Eichel R., & Tanne D.:NASIS Investigators. (2009). Prior use of statins improves outcome in patients with intracerebral hemorrhage: prospective data from the National Acute Stroke Israeli Surveys (NASIS). *Stroke*, 40(7), (Jul 2009), pp. 2581-2584

Li W., Liu M., Wu B., Liu H., Wang L.C., & Tan S. (2008). Serum lipid levels and 3-month prognosis in Chinese patients with acute stroke. Adv Ther, 25(4), (Apr 2008), pp. 329-341

Longcope C., Herbert P.N., McKinlay S.M., & Goldfield S.R. (1990). The relationship of total and free estrogens and sex hormone-binding globulin with lipoproteins in women. *J Clin Endocrinol Metab*, 71(1), (Jul 1990), pp. 67-72

Lynch J.R., Wang H., McGirt M.J., Floyd J., Friedman A.H., Coon A.L., Blessing R., Alexander M.J., Graffagnino C., Warner D.S., & Laskowitz D.T. (2005). Simvastatin reduces vasospasm after aneurysmal subarachnoid hemorrhage: results of a pilot randomized clinical trial. *Stroke*, 36(9), (Sep 2005), pp. 2024-2026

Makihara N., Okada Y., Koga M., Shiokawa Y., Nakagawara J., Furui E., Kimura K., Yamagami H., Hasegawa Y., Kario K., Okuda S., Naganuma M., & Toyoda K.

(2010). Effects of statin use on intracranial hemorrhage and clinical outcome after intravenous rt-PA for acute ischemic stroke: SAMURAI rt-PA registry. (Article in Japanese). *Rinsho Shinkeigaku*, 50(4), (Apr 2010), pp. 225-231

Mangravite L.M. & Krauss R.M. (2007). Pharmacogenomics of statin response. *Curr Opin Lipidol*, 18(4), (Aug 2007), pp. 409-414

Mangravite L.M., Wilke R.A., Zhang J., & Krauss R.M. (2008). Pharmacogenomics of statin response. *Curr Opin Mol Ther*, 10(6), (Dec 2008), pp. 555-561

Mariucci G., Taha E., Tantucci M., Spaccatini C., Tozzi A., & Ambrosini M.V. (2011). Intravenous administratin of pravastatin immediately after middle cerebral artery occlusion reduces cerebral oedema in spontaneously hypertensive rats. *Eur J Pharmacol*, 660(2-3), (Jun 2011), pp. 381-386

Marti-Fabregas J., Gomis M., Arboix A., Aleu A., Pagonabarraga J., Belvis R., Cocho D., Roquer J., Rodriguez A., Garcia M.D., Molina-Porcel L., Diaz-Manera J., & Marti-Vilalta J.L. (2004). Favorable outcome of ischemic stroke in patients pretreated with statins. *Stroke*, 35(5), (May 2004), pp. 1117-1121

Meier N., Nedeltchev K., Brekenfeld C., Galimanis A., Fischer U., Findling O., Remonda L., Schroth G., Mattle H.P., & Arnold M. (2009). Prior statin use, intracranial hemorrhage, and outcome after intra-arterial thrombolysis for acute ischemic stroke. Stroke, 40(5), (May 2009), pp. 1729-1737

Mendez I., Hachinski V., & Wolfe B. (1987). Serum lipids after stroke. *Neurology*, 37(3), (Mar 1987), pp. 507-511

Miedema I., Uyttenboogaart M., Koopman K., DeKeyser J., & Luijckx G.J. (2010). Statin use and functional outcome after tissue plasminogen activator treatmeknt in acute ischaemic stroke. *Cerebrovasc Dis*, 29(3), (Feb 2010), pp. 263-267

Misirli H., Somay G., Ozbal N., & Yasar Erenoglu N. (2002). Relation of lipid and lipoprotein (a) to ischaemic stroke. *J Clin Neurosci*, 9(2), (Mar 2002), pp. 127-132

Montaner J., Chacon P., Krupinski J., Rubio F., Millan M., Molina C.A., Hereu P., Quintana M., & Alvarez-Sabin J. (2008). Simvastatin in the acute phase of ischemic stroke: a safety and efficacy pilot trial. *Eur J Neurol*, 15(1), (Jan 2008), pp. 82-90

Moonis M., Kane K., Schwiderski U, Sandage B.W., & Fisher M. (2005). HMG-CoA reductase inhibitors improve acute ischemic stroke outcome. *Stroke*, 36(6), (Jun 2005), pp. 1298-1300

Nakata S., Tsutsui M., Shimokawa H., Yamashita T., Tanimoto A., Tasaki H., Ozumi K., Sabani K., Morishita T., Suda O., Hirano H., Sasaguri Y., Nakashima Y., & Yanagihara N. (2007). Statin treatment upregulates vascular neuronal nitric oxide synthase through Akt/NF-kappa B pathway. *Arterioscler Thromb Vasc Biol*, 27(1), (Jan 2007), pp. 92-98

Nicholas J.S., Swearingen C.J., Thomas J.C., Rumboldt Z., Tummirello P., & Patel S.J. (2008). The effect of statin pretreatment on infarct volume in ischemic stroke. *Neuroepidemiology*, 31(1), (2008), pp. 48-56

Ni Chroinin D, Callaly E.L., Duggan J., Merwick A., Hannon N., Sheehan O, Marnane M., Horgan G., Williams E.B., Harris D., Kyne L., McCormack P.M., Moroney J., Grant T., Williams D., Daly L., & Kelly P.J. (2011). Association between acute statin therapy, survival, and improved functional outcome after ischemic stroke: the North Dublin Population Stroke Study. *Stroke*, 42(4), (Apr 20011), pp. 1021-1029

Nishiyama Y., Ueda M., Otsuka T., Katsura K., Abe A., Nagayama H., & Katayama Y. (2011). Statin treatment decreased serum asymmetric dimethylarginine (ADMA) levels in ischemic stroke patients. *J Atheroscler Thromb*, 18(2), (2011), pp. 131-137

Olsen T.S., Christensen R.H., Kammersgaard L.P., & Andersen K.K. (2007). Higher total serum cholesterol levels are associated with less severe strokes and lower all-cause mortality: ten-year follow-u of ischemic strokes in the Copenhagen Stroke Study. *Stroke*, 38(10), (Oct 2007), pp. 2646-2651

Pan S.L., Lien I.N., Chen T.H. (2010). Is higher serum total cholesterol level associated with better long-term functional outcomes after noncardioembolic ischemic stroke? *Arch Phys Med Rehabil*, 91(6), (Jun 2010), pp. 913-918

Prinz V., Laufs U., Gertz K., Kronenberg G., Balkaya M., Leithner C., Lindauer U., & Endres M. (2008). Intravenous rosuvastatin for acute stroke treatment: an animal study. *Stroke*, 39(2), (Feb 2008), pp. 433-438

Puccetti L., Acampa M., & Auteri A. (2007). Pharmacogenetics of statins therapy. *Recent Pat Cardiovasc Drug Discov*, 2(3), (Nov 2007), pp. 228-236

Ramirez-Moreno J.M., Casado-Naranjo I., Portilla J.C., Calle M.L., Tena D., Falcon A., & Serrano A. (2009). Serum cholesterol LDL and 90-day mortality in patients with intracerebral hemorrhage. *Stroke*, 40(5), (May 2009), pp. 1917-1920

Reeves M.J., Gargano J.W., Luo Z., Mullard A.J., Jacobs B.S., & Majid A.: Paul Coverdell National Stroke Registry Michigan Prototype Investigators. (2008). Effect of pretreatment with statins on ischemic stroke outcomes. *Stroke*, 39(6), (Jun 2008), pp. 1779-1785

Restrepo L., Bang O.Y., Ovbiagele B, Ali L., Kim D., Liebeskind D.S., Starkman S., Vinuela F., Duckwiler G.R., Jahan R., & Saver J.L. (2009). Impact of hyperlipidemia and statins on ischemic stroke outcomes after intra-arterial fibrinolysis and percutaneous mechanical embolectomy. *Cerebrovasc Dis*, 28(4), (2009), pp. 384-390

Ribo M., Montaner J., Molina C.A., Arenillas J.F., Santamarina E., Quintana M., & Alvarez-Sabin J. (2004). Admission fibrinlolytic profile is associated with symptomatic hemorrhagic transformation in stroke patients treated with tissue plasminogen activator. *Stroke*, 35(9), (Sep 2004), pp. 2123-2127

Rueckschloss U., Galle J., Holtz J., Zerkowski H.R., & Morawietz H. (2001). Induction of NAD(P)H oxidase by oxidized low-density lipoprotein in human endothelial cells: antioxidative potential of hydroxymethylglutaryl coenzyme A reductase inhibitor therapy. *Circulation*, 104(15), (Oct 2001), pp. 1767-1772

Russman A.N., Schultz L.R., Zaman I.F., Rehman M.F., Silver B., Mitsias P., & Nerenz D.R. (2009). A significant temporal and quantitative relationship exists between high-density lipoprotein levels and acute ischemic stroke presentation. *J Neurol Sci*, 279(1-2), (Apr 2009), pp. 53-56

Sacco R.L., Benson R.T., Kargman D.E., Boden-Albala B., Tuck C., Lin I.F., Cheng J.F., Paik M.C., Shea S., & Berglund L. (2001). High-density lipoprotein cholesterol and ischemic in the elderly: the Northern Manhattan Stroke Study. *JAMA*, 285(21), (Jun 2001), pp. 2729-2735

Sadowitz B., Maier K.G., & Gahtan V. (2010). Basic science review: Statin therapy-Part 1: the pleiotropic effects of statins in cardiovascular disease. *Vasc Endovascular Surg*, 44(4), (May 2010), pp. 241-251

Sadowitz B., Seymour K., Costanza M.J., & Gahtan V. (2010). Statin therapy-Part 2: Clinical considerations for cardiovascular disease. *Vasc Endovascular Surg*, 44(6), (Aug 2010), pp. 421-433

Seki Y., Takahashi H., Shibata A., & Aizawa Y. (1997). Plasma levels of thrombomodulin and lipoprotein (a) in patients with cerebral thrombosis. *Blood Coagul Fibrinolysis*, 8(7), (Oct 1997), pp. 391-396

Shie F.S., Neely M.D., Maezawa I., Wu H, Olson S.J., Jurgens G., Montine K.S., & Montine T.J. (2004). Oxidized low-density lipoprotein is present in astrocytes surrounding cerebral infarcts and stimulates astrocyte interleukin-6 secretion. *Am J Pathol*, 164(4), (Apr 2004), pp. 1173-1181

Sierra S., Ramos M.C., Molina P., Esteo C., Vazquez J.A., & Burgos J.S. (2011). Statins as neuroprotectants: a comparative in vitro study of lipophilicity, blood-brain-barrier penetration, lowering of brain cholesterol, and decrease of neuron cell death. *J Alzheimers Dis*, 23(2), (2011), pp. 307-318

Sillberg V.A., Wells G.A., & Perry J.J. (2008). Do statins improve outcomes and reduce the incidence of vasospasm after aneurysmal subarachnoid hemorrhage: a meta-analysis. *Stroke*, 39(9), (Sep 2008), pp. 2622-2626

Simundic A.M., Nikolac N., Topic E., Basic-Kes V., & Demarin V. (2008). Are serum lipids measured on stroke admission prognostic? *Clin Chem Lab Med*, 46(8), (2008), pp. 1163-1167

Sironi L., Cimino M., Guerrini U., Calvio A.M., Lodetti B., Asdente M., Balduini W., Paoletti R., & Tremoli E. (2003). Treatment with statins after induction of focal ischemia in rats reduces the extent of brain damage. *Arterioscler Thromb Vasc Biol*, 23(2), (Feb 2003), pp. 322-327

Stead L.G., Vaidyanathan L., Kumar G., Bellolio M.F., Brown R.D. Jr., Suravaram S, Enduri S., Gilmore R.M., & Decker W.W. (2009). Statins in ischemic stroke: just low-density lipoprotein lowering or more? J *Stroke Cerebrovasc Dis*, 18(2), (Mar-Apr 2009), pp. 124-127

Tepia-Perez H., Sanchez-Aguilar M., Torres-Corzo J.G., Rodriguez-Leyva I., Gonzalez-Aguirre D., Gordillo-Moscoso A., & Chalita-Williams C. (2009). Use of statins for the treatment of spontaneous intracerebral hemorrhage: results of a pilot study. *Cen Eur Neurosurg*, 70(1), (Feb 2009), pp. 15-20

Tseng M.Y., Czosnyka M., Richards H., Pickard J.D., & Kirkpatrick P.J. (2005). Effects of acute treatment with pravastatin on cerebral vasospasm, autoregulation, and a delayed ischemic deficits after aneurysmal subarachnoid hemorrhage: a phase II randomized placebo-controlled trial. *Stroke*, 36(6), (Aug 2005), pp. 1627-1632

Uno M., Kitazato K.T., Nishi K., Itabe H., & Nagahiro S. (2003). Raised plasma oxidised LDL in acute cerebral infarction. *J Neurol Neurosurg Psychiatry*, 74(3), (Mar 2003), pp. 312-316

Uno M., Harada M., Takimoto O., Kitazato K.T., Suzue A., Yoneda K., Morita N., Itabe H., & Nagahiro S. (2005). Elevation of plasma oxidized LDL in acute stroke patients is associated with ischemic lesions depicted by DWI and predictive of infarct enlargement. *Neurol Res*, 27(1), (Jan 2005), pp. 94-102

Uyttenboogaart M, Koch M.W., Koopman K., Vroomen P.C., Luijckx G.J., DeKeyser J. (2008). Lipid profile, statin use, and outcome after intravenous thrombolysis for acute ischaemic stroke. J *Neurol*, 255(6), (Jun 2008), pp. 875-880 van Kooten F., van Krimpen J., Dippel D.W., Hoogerbrugge N., & Koudstaal P.J. (1996). Lipoprotein(a) in patients with acute cerebral ischemia. *Stroke*, 27(7), (Jul 1996), pp. 1231-1235

Vauthey C., de Freitas G.R., van Melle G., Devuyst G., Bogousslavsky J. (2000). Better outcome after stroke with higher serum cholesterol levels. *Neurology*, 54(10), (May 2000), pp. 1944-1949

Vergouwen M.D., Meijers J.C., Geskus R.B., Coert B.A., Horn J., Stroes E.S., van der Poll T., Vermeulen M., & Roos Y.B. (2009). Biologic effects of simvastatin in patients with aneurysmal subarachnoid hemorrhage: a double-blind, placebo-controlled randomized trial. *J Cereb Blood Flow Metab*, 28(8), (Aug 2009), pp. 1444-1453

von Budingen H.C., Baumgartner R.W., Baumann C.R., Rousson V., Siegel A.M., & Georgiadis DK. (2008). Serum cholesterol levels do not influence outcome or recovery in acute ischemic stroke. *Neurol Res*, 30(1), (Feb 2008), pp. 82-84

Welch K.M. (2009). Review of the SPARCL trial and its subanalysis. *Curr Atheroscler Rep*, 11(4), (Jul 2009), pp. 315-321

Woo J., Lam C.W., Kay R., Wong H.Y., Teoh R., & Nicholls M.G. (1990). Acute and long-term changes in serum lipids after acute stroke. *Stroke*, 21(10), (Oct 1990), pp. 1407-1411

Yingdong Z. & Xiuling L. (1999). Apolipoprotein (a) and cortical cerebral infarction. *Chin Med Sci J*, 14(4), (Dec 1999), pp. 249-254

Xu G., Fitzgerald M.E., Wen Z., Fain S.B., Alsop D.C., Carroll T., Ries M.L., Rowley H.A., Sager M.A., Asthana S., Johnson S.C., & Carlsson C.M. (2008). Atorvastatin therapy is associated with greater and faster cerebral hemodynamic response. *Brain Imaging Behav*, 2(2), (Jun 2008), pp. 94

Yagi S., Akaike M., Aihara K., Ishikawa K., Iwase T., Ikeda Y., Soeki T., Yoshida S., Sumitomo-Ueda Y., Matsumoto T., & Sata M. (2010). Endothelial nitric oxide synthase-independent protective action of statin against angiotensin II-induced atrial remodeling via reduced oxidant injury. *Hypertension*, 55(4), (Apr 2010), pp. 918-923

Ye Y., Martinez J.D., Perez-Polo R.J., Lin Y., Uretsky B.F., & Birnbaum Y. (2008). The role of eNOS, iNOS, and NF-kappaB in upregulation and activation of cyclooxygenase-2 and infarct size reduction by atorvastatin. *Am J Physiol Heart Circ Physiol*, 295(1), (Jul 2008), H343-351.

Yoon S.S., Dambrosia J., Chalela J., Ezzeddine M., Warach S., Haymore J., Davis L., & Baird A.E. (2004). Rising statin use and effect on ischemic stroke outcome. *BMC Med*, 2, (Mar 2004), pp. 4

Yrjanheikki J., Koistinaho J., Kettunen M., Kauppinen R.A., Appel K., Hull M., & Fiebich B.L. (2005). Long-term protective effect of atorvastatin in permanent focal cerebral ischemia. *Brain Res*, 1052(2), (Aug 2005), pp. 174-179

Endovascular Management of Acute Ischemic Stroke

Stavropoula I. Tjoumakaris,
Pascal M. Jabbour, Aaron S. Dumont,
L. Fernando Gonzalez and Robert H. Rosenwasser
Thomas Jefferson University, Philadelphia, USA

1. Introduction

Stroke is a major cause of serious, long-term disability and the third leading cause of death in the United States[1]. According to the World Health Organization, 15 million people suffer a stroke worldwide annually. Of those, one third do not survive and another third is left with a significant neurological deficit. The majority of these events are ischemic (87%), as opposed to intracerebral (10%) and subarachnoid hemorrhages (3%)[1]. Management of acute ischemic stroke was previously geared toward prevention, supportive care, and rehabilitation. Over the past few decades, however, the medical management of stroke has progressed exponentially, beginning with the US Food and Drug Administration (FDA) approval of tissue plasminogen activator (r-TPA, alteplase) in 1996. Intravenous administration of r-TPA within a limited 3-hour window from symptom onset has shown a significant improvement in patient outcome at 3 months and at one year following an acute cerebrovascular event.[2] Current stroke guidelines have extended the therapeutic r-TPA administration window to 4.5 hours.

The intra-arterial (IA) injection of therapeutic agents was first published nearly 60 years ago, when Sussman and Fitch described the IA treatment of acute carotid occlusion with fibrinolysin injection in 1958.[3] It was not until the late 1990's that the endovascular management of acute stroke experienced exponential progress and development. Recent advances in endovascular techniques have increased the therapeutic window of r-TPA administration and introduced new agents such as reteplase and abciximab. Furthermore, the use of IA devices for clot retrieval and vessel recanalization has revolutionized the neuroendovascular management of acute ischemic stroke.

2. Patient selection

The goal of endovascular management of acute ischemic stroke is to enhance the survival of local ischemic brain tissue (penumbra) and limit the extent of infarcted brain parenchyma. An initial evaluation with a non-contrast computerized tomography (CT) head scan is necessary. In a retrospective review of 85 patients from the Penumbra Pivotal

Stroke Trial, Goyal and colleagues found that a baseline CT scan by ASPECTS score>7 (Alberta Stroke Program Early CT Scale) had a 50% chance of a favorable clinical outcome with early recanalization ($p=0.0001$). In addition, ASPECTS scores of less than 4 did not show clinical improvement regardless of endovascular recanalization[4]. Patients with large territorial infarcts on CT scan are at a higher risk for hemorrhagic conversion following treatment and are therefore poor candidates for endovascular therapy.[5] In addition, the presence of an intra-parenchymal hematoma is a contraindication to endovascular recanalization. Lastly, the presence of a hyperdense MCA sign on the initial head CT does not have a significant prognostic value in patient outcome and vessel recanalization rates.[6-8]
Over the past decade, the clinical application of CT perfusion scans has facilitated the pre-treatment evaluation of "salvageable" tissue. A scan consistent with a mismatch between cerebral blood volume (CBV, "core" cerebral lesion volume) and cerebral blood flow or mean transient time (CBF or MTT, "penumbra" lesion volume) is a favorable patient selection criterion.[9] In our institution, a favorable CT perfusion scan may overcome the six-hour post-symptom onset time restriction.
Although patient age and initial National Institutes of Health Stroke Scale score (NIHSS) do not show statistically significant correlation with post-treatment intracranial hemorrhage (ICH), careful attention should be paid to both.[5] In a recent retrospective review of 156 patients, Zacharatos and colleagues found that thrombolytic therapy (chemical or mechanical) showed a favorable clinical outcome versus supportive management in the 80 years and older age group[10]. However, patient co-morbidities are evaluated prior to treatment. Specifically, the presence of hyperglycemia, defined as blood sugar levels greater than 200mg/dl within 24 hours from presentation, can significantly increase the likelihood of post-thrombolysis hemorrhagic conversion.[5]
Previous administration of intravenous tPA is not a contraindication to IA intervention. However, the hemorrhagic complications in these patients are significantly higher, especially if urokinase was the arterial agent.[5] One must therefore clearly explain the risks and benefits of the procedure to the family and include them in the decision making process. Overall, endovascular intervention is an invaluable tool in the management of acute ischemic stroke. However, the duration of ischemia and the presence of viable ischemic tissue in excess of irreversibly damaged tissue are both critical factors in the successful management of acute stroke.

3. Angiographic evaluation

Initial angiographic evaluation of the patient's vasculature is of paramount importance for the establishment of the ischemic etiology and initiation of treatment. Thus far, the use of general anesthesia is preferred due to motion elimination contributing to procedural safety and efficacy[11]. However, newer studies suggest that conscious sedation or local anesthesia may lead to more favorable radiographic and clinical outcomes by decreasing time delay and cerebral ischemia from hypoperfusion[11-13]. Femoral access is established in the symptomatic lower extremity, if no vascular contraindications exist. A thorough examination of the cerebrovascular anatomy begins with the aortic arch. The brachiocephalic vessels are visualized and any proximal stenosis, irregularities or occlusion noted. Proximal vessel disease may require immediate treatment with balloon angioplasty and/or stenting to allow access to the intracranial pathology or may itself be the cause of the acute ischemic event.

Based on the patient symptomatology and pre-procedure imaging, selective catheterization of the carotid or vertebrobasilar circulation supplying the affected territory is performed. Attention is paid to the extracranial collateral circulation, the leptomeningeal anatomy, the circle of Willis, and overall global cerebral perfusion. Recent data showed that the grade of angiographic collaterals is a decisive factor for the degree of reperfusion and clinical improvement following endovascular intervention in acute ischemic stroke[14].

The modality of treatment (for example IA thrombolysis, balloon angioplasty, stenting, clot retrieval mechanisms) is tailored to each individual case. At times, advanced age or significant atherosclerotic disease may limit treatment options.

4. Intra-arterial chemical thrombolysis

Over the past decade, several agents have been investigated for IA thrombolysis with variable dosages and administration routes. Overall, these drugs act by activating plasminogen to plasmin, which in turn degrades fibrin and its associated derivatives. Although studies targeting direct comparisons of the different agents have not yet been published, fibrin-specific agents, such as recombinant tissue plasminogen activator (r-tPA) and recombinant pro-urokinase (rpro-UK) have been widely studied and used most frequently.[15]

First-generation agents, such as streptokinase and urokinase, are non-fibrin selective and could therefore have greater systemic complications.[16] Streptokinase, a protein derivative from group C beta-hemolytic streptococci, has a half-life of 16-90 minutes. It has an increased association with intracranial and systemic hemorrhages, and was therefore removed from the chemical armamentarium for the management of acute ischemic stroke.[17] Urokinase, a serine protease, has a half-life of 14 minutes and dosage range of 0.02-2 million units.[18]

Second-generation agents have a higher fibrin-specificity and are most commonly studied in IA stroke management studies. Alteplase (r-tPA), also a serine protease, has a half-life of 3.5 minutes and a dosage range of 20-60 mg.[18] The precursor of urokinase (rpro-UK) has a half-life of 7 minutes and may be favorable to r-tPA due to decreased side effects. Kaur and colleagues published potential neurotoxic properties of alteplase, such as activation of NMDA receptor in the neuronal cell-death pathway, amplification of calcium conductance, and activation of extracellular matrix metalloproteinases.[19] These effects may facilitate exacerbation of cerebral edema, disturbance of the blood brain barrier, and development of ICH.

Third-generation agents, such as reteplase and tenecteplase, have longer half-lives (15-18 minutes) and theoretically favorable vessel recanalization and local recurrence rates.[16] Newer -generation agents are genetically engineered, such as Desmoteplase and Microplasmin (Thrombogenics, Heverlee, Belgium).

Besides their fibrinolytic properties, the aforementioned agents have prothrombotic effects by the production of thrombin during thrombolysis, and subsequent activation of platelets and fibrinogen.[16] As a result, concomitant use of systemic anticoagulation during IA thrombolysis is recommended with caution to risk of ICH. The most widely used adjuvant systemic agent is heparin. Newer generation agents under the category of glycoprotein (GP) IIIb/IIa antagonist, such as Reopro (abciximab) and Integrilin (eptifibatide) are currently under investigation. Memon and colleagues reviewed 35 cases of adjunctive use of eptifibatide in salvage reocclusion and thrombolysis of distal thrombi with a single bolus of 180μg/kg. They reported a partial to complete recanalization of 77%. However, incidence of post-operative hemorrhage was 37% and symptomatic in 14% of patients[20].

4.1 Anterior circulation

4.1.1 Middle cerebral artery

Three major clinical trials evaluated the efficacy of IA thrombolysis in the Middle Cerebral Artery (MCA) circulation, specifically the PROACT I and II (Prolyse in Acute Cerebral Thromboembolism), and MELT trials (Middle Cerebral Artery Local Fibrinolytic Intervention Trial). Although IA thrombolysis shows a favorable outcome in the setting of acute ischemic injury, FDA approval has thus far been granted for its intravenous counterpart alone.[21]

In 1998, del Zoppo and colleagues presented a phase II clinical trial investigating the safety and efficacy of IA delivery of recombinant-pro-urokinase (rpro-UK) in acute MCA stroke, PROACT I.[22] Following the exclusion of intracranial hemorrhage with a non-contrast head CT, 40 patients were randomized for treatment of acute ischemic stroke within 6 hours of symptom onset. Cerebral angiography was performed, and M1 or M2 occlusions were treated with 6 mg of rpro-UK (n=26) or placebo (n=14). All patients received a concomitant heparin bolus followed by a 4-hour infusion. The final endpoints were recanalization efficacy at the end of the infusion period and neurological deterioration from intracranial hemorrhage (ICH) within 24 hours of treatment. Rpro-UK treated patients had higher vessel recanalization rates compared to placebo (57.7% versus 14.3%). Furthermore, the incidence of ICH was higher in the rpro-UK group (15.4% versus 7.1%). Overall, PROACT I was the first organized trial proving the safety and efficacy of IA thrombolysis for the management of acute ischemic stroke.

PROACT II was a subsequent phase III clinical trial that studied the safety and efficacy of rpro-UK in a larger patient population (n=180).[23] This randomized, controlled clinical trial treated patients with MCA occlusion within 6 hours of symptom onset with either 9 mg of IA rpro-UK and heparin infusion (n=121) or heparin infusion alone (n-59). The study's primary endpoint was the 90-day patient neurological disability based on the modified Rankin score scale. Secondary outcomes included mortality, vessel recanalization, and neurological deterioration from the development of ICH. Patients who received IA rpro-UK had significantly lower Rankin scores at the 90-day endpoint compared to heparin only treated patients. Furthermore, the MCA racanalization and mortality rates favored the rpro-UK group as opposed to the control group (66% versus 18%). Albeit a higher incidence of ICH in the rpro-UK group (10% as opposed to 2% in the control group), the PROACT II multicenter trial demonstrated that the use of IA chemical thrombolysis in acute ischemia of the anterior circulation leads to radiographic and clinical improvement.

Recently, the MELT Japanese study group investigated the IA administration of UK in the setting of MCA stroke within 6 hours of onset.[24] Although the study showed favorable 90-day functional outcome in the UK-treated patients with respect to controls, results did not reach statistical significance. Unfortunately, the investigation was aborted prematurely following the approval of intravenous r-TPA in Japan for the treatment of acute ischemic stroke.

The optimal window for IA thrombolysis in the anterior circulation has been investigated in multiple clinical trials. Overall, results show that IA treatment of acute MCA infarction outweighs potential hemorrhagic risks when implemented within a 6-hour window from symptom onset.[15] Theron et al investigated the efficacy of IA thrombolysis in patients with acute internal carotid artery (ICA) occlusion as it related to the timing of treatment and angiographic location.[25] Based on his work, IA fibrinolysis of the MCA should be performed within 6 hours from ischemia onset, when the occlusion involves the horizontal segment of the MCA extending into the lenticulostriate arteries. Treatment complications, mainly hemorrhagic incidence, increase significantly beyond this optimal time-frame. However, if the occlusion does not involve the horizontal MCA segment and the lenticulostriate arteries, then the treatment window can be extended to 12 hours following symptoms.[15] The paucity of collateral circulation in the lenticulostriate arteries, as well as their distal distribution, both contribute to their sensitivity to ischemia in the setting of acute stroke. When initiating endovascular intra-arterial thrombolysis, the operator should account for time required to perform the procedure. Considering that the average intervention time varies from 45 to 180 minutes, high-risk patients should be treated within 4-5 hours from ischemia onset.[26-28]

4.1.2 Internal carotid artery

Occlusions of the proximal ICA (extra-cranial) generally have a better prognosis than intracranial occlusions. The presence of external-internal carotid collateral flow and the anastomosis at the circle of Willis account for this observation. Patients with insufficient extracranial-intracranial anastomoses or an incomplete circle of Willis may be predisposed to developing significant neurological symptoms. These patients are potential candidates for IA intervention. In these cases, mechanical thrombolysis, in addition to pharmacological thrombolysis, is of paramount importance for recanalization. In a 25-patient series, Jovin and colleagues demonstrated successful revascularization in 92 % of patients following thrombolysis and ICA stenting.[29]

Intracranial ICA acute occlusions have a dismal natural history and overall prognosis. Negative prognostic factors include distal ICA distribution involving the M1 and A1 segments ("T" occlusion) and poor neurological presentation. Furthermore, as observed by Bhatia et al, recanalization following IV r-tPA in patients with T occlusion is the lowest at 4.4%[30]. Arnold and colleagues presented a series of 24 patients with distal ICA occlusions treated with IA urokinase. Favorable 3-month functional outcome was present in only 16% of patients, and the mortality rate was approximately 42%.[31] Adjuvant mechanical assistance with devices for balloon angioplasty, clot retrieval, and vessel stenting enhance the probability of vessel recanalization (Fig. 1). Flint et al published a series of 80 patients with ICA occlusion who were treated with combinations of the Merci retriever (Concentric Medical, Mountain View, California) with or without adjunctive endovascular therapy. Recanalization rates were higher in the combination group (63%) as opposed to the Merci group (53%). At a 3-month follow-up, 25% of patients had a good neurological outcome, with their age being a positive predictive indicator.[32] Overall, these results are encouraging, and IA intervention in select cases of acute ICA occlusion should be considered.

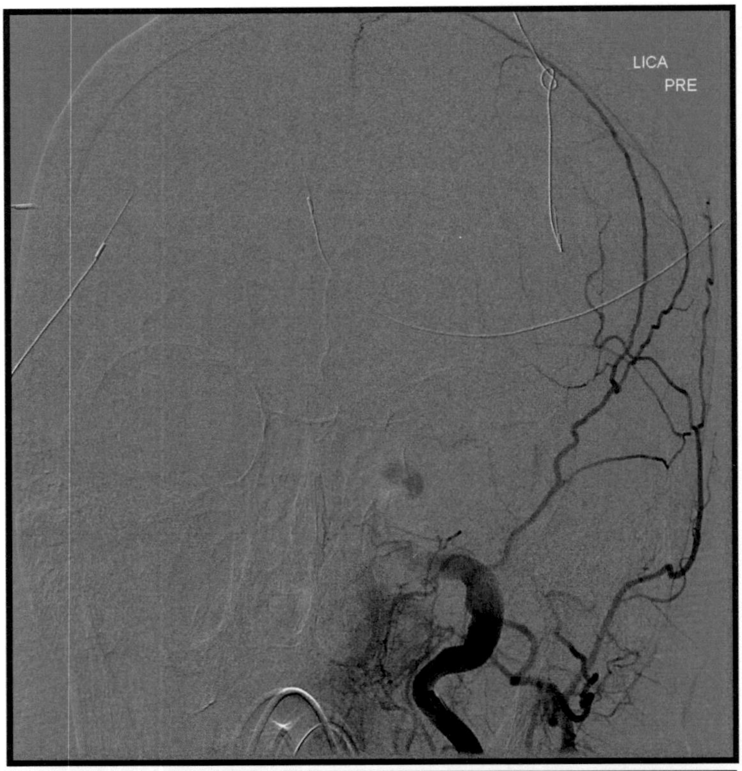

1.A.

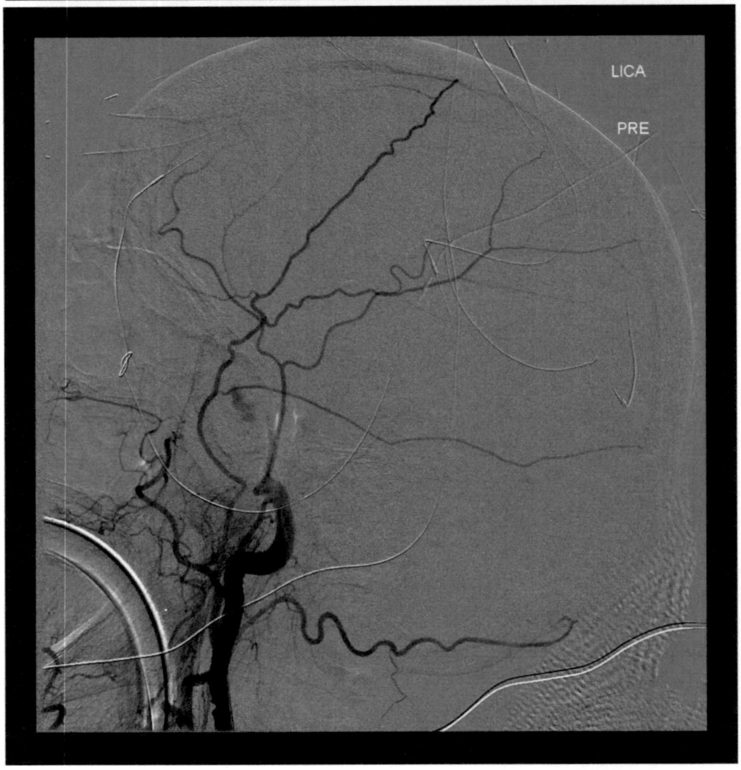

1.B.

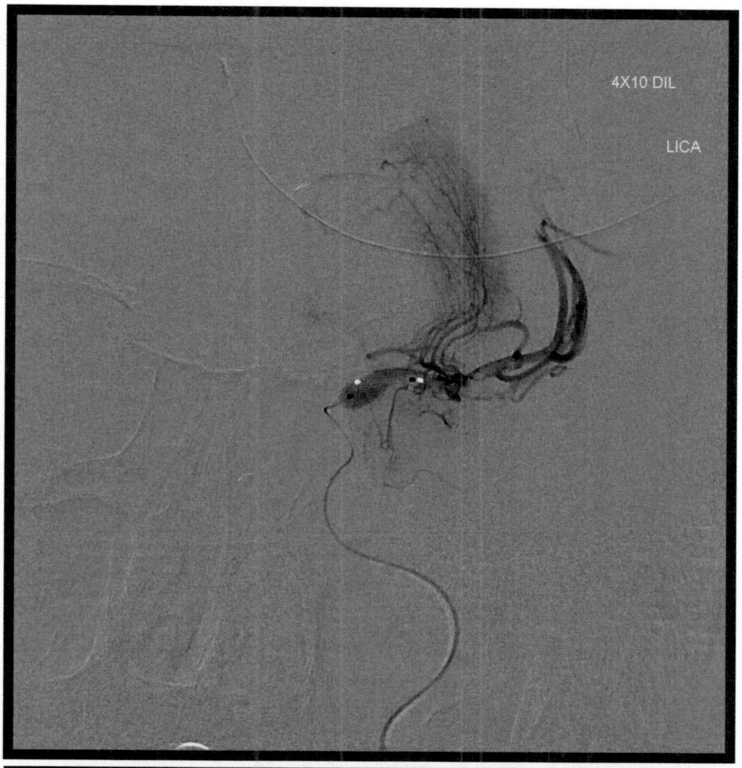
4X10 DIL
LICA

1.C.

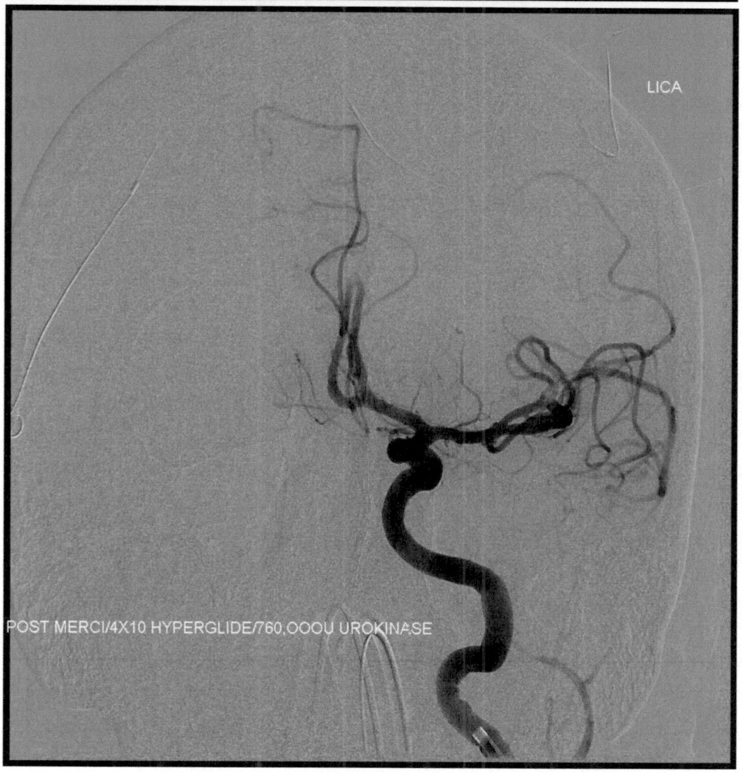
LICA
POST MERCI/4X10 HYPERGLIDE/760,OOOU UROKINASE

1.D.

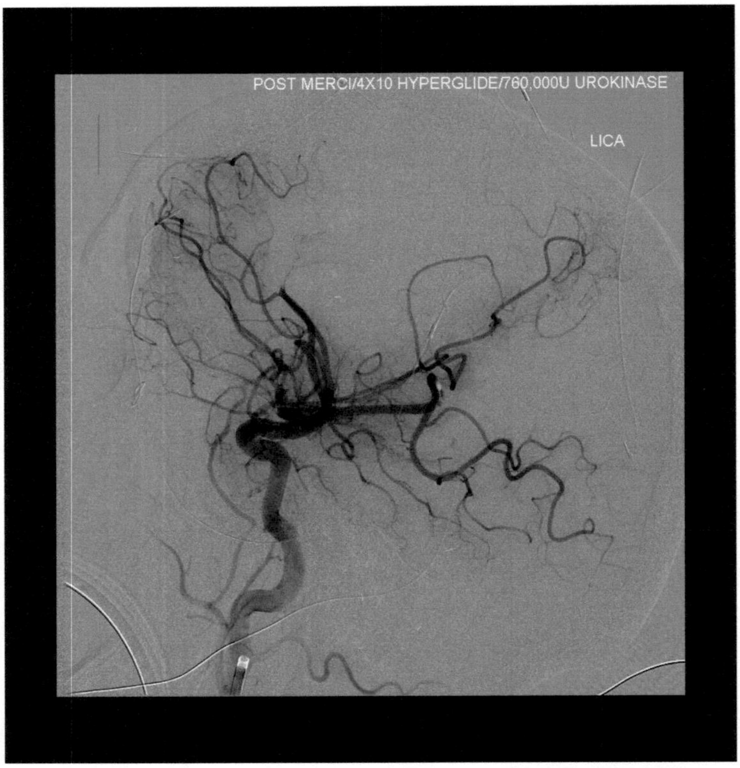

1.E.

Fig. 1. **A-E.** Acute left ICA occlusion. The patient presented 6 hours following onset of global aphasia and R hemiplegia. **A-B.** Mid-arterial digital subtraction angiogram of left ICA artery showing complete occlusion of the distal ICA (T occlusion), frontal and lateral views.
C. Frontal view of balloon angioplasty and recanalization of the distal left ICA.
D-E. Frontal and lateral views of left ICA angiograms following mechanical and chemical recanalization with balloon angioplasty, Merci device, and administration of of Urokinase.

4.1.3 Central retinal artery

Occlusion of the Central Retinal Artery (CRA) is an ophthalmologic emergency with a natural history that leads to loss of vision. Conventional medical therapy includes ocular massage, carbohydrate inhibitors, inhalation of carbogen mixture, paracentesis, topical beta-blockers, aspirin, and intravenous heparin.[15] However, the limited efficacy of all these therapies made acute CRA occlusion a potential candidate for endovascular management.
Several studies have documented successful vessel recanalization with visual improvement compared to controls. In most studies, IA alteplase is most commonly used within 4-6 hours from symptom onset. The agent is infused via supraselective catheterization of the ophthalmic artery. Padolecchia and colleagues showed that intervention within 4.5 hours of ischemic onset leads to visual improvement in all patients.[33] Studies performed by Arnold, Aldrich, Noble and their colleagues showed visual improvement in a significant amount of patients treated with IA thrombolysis that ranged from 22% to 93% compared to much lower conventionally-treated controls [34-36]. The IA agent was r-tPA or urokinase and the treatment time varied from 6 to 15 hours from symptom onset. Ischemic and hemorrhagic complications were either not present (Arnold, Aldrich) or occurred at significantly low rates (Noble).

4.2 Posterior circulation

Acute basilar artery (BA) occlusion is a life-threatening event that poses a significant therapeutic challenge. The natural progression of untreated BA occlusion has mortality rates ranging from 86% to 100%.[15] The rare incidence of this disease, less than 10% of acute ischemic strokes, could account for the lack of significant randomized controlled studies in the topic. Several meta-analyses of case reports and case series reflect the severity of the disease. In a series of nearly 300 patients, Furlan and Higashida reported an IA recanalization rate of 60%, and mortality rates of 31% in at least partially recanalized patients as opposed to 90% in non-recanalized patients.[37] Lindsberg and Mattle compared BA occlusion treatment with IV or IA thrombolysis. They found that although recanalization rates were higher with IA treatement (65% versus 53%), dependency or death rates were equal between the two groups (76-78%). Overall, 22% of treated patients had good outcomes, as opposed to only 2% of untreated individuals. Therefore, emergent thrombolysis via either technique is of paramount importance to the survival of this patient population.

The timing of treatment initiation in relation to symptom onset is a controversial topic. Theoretically, the same treatment restrictions apply as in the anterior circulation, however, in practice, the therapeutic window can be successfully extended beyond 6 hours. In our institution, we have achieved favorable clinical outcomes in patients treated up to 12 hours from symptom onset. Between 12 and 18 hours, incidence of hemorrhagic conversion is more significant, and treatment is rarely extended beyond the 24-hour window. In the Basilar Artery International Cooperation Study (BASICS), 624 patients with radiographically confirmed occlusion of the BA were enrolled in nearly 50 centers over a 5-year period.[38] All patients (n=41) treated with IA or IV thrombolytics beyond 9 hours from symptom onset had a poor reported outcome.

2.A. 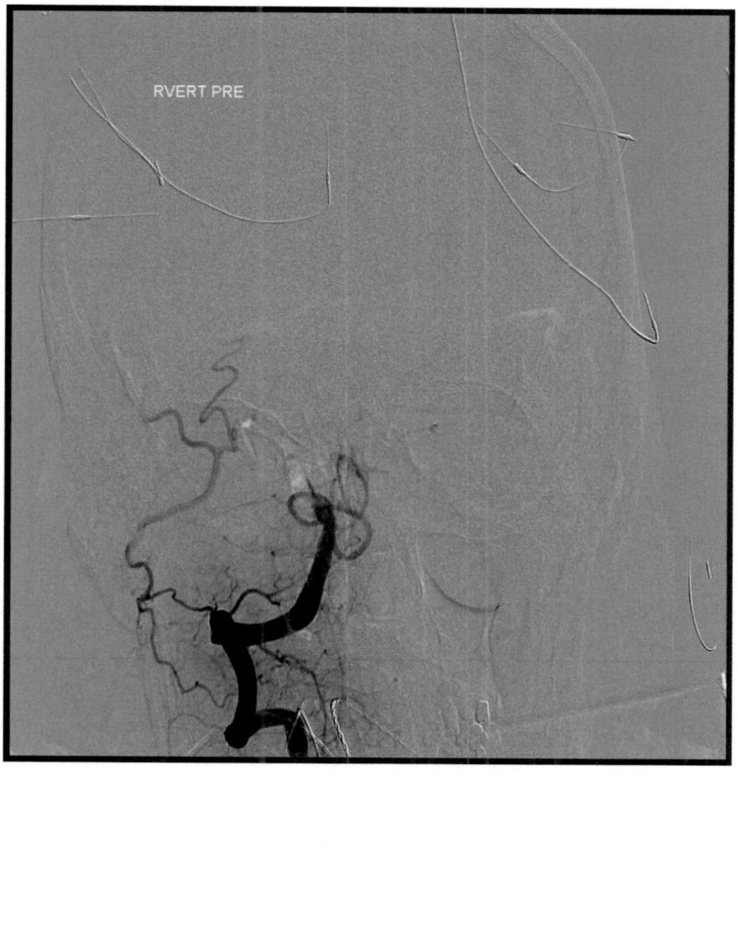

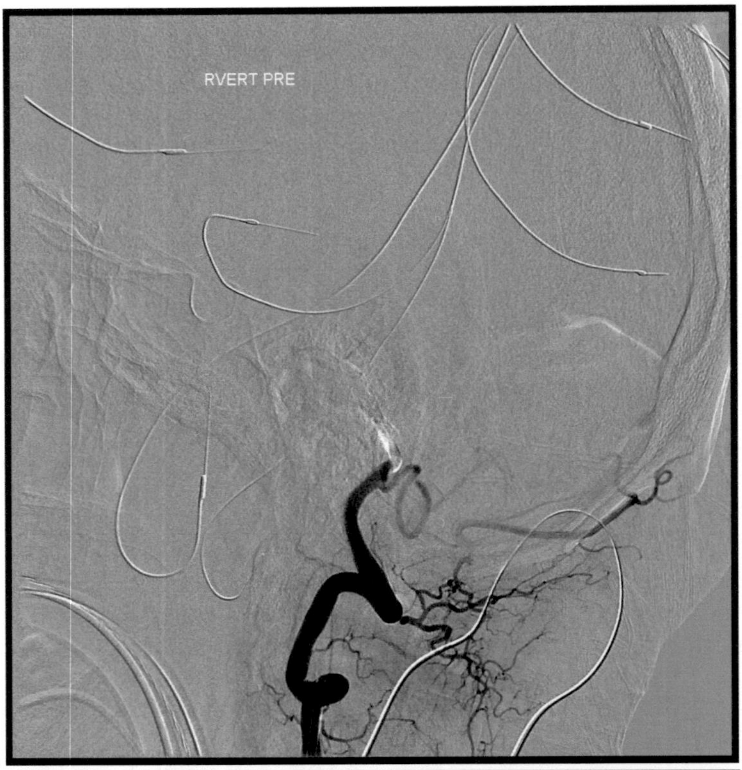

2.B.

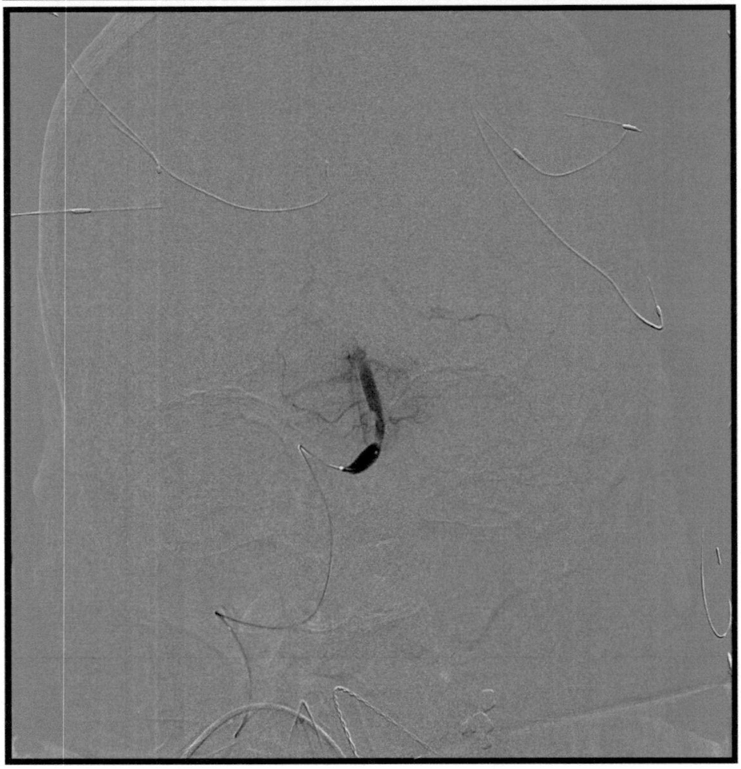

2.C.

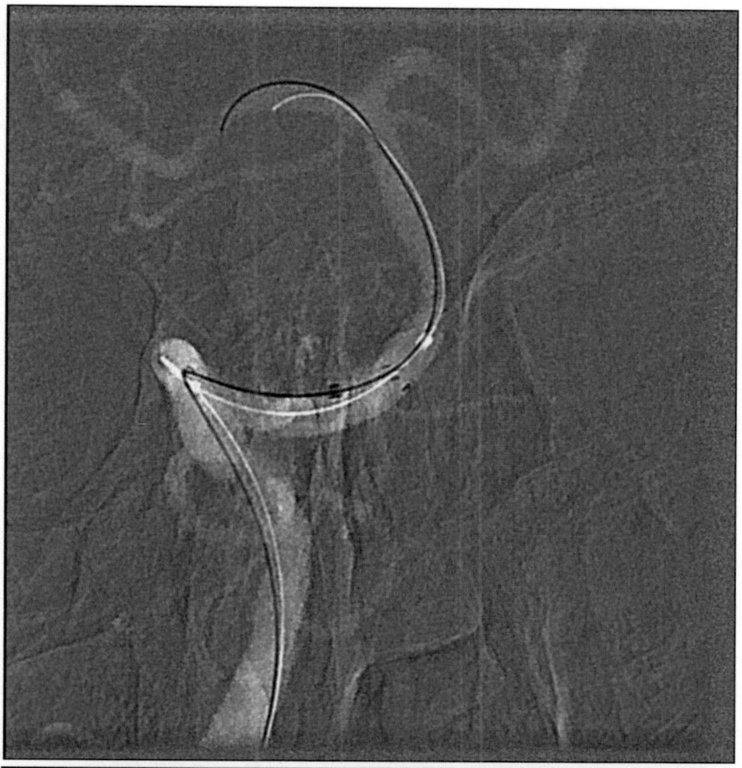

2.D.

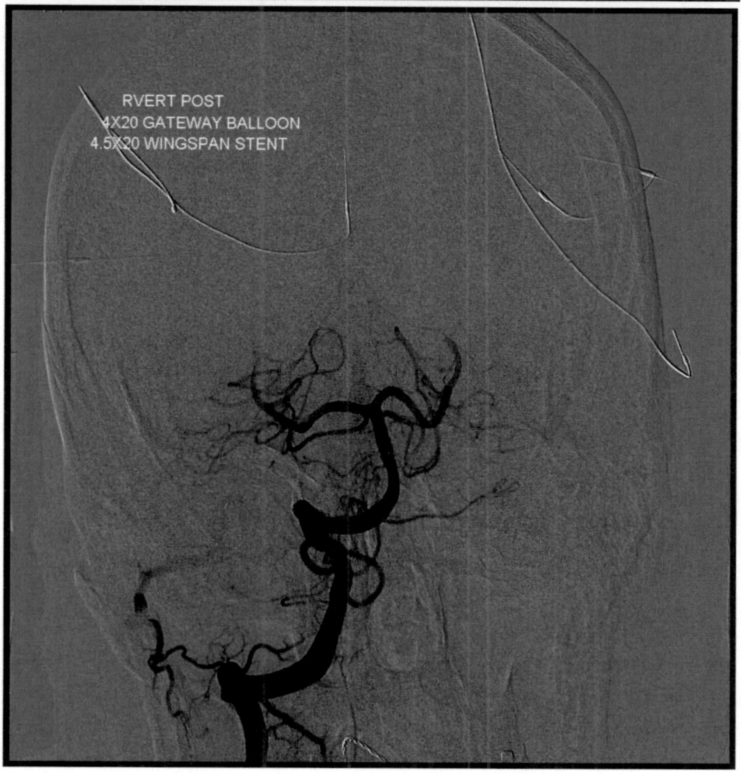

2.E.

2.F.

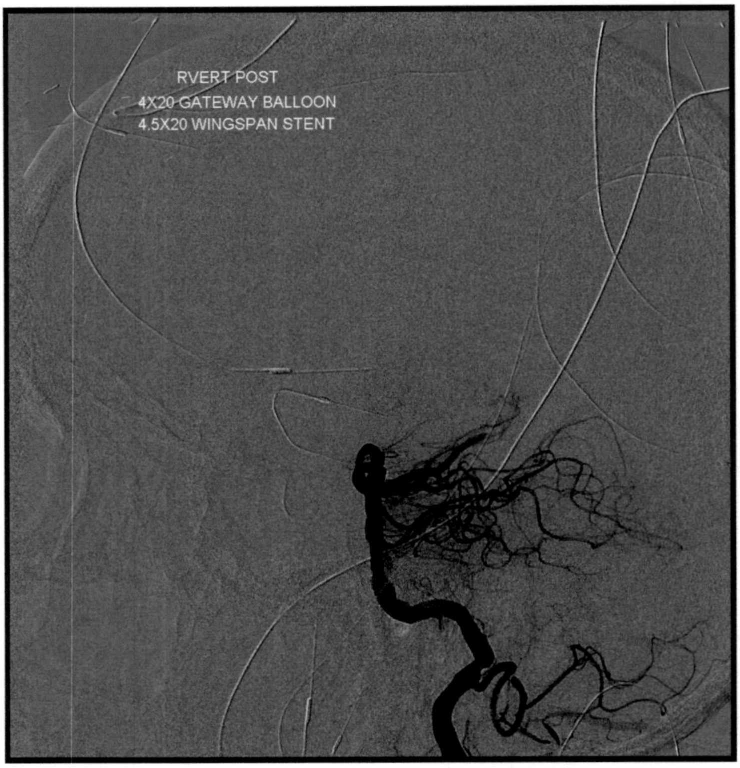

Fig. 2. **A-F.** Acute right vertebro-basilar occlusion. **A-B.** Mid-arterial digital subtraction angiogram of the right vertebral artery (dominant) showing complete occlusion with no distal filling of the basilar artery, frontal and lateral views. **C.** Frontal view of balloon angioplasty of the right vertebro-basilar junction. **D.** Road map during deployment of Wingspan stent at the vertebro-basilar level. **E-F.** Frontal and lateral views of right vertebral artery mid-arterial angiograms depicting vessel recanalization following mechanical thrombolysis.

Recent advances in mechanical and pharmacological approaches to endovascular therapies may increase BA recanalization rates and improve patient outcome (Fig. 2). In a meta-analysis of 164 patients with BA occlusion over a 10-year period, Levy et al reported several predictive factors in treatment consideration.[39] Factors with a negative prognostic value were coma at initial presentation, failure of vessel recanalization, and proximal vessel occlusion. Distal BA occlusions are more commonly embolic in nature and therefore have a better response to thrombolytic agents.

5. Intra-arterial mechanical thrombolysis

The use of mechanical endovascular devices for thrombolysis is emerging as a powerful adjuvant, or even an alternative to chemical thrombolysis. In their multi-center review, Gupta and colleagues have demonstrated that multimodality approach with chemical and mechanical thrombolysis leads to higher recanalization rates[40]. The mechanical disruption of the arterial clot has several advantages to IA management of acute stroke.[16] First, it increases the working surface area for thrombolytic agents thereby enhancing their efficacy. Even partial removal of clot via retrieval or thromboaspiration techniques lessens the concentration of IA agent required to dissolve the remainder pieces. As a result, the risk of ICH is further decreased and the treatment window could be extended beyond the 6-hour limit. Mechanical thrombolysis provides patients with contraindications to anticoagulation with a reasonable alternative to endovascular therapy.

The use of mechanical thrombolysis is associated with several associated risks. The endovascular trauma to the blood vessel could cause endothelial damage, permanent vascular injury, and ultimately vessel rupture, especially in old friable vessels. The technical skills needed for the endovascular navigation of such devices, especially through severely occluded segments, are substantial, and require rigorous training. Finally, the dislodged clot material could become an embolic source, exposing the already compromised distal circulation to additional ischemic risks.

Overall, the multiple advantages of mechanical endovascular devices have revolutionized current therapies of acute ischemic stroke, and are safe adjuvant and/or alternatives to chemical thrombolysis in experienced hands. The conceptual basis of such devices can be broadly categorized into the following categories: thrombectomy, thromboaspiration, thrombus disruption, augmented fibrinolysis, and thrombus entrapment.[16]

5.1 Endovascular thrombectomy

Devices under this category apply a constant force to the clot material at its proximal or distal end and facilitate clot removal. Proximal end forces are applied through grasp-like attachments, whereas distal end forces are applied via basket-like devices. The advantage of these devices is their decreased association with embolic material since there is no attempt for mechanical clot disruption. Some of the most widely used examples are the Merci retriever (Concentric Medical, Mountain View, California), the Neuronet device (Guidant, Santa Clara, California), the Phenox clot retriever (Phenox, Bochum, Germany), the Catch thrombectomy device (Balt Extrusion, Montmorency, France), and the Alligator retrieval device (Chestnut Medical Technologies, Menlo Park, California).[16] The Merci device became FDA-approved in 2004 for the endovascular clot retrieval in acute ischemic stroke.[41] It is a flexible nitinol wire with coil loops that incorporate into the clot and facilitate retrieval. Recent analysis of the Mechanical Embolus Removal in Cerebral Ischemia (MERCI) and Multi Merci trials showed that patients with M2 occlusions had higher recanalization rates, decreased procedure duration and similar complication rates with M1 occlusion patients[42]. In a recent study that investigated the efficacy of current thrombectomy mechanisms, the Merci, Phenox, and Catch devices presented equal results with clot mobilization and retrieval.[43]

5.2 Endovascular thromboaspiration

The functioning mechanism in this category utilizes an aspiration technique, which is suited for fresh non-adhesive clots. These devices also have the advantage of fewer embolic material and decreased vasospasm. Some examples in this category are the Penumbra system (Penumbra, Alameda, California) and the AngioJet system (Possis Medical, Minneapolis, Minnesota).[16] The Penumbra system includes a reperfusion catheter that aspirates the clot and a ring-shaped retriever (Fig. 3). The favorable results of a prospective multi-center trial conducted in the United States and Europe led to the approval of the device by the FDA for the endovascular treatment of acute ischemic stroke in 2008.[44] The AngioJet system uses a high-pressure saline jet for clot agitation and an aspiration catheter for retrieval. Technical difficulties with endovascular navigation resulting in vessel injury led to the premature discontinuation of its trial in acute ischemic stroke patients.[45]

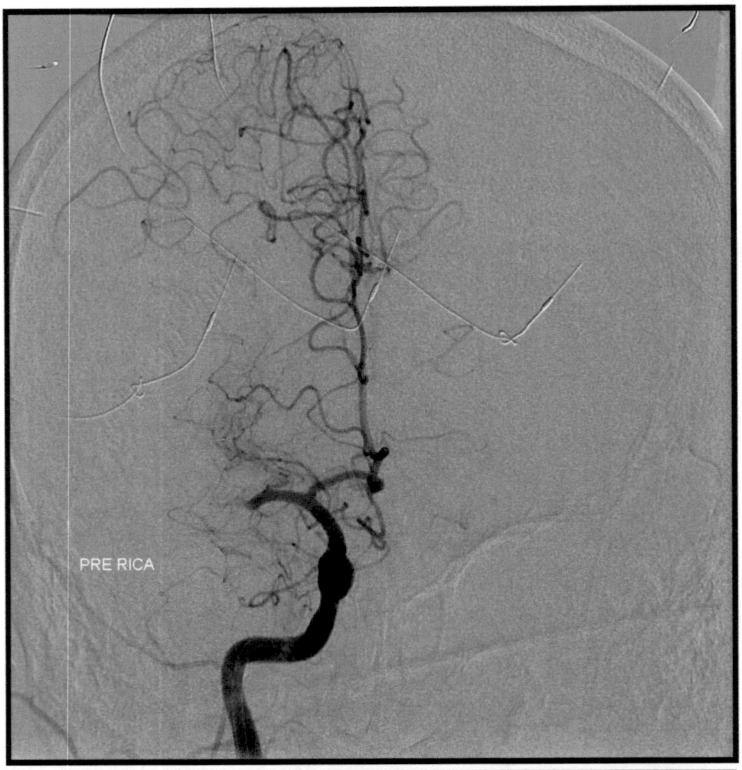

3.A.

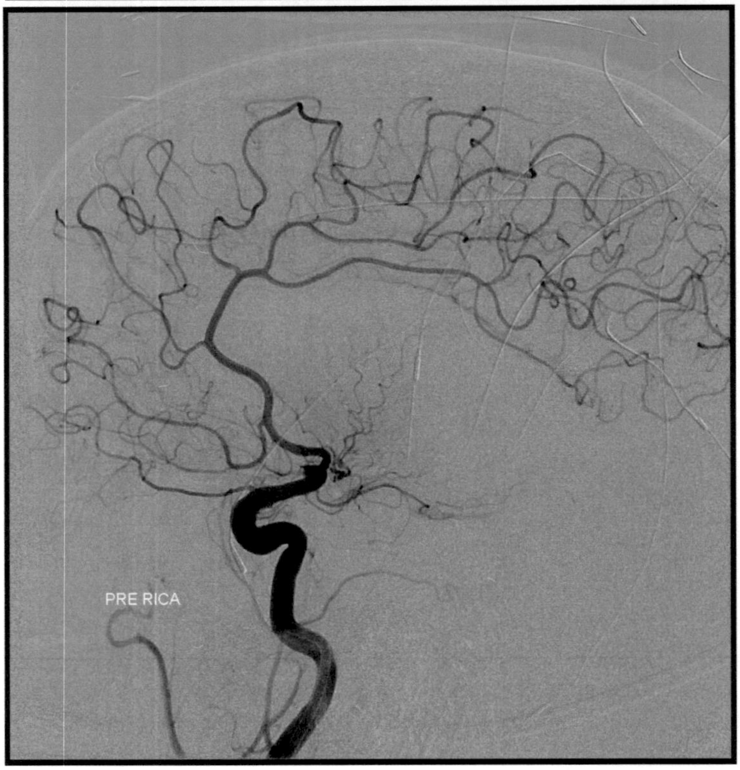

3.B.

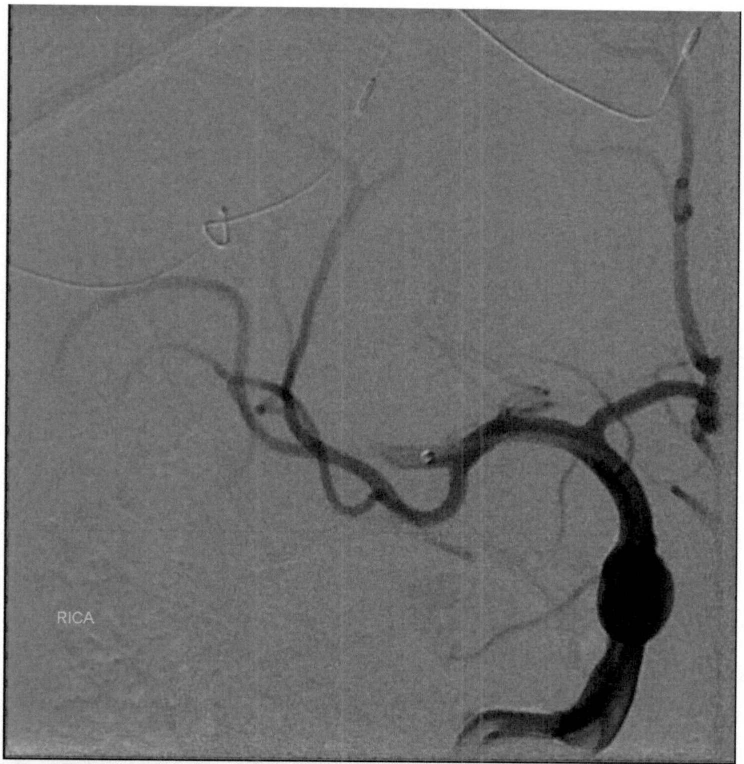

3.C.

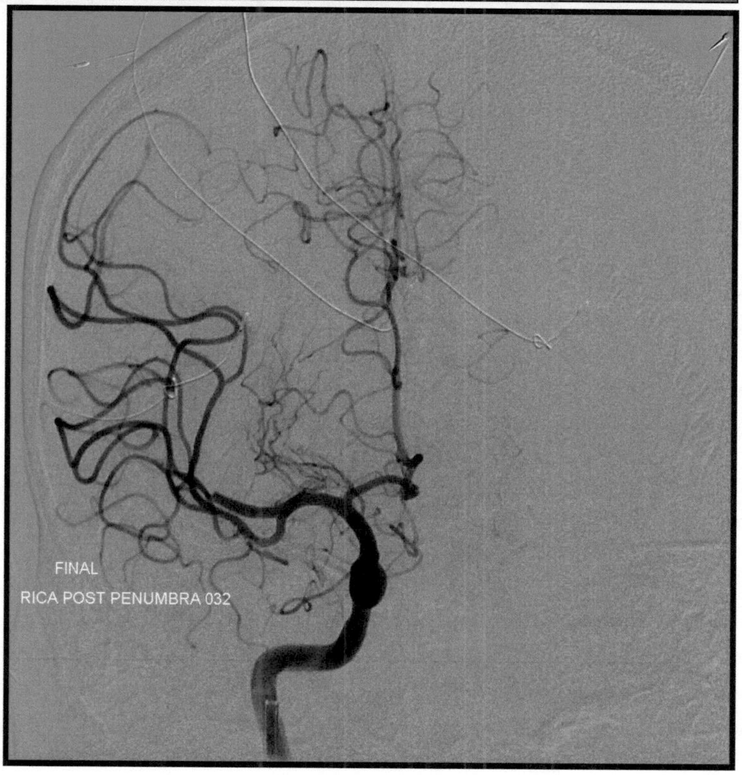

3.D.

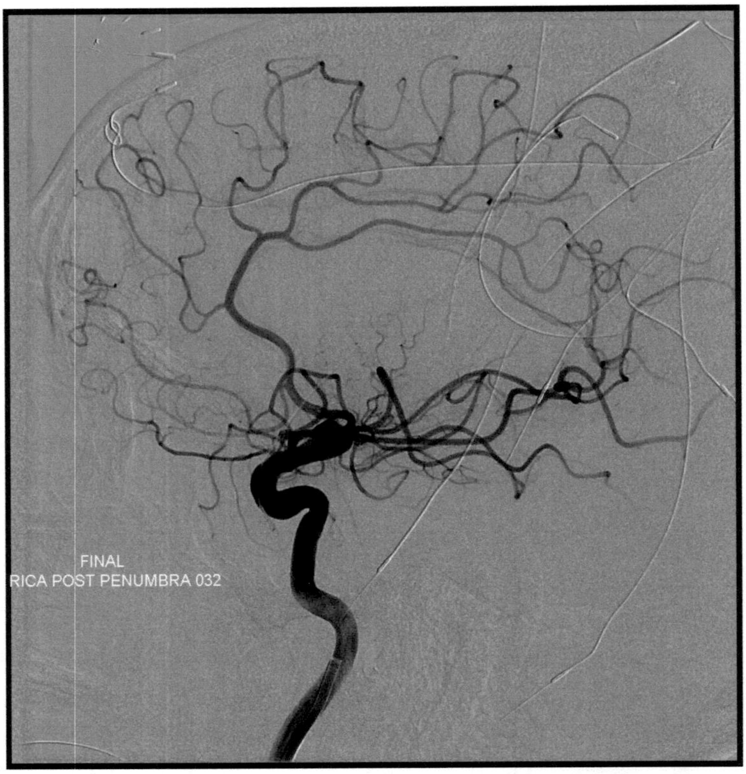

3.E.

Fig. 3. **A-E.** Acute right MCA occlusion. The patient presented 4 hours after an acute event of MCA occlusion. **A-B.** Mid-arterial digital subtraction angiogram of right ICA shows complete MCA occlusion at the level of the bifurcation, frontal and lateral views.
C. Mechanical thrombolysis with Penumbra device showing recanalization of the superior M2 division in a frontal high magnification view. **D-E.** Frontal and lateral views of right ICA angiograms following MCA mechanical recanalization.

5.3 Thrombus disruption

In this category, mechanical disruption of the clot is accomplished via a microguidewire or a snare. Some devices utilizing this mechanism are the EPAR (Endovasix, Belmont, California) and the LaTIS laser device (LaTIS, Minneapolis, Minnesota).[16] The potential endothelial damage with resultant vessel injury, and genesis of embolic material make these devices less favorable in the setting of acute ischemic stroke.

Traditional balloon inflation techniques could also cause central intra-arterial clot disruption and vessel recanalization (Fig. 4). The balloon is positioned across the vascular filling defect and gently inflated. Typically, a Hyperglide balloon (ev3 Neurovascular, Toledo, CA) is utilized for this technique. The final revascularization result and residual clot burden determine the possibility of additional stenting across the lesion.

5.4 Augmented fibrinolysis

These devices, such as the MicroLysUS infusion catheter (EKOS, Bothell, Washington), utilize a sonographic micro-tip to facilitate thrombolysis through ultrasonic vibration.[16] As a result, clot removal is augmented without any additional fragment embolization to the distal circulation. Recent studies show a favorable outcome with the use of such devices for the endovascular management of acute ischemic stroke.[46, 47]

5.5 Thrombus entrapment

The underlying mechanism of these devices utilizes a stent to recanalize the occluded vessel and therefore trap the clot between the stent and vessel wall. Besides their use at the site of occlusion, stents could recanalize proximal vessels (such as the extracranial ICA) to allow device navigation to the site of pathology. Stents can be deployed via a balloon mechanism or could be self-expandable. The latter are becoming increasingly popular due to their flexibility and ease of navigation. They include the Neuroform stent (Boston Scientific, Natick, Massachusetts), the Enterprise stent (Cordis, Miami Lakes, Florida), the LEO stent (Balt Extrusion, Montmorency, France), the Solitaire/Solo stent (ev3, Irvine, California), and the Wingspan stent (Boston Scientific). The first 4 stents are utilized in stent-assisted coiling of wide-neck aneurysms, whereas the Wingspan is the only stent approved for intracranial treatment of atherosclerotic disease.[16]Their use in acute ischemic events has been investigated in several trials[48-50]. Kim and colleagues reported recanalization rates as high as 71.4% in acute ischemic stroke with the use of Neuroform stent in 14 patients[48]. In two studies investigating the Neuroform and Wingspan stents, recanalization rates ranged from 67% to 89% and early follow-up (mean of 8 months) showed small (5%) or no restenosis rates.[51, 52]

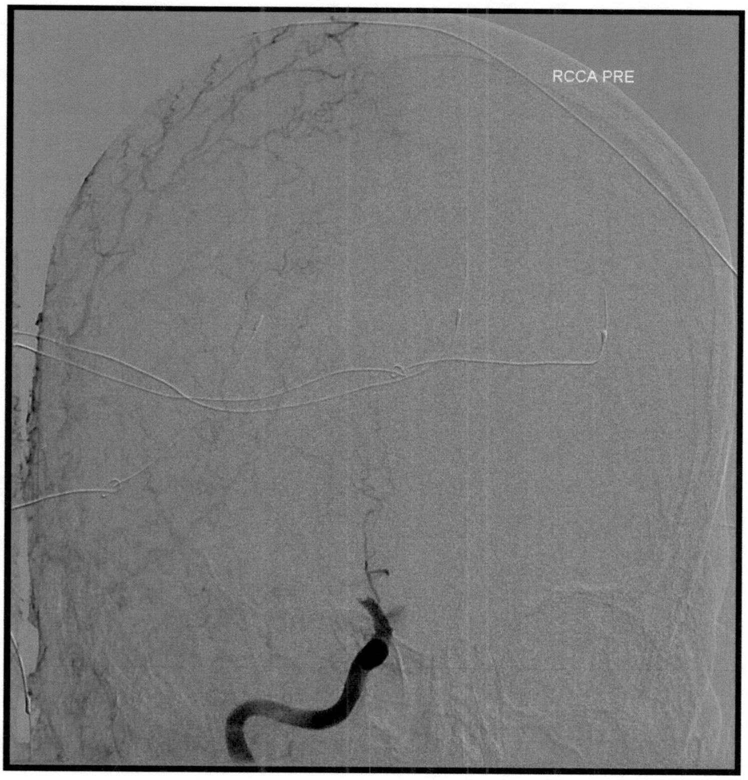

4.A.

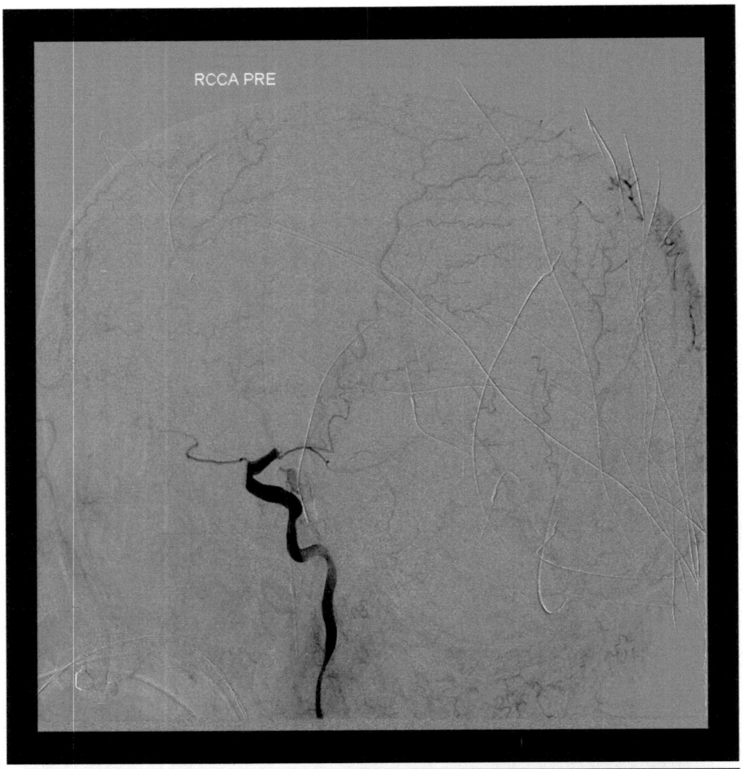

4.B.

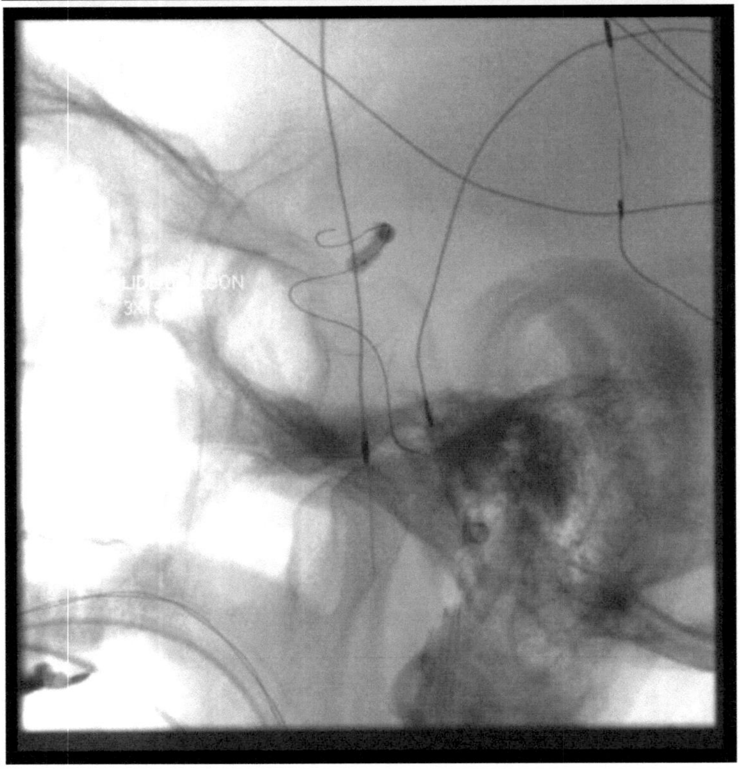

4.C.

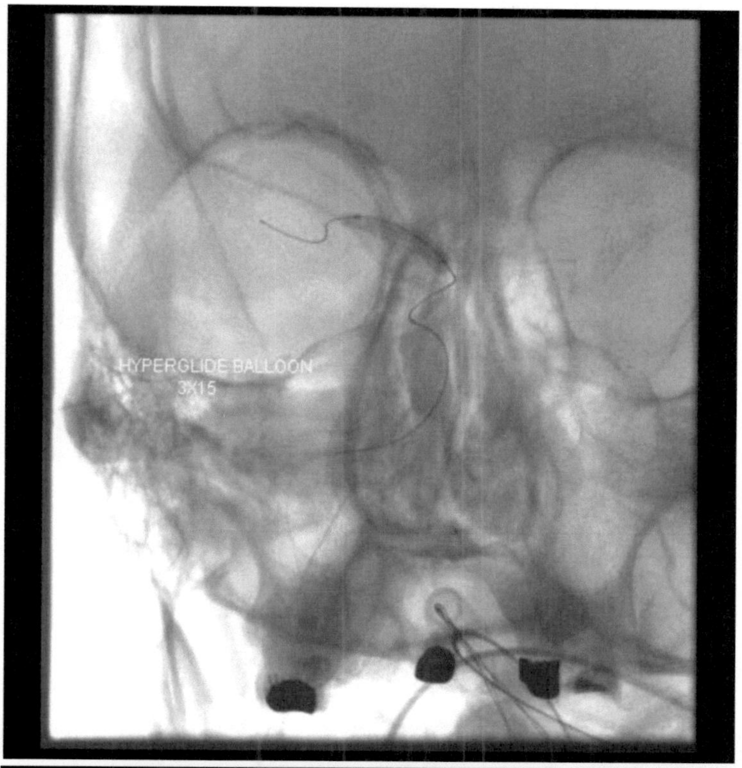

4.D.

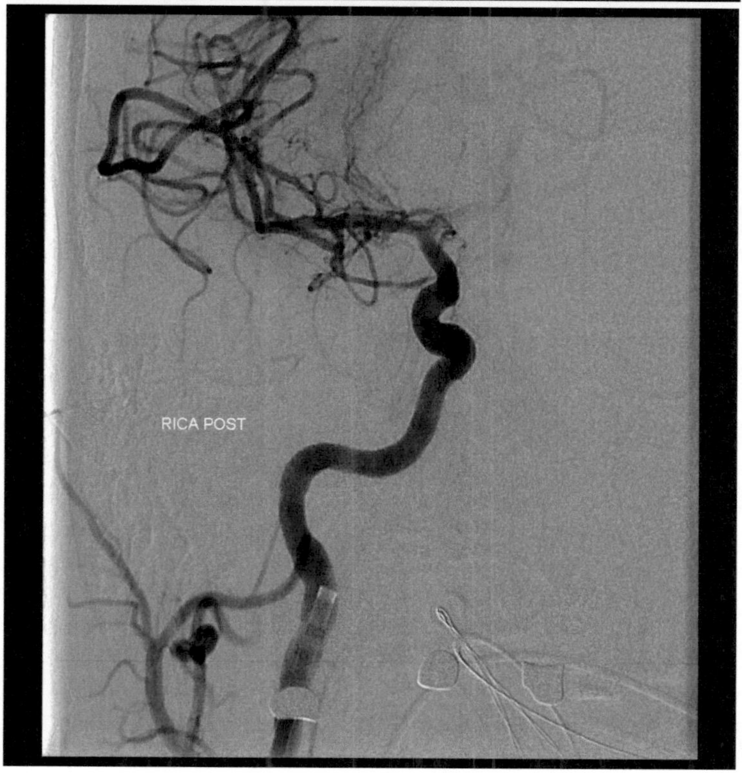

4.E.

4.F.

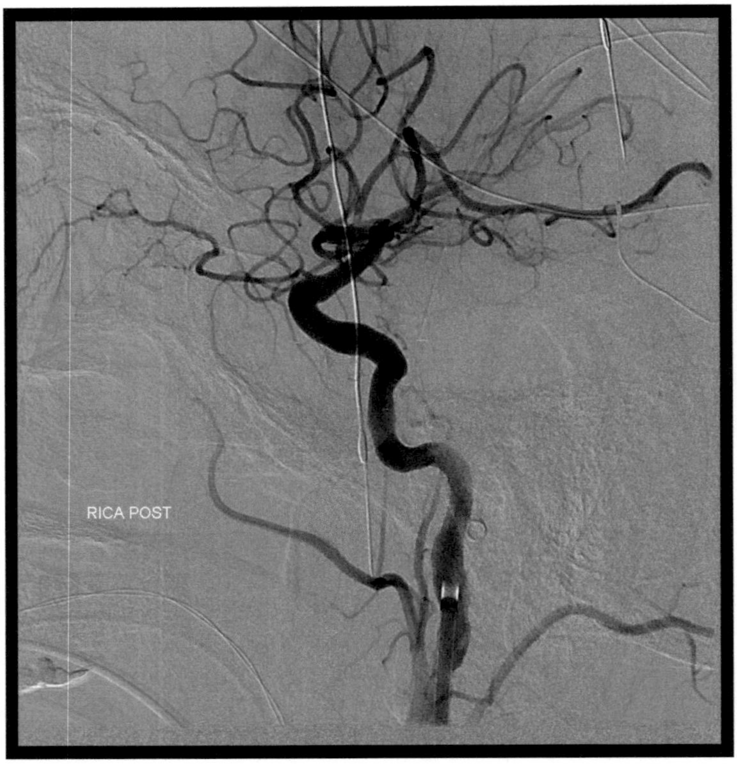

Fig. 4. **A-F.** Acute right ICA occlusion. The patient presented 5 hours after an acute event of left hemiplegia. **A-B.** Mid-arterial digital subtraction angiogram of right CCA shows complete ICA occlusion at the level of the ophthalmic artery, frontal and lateral views. **C-D.** Balloon angioplasty across the lesion with a Hyperglide 3x15mm balloon, frontal and lateral native angiographic views. **E-F.** Frontal and lateral views of right ICA angiograms following ICA mechanical recanalization.

6. Alternative reperfusion strategies

Cerebral reperfusion during acute ischemic stroke can be augmented via alternative strategies that utilize an anterograde or retrograde route. Anterograde reperfusion can be facilitated systemically with vasopressors leading to global reperfusion by increasing the mean arterial blood pressure. Retrograde reperfusion can be facilitated with a transarterial or transvenous approach. The transarterial approach involves the endovascular deployment of the NeuroFlo device (CoAxia, Maple Grove, Minnesota). This dual balloon catheter allows for partial occlusion of the aorta above and below the level of the renal arteries, therefore diverting flow away from the systemic and toward the cerebral circulation.[53] Several clinical trials are currently underway investigating the safety and efficacy of NeuroFlo and similar devices.

Transvenous retrograde reperfusion is an experimental technique with potential benefit in acute ischemic stroke. Animal studies suggest that diversion of blood from the femoral artery into the transverse venous sinuses via transvenous catheters could lower infarction size and improve neurological outcome in the setting of acute cerebrovascular ischemia.[54] Further investigational human trials are required prior to introducing such a novel concept to current stroke therapies.

7. Future directions

Advances in knowledge about pharmacology, endovascular biomechanics, and endothelial properties are stimulating research on new diagnostic and therapeutic tools in the management of acute ischemic stroke. Currently there are several clinical trials targeting neuroendovascular therapy.[21] The Interventional Management of Stroke Study III (IMS III) is a phase III multicenter clinical trial that continues the investigation of combined IA and IV therapies in the management of acute stroke. The SYNTHESIS Expansion trial is a phase III clinical study that compares the safety and efficacy of IV thrombolysis to IA chemical and mechanical thrombolysis. Future studies may include the individual comparison of mechanical devices versus intravenous thrombolytics[55].

Multiple studies are investigating the safety and efficacy of new generation endovascular devices, such as the Safety and Efficacy of NeuroFlo Technology in Ischemic Stroke (SENTIS). The neurological outcomes of optimal medical management versus IA thrombolysis are examined in clinical trials such as RETRIEVE (Randomized Trial of Endovascular treatment of Acute Ischemic Stroke Versus Medical Management) and PISTE (Pragmatic Ischemic Stroke Thrombectomy Evaluation). Extending the timing of endovascular intervention is being evaluated in conjunction with new radiographic techniques. Examples include the DWI and CTP Assessment in the Triage of Wake-Up and Late Presenting Strokes Undergoing Neurointervention Trial, and the MR Imaging and Recanalization of Stroke Clots During Embolectomy Trial.[21]

These and several other upcoming trials will hopefully provide sufficient clinical data for the FDA approval of IA agents, the introduction of new endovascular devices, and other adjunctive therapies for the management of the acute stroke patient.

8. Conclusion

Over the past decade, endovascular intervention has become a mainstay treatment in the setting of acute ischemic stroke. Innovative techniques in both chemical and mechanical intraarterial thrombolysis increase the safety and efficacy of endovascular management and expand its indications in acute cerebral infarction. Additional larger clinical trials are warranted for the improvement of the endovascular care of stroke patients resulting in faster and safer reperfusion mechanisms.

9. References

[1] AHA. Heart and Stroke Update. 2010.

[2] Fagan SC, Morgenstern LB, Petitta A, et al. Cost-effectiveness of tissue plasminogen activator for acute ischemic stroke. NINDS rt-PA Stroke Study Group. In: Neurology; 1998:883-90.

[3] Sussman BJ, Fitch TS. Thrombolysis with fibrinolysin in cerebral arterial occlusion. In: Journal of the American Medical Association; 1958:1705-9.

[4] Goyal M, Menon BK, Coutts SB, Hill MD, Demchuk AM, Penumbra Pivotal Stroke Trial Investigators CSP, and the Seaman MR Research Center. Effect of baseline CT scan appearance and time to recanalization on clinical outcomes in endovascular thrombectomy of acute ischemic strokes. In: Stroke; 2011:93-7.

[5] Vora NA, Gupta R, Thomas AJ, et al. Factors predicting hemorrhagic complications after multimodal reperfusion therapy for acute ischemic stroke. In: AJNR American journal of neuroradiology; 2007:1391-4.

[6] Gönner F, Remonda L, Mattle H, et al. Local intra-arterial thrombolysis in acute ischemic stroke. In: Stroke; 1998:1894-900.

[7] von Kummer R, Meyding-Lamadé U, Forsting M, et al. Sensitivity and prognostic value of early CT in occlusion of the middle cerebral artery trunk. In: AJNR American journal of neuroradiology; 1994:9-15; discussion 6-8.

[8] Wolpert SM, Bruckmann H, Greenlee R, Wechsler L, Pessin MS, del Zoppo GJ. Neuroradiologic evaluation of patients with acute stroke treated with recombinant tissue plasminogen activator. The rt-PA Acute Stroke Study Group. In: AJNR American journal of neuroradiology; 1993:3-13.

[9] Konstas AA, Goldmakher GV, Lee TY, Lev MH. Theoretic basis and technical implementations of CT perfusion in acute ischemic stroke, part 1: Theoretic basis. In: AJNR American journal of neuroradiology; 2009:662-8.

[10] Zacharatos H, Hassan AE, Vazquez G, et al. Comparison of acute nonthrombolytic and thrombolytic treatments in ischemic stroke patients 80 years or older. In: The American journal of emergency medicine; 2011.

[11] McDonagh DL, Olson DM, Kalia JS, Gupta R, Abou-Chebl A, Zaidat OO. Anesthesia and Sedation Practices Among Neurointerventionalists during Acute Ischemic Stroke Endovascular Therapy. In: Frontiers in neurology; 2010:118.

[12] Gupta R. Local is better than general anesthesia during endovascular acute stroke interventions. In: Stroke; 2010:2718-9.

[13] Jumaa MA, Zhang F, Ruiz-Ares G, et al. Comparison of safety and clinical and radiographic outcomes in endovascular acute stroke therapy for proximal middle cerebral artery occlusion with intubation and general anesthesia versus the nonintubated state. In: Stroke; 2010:1180-4.

[14] Bang OY, Saver JL, Kim SJ, et al. Collateral flow predicts response to endovascular therapy for acute ischemic stroke. In: Stroke; 2011:693-9.

[15] Berenstein Alejandro, Lasjaunias Pierre, G. ter Brugge Karel. Surgical neuroangiography. Vol. 2, Clinical and endovascular treatment .... In.

[16] Nogueira RG, Schwamm LH, Hirsch JA. Endovascular approaches to acute stroke, part 1: Drugs, devices, and data. In: AJNR American journal of neuroradiology; 2009:649-61.

[17] Cornu C, Boutitie F, Candelise L, et al. Streptokinase in acute ischemic stroke: an individual patient data meta-analysis : The Thrombolysis in Acute Stroke Pooling Project. In: Stroke; 2000:1555-60.

[18] Lisboa RC, Jovanovic BD, Alberts MJ. Analysis of the safety and efficacy of intra-arterial thrombolytic therapy in ischemic stroke. In: Stroke; 2002:2866-71.

[19] Kaur J, Zhao Z, Klein GM, Lo EH, Buchan AM. The neurotoxicity of tissue plasminogen activator? In: J Cereb Blood Flow Metab; 2004:945-63.

[20] Memon MZ, Natarajan SK, Sharma J, et al. Safety and feasibility of intraarterial eptifibatide as a revascularization tool in acute ischemic stroke. In: J Neurosurg; 2010.

[21] Nogueira RG, Yoo AJ, Buonanno FS, Hirsch JA. Endovascular approaches to acute stroke, part 2: a comprehensive review of studies and trials. In: AJNR American journal of neuroradiology; 2009:859-75.

[22] del Zoppo GJ, Higashida RT, Furlan AJ, Pessin MS, Rowley HA, Gent M. PROACT: a phase II randomized trial of recombinant pro-urokinase by direct arterial delivery

in acute middle cerebral artery stroke. PROACT Investigators. Prolyse in Acute Cerebral Thromboembolism. In: Stroke; 1998:4-11.

[23] Furlan A, Higashida R, Wechsler L, et al. Intra-arterial prourokinase for acute ischemic stroke. The PROACT II study: a randomized controlled trial. Prolyse in Acute Cerebral Thromboembolism. In: JAMA; 1999:2003-11.

[24] Ogawa A, Mori E, Minematsu K, et al. Randomized trial of intraarterial infusion of urokinase within 6 hours of middle cerebral artery stroke: the middle cerebral artery embolism local fibrinolytic intervention trial (MELT) Japan. In: Stroke; 2007:2633-9.

[25] Theron J, Courtheoux P, Casasco A, et al. Local intraarterial fibrinolysis in the carotid territory. In: AJNR American journal of neuroradiology; 1989:753-65.

[26] Brott T. Thrombolytic therapy. In: Neurologic clinics; 1992:219-32.

[27] Levine SR, Brott TG. Thrombolytic therapy in cerebrovascular disorders. In: Progress in cardiovascular diseases; 1992:235-62.

[28] Barnwell SL, Clark WM, Nguyen TT, O'Neill OR, Wynn ML, Coull BM. Safety and efficacy of delayed intraarterial urokinase therapy with mechanical clot disruption for thromboembolic stroke. In: AJNR American journal of neuroradiology; 1994:1817-22.

[29] Jovin TG, Gupta R, Uchino K, et al. Emergent stenting of extracranial internal carotid artery occlusion in acute stroke has a high revascularization rate. In: Stroke; 2005:2426-30.

[30] Bhatia R, Hill MD, Shobha N, et al. Low rates of acute recanalization with intravenous recombinant tissue plasminogen activator in ischemic stroke: real-world experience and a call for action. In: Stroke; 2010:2254-8.

[31] Arnold M, Nedeltchev K, Mattle HP, et al. Intra-arterial thrombolysis in 24 consecutive patients with internal carotid artery T occlusions. In: J Neurol Neurosurg Psychiatr; 2003:739-42.

[32] Flint AC, Duckwiler GR, Budzik RF, Liebeskind DS, Smith WS, Committee MaMMW. Mechanical thrombectomy of intracranial internal carotid occlusion: pooled results of the MERCI and Multi MERCI Part I trials. In: Stroke; 2007:1274-80.

[33] Padolecchia R, Puglioli M, Ragone MC, Romani A, Collavoli PL. Superselective intraarterial fibrinolysis in central retinal artery occlusion. In: AJNR American journal of neuroradiology; 1999:565-7.

[34] Arnold M, Koerner U, Remonda L, et al. Comparison of intra-arterial thrombolysis with conventional treatment in patients with acute central retinal artery occlusion. In: J Neurol Neurosurg Psychiatr; 2005:196-9.

[35] Aldrich EM, Lee AW, Chen CS, et al. Local intraarterial fibrinolysis administered in aliquots for the treatment of central retinal artery occlusion: the Johns Hopkins Hospital experience. In: Stroke; 2008:1746-50.

[36] Noble J, Weizblit N, Baerlocher MO, Eng KT. Intra-arterial thrombolysis for central retinal artery occlusion: a systematic review. In: Br J Ophthalmol; 2008:588-93.

[37] Furlan A, Higashida, R. Intra-arterial thrombolysis in acute ischemic stroke. In: Stroke: Pathophysiology, Diagnosis, and Management. 4th ed. Philadelphia: Churchill Livingstone; 2004:943-51.

[38] Schonewille WJ, Wijman CA, Michel P, Algra A, Kappelle LJ, Group BS. The basilar artery international cooperation study (BASICS). In: International journal of stroke : official journal of the International Stroke Society; 2007:220-3.

[39] Levy EI, Firlik AD, Wisniewski S, et al. Factors affecting survival rates for acute vertebrobasilar artery occlusions treated with intra-arterial thrombolytic therapy: a meta-analytical approach. In: Neurosurgery; 1999:539-45; discussion 45-8.

[40] Gupta R, Tayal AH, Levy EI, et al. Intra-arterial thrombolysis or Stent Placement during Endovascular Treatment for Acute Ischemic Stroke Leads to the Highest Recanalization Rate: Results of a Multi-center Retrospective Study. In: Neurosurgery; 2011.
[41] Smith WS, Sung G, Starkman S, et al. Safety and efficacy of mechanical embolectomy in acute ischemic stroke: results of the MERCI trial. In: Stroke; 2005:1432-8.
[42] Shi Z-S, Loh Y, Walker G, Duckwiler GR, Investigators MaM-M. Clinical outcomes in middle cerebral artery trunk occlusions versus secondary division occlusions after mechanical thrombectomy: pooled analysis of the Mechanical Embolus Removal in Cerebral Ischemia (MERCI) and Multi MERCI trials. In: Stroke; 2010:953-60.
[43] Liebig T, Reinartz J, Hannes R, Miloslavski E, Henkes H. Comparative in vitro study of five mechanical embolectomy systems: effectiveness of clot removal and risk of distal embolization. In: Neuroradiology; 2008:43-52.
[44] Bose A, Henkes H, Alfke K, et al. The Penumbra System: a mechanical device for the treatment of acute stroke due to thromboembolism. In: AJNR American journal of neuroradiology; 2008:1409-13.
[45] Nesbit GM, Luh G, Tien R, Barnwell SL. New and future endovascular treatment strategies for acute ischemic stroke. In: Journal of vascular and interventional radiology : JVIR; 2004:S103-10.
[46] Mahon BR, Nesbit GM, Barnwell SL, et al. North American clinical experience with the EKOS MicroLysUS infusion catheter for the treatment of embolic stroke. In: AJNR American journal of neuroradiology; 2003:534-8.
[47] Investigators IIT. The Interventional Management of Stroke (IMS) II Study. In: Stroke; 2007:2127-35.
[48] Kim SM, Lee DH, Kwon SU, Choi CG, Kim SJ, Suh DC. Treatment of acute ischemic stroke: feasibility of primary or secondary use of a self-expanding stent (Neuroform) during local intra-arterial thrombolysis. In: Neuroradiology; 2011.
[49] Mourand I, Brunel H, Vendrell J-F, Thouvenot E, Bonafé A. Endovascular stent-assisted thrombolysis in acute occlusive carotid artery dissection. In: Neuroradiology; 2010:135-40.
[50] Prince EA, Jayaraman MV, Haas RA. Use of self-expanding intracranial stents in the treatment of acute ischemic stroke. In: Journal of vascular and interventional radiology : JVIR; 2010:1755-9.
[51] Levy EI, Mehta R, Gupta R, et al. Self-expanding stents for recanalization of acute cerebrovascular occlusions. In: AJNR American journal of neuroradiology; 2007:816-22.
[52] Zaidat OO, Wolfe T, Hussain SI, et al. Interventional acute ischemic stroke therapy with intracranial self-expanding stent. In: Stroke; 2008:2392-5.
[53] Lylyk P, Vila JF, Miranda C, Ferrario A, Romero R, Cohen JE. Partial aortic obstruction improves cerebral perfusion and clinical symptoms in patients with symptomatic vasospasm. In: Neurol Res; 2005:S129-35.
[54] Frazee JG, Luo X, Luan G, et al. Retrograde transvenous neuroperfusion: a back door treatment for stroke. In: Stroke; 1998:1912-6.
[55] Mazighi M, Amarenco P. Reperfusion therapy in acute cerebrovascular syndrome. In: Curr Opin Neurol; 2011:59-62.
[56] Neurology WGftAAo, Section ACC, Surgery SoN, et al. Performance and training standards for endovascular ischemic stroke treatment. In: AJNR American journal of neuroradiology; 2010:E8-11.

7

Microemboli Monitoring in Ischemic Stroke

Titto Idicula and Lars Thomassen
*University of Bergen,
Norway*

1. Introduction

Circulating microemboli in the arterial system were detected using ultrasound as early as 1969 (Spencer, Lawrence et al. 1969) (Fig 1). Microemboli to brain can be detected with high sensitivity using trancranial Doppler by insonating the middle cerebral arteries.

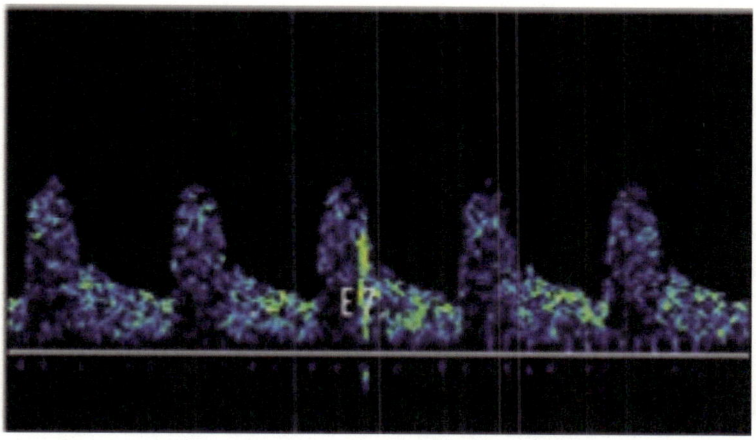

Fig. 1. Microemboli from middle cerebral artery detected by TCD.

The detection is made possible because of the acoustic impedance between microemboli and blood, which increases the ultrasound intensity. Microemboli are transient (<100ms), high intensity (> 3dB) and unidirectional signal which are accompanied by a characteristic click or chirp sound (Ringelstein, Droste et al. 1998). The origin of microemboli are usually from an atheromatous plaque in the carotid artery or the aorta, from the heart chambers in patients with atrial fibrillation, or from prosthetic heart valves.

2. Characteristics of microemboli

The detected signals are either of gaseous or solid embolic material (Russell, Madden et al. 1991). Solid microemboli consist of platelet aggregates, thrombus or whole blood (Markus and Brown 1993). Platelet aggregates are usually ruptured off an atheromatous plaque because of the shear stress on vessel wall (Kessler 1992). Postmortem studies have shown that solid microemboli contain lipids in addition to small birefrigent particles (Brown, Moody et al. 1996). The gaseous microemboli usually originates from a prosthetic heart valve. It is created by mechanically induced cavitations. A reliable differentiation between gaseous and solid microemboli is not possible with single frequency probe that are being currently used in most centers (Dittrich, Ritter et al. 2002). Newly available dual frequency probes can reliably differentiate between solid and gaseous microemboli. However, such differentiation is not of much significance in most patient subgroups.

3. Impact of microemboli on brain

Solid microemboli are much bigger than gaseous microemboli, having an approximate diameter of 100 µm and 4µm respectively. The larger size of solid microemboli compared to capillaries (diameter 7-10 µm) can cause blockade of microcirculation. Solid microemboli, which predominantly arises from atheromatous plaque, can cause injury to the brain, which may manifest as cognitive impairement. Histological studies have shown that such microemboli leads to loss of enzymatic activities of endothelial cells leading to degeneration of capillaries (Brown, Moody et al. 1996). These microemboli usually disappear from brain within two weeks, but can persist there for up to 6 months. In contrast gaseous microemboli, predominantly seen in patients with prosthetic valve, have no deleterious effect on brain (Kaps, Hansen et al. 1997).

4. Prevalence

Prevalence of microemboli varies in different patient sub-groups. An estimated prevalence of 1-5% is estimated in the general population based on small control groups from different studies(Daffertshofer, Ries et al. 1996) (Georgiadis, Lindner et al. 1997). The prevalence is higher in high-risk patients who are vulnerable to thromboembolic events.

4.1 Prevalence in acute ischemic stroke

A large proportion of ischemic stroke is of embolic etiology. Therefore, assessing the prevalence of microemboli following ischemic stroke is of great interest. Very few studies have assessed the prevalence of microemboli in the acute phase of stroke because of the technical difficulties. The available studies in the acute phase of stroke (<24 hours) have shown the prevalence of microemboli to be between 19-49% (Sliwka, Lingnau et al. 1997; Delcker, Schnell et al. 2000; Iguchi, Kimura et al. 2008; Idicula, Naess et al. 2010). However monitoring beyond the first 24 hours after stroke shows a lower prevalence ranging from 6 to 32% (Tong and Albers 1995; Del Sette, Angeli et al. 1997; Koennecke, Mast et al. 1998; Valton, Larrue et al. 1998; Kaposzta, Young et al. 1999; Lund, Rygh et al. 2000; Serena, Segura et al. 2000; Gucuyener, Uzuner et al. 2001; Poppert, Sadikovic et al. 2006). The prevalence of microemboli in the largest of those studies (n=653) was less than 6% (Poppert, Sadikovic et al. 2006). It seems like there is an inverse relationship between timing of monitoring and the prevalence of microemboli following acute ischemic stroke. Table 1 shows the prevalence of microemboli following ischemic stroke in various studies.

Author	Monitoring	n	Prevalence(%)
Iguchi	< 24 hrs	125	49
Delcker	< 24 hrs	61	43
Sliwka	< 24 hrs	100	19
Idicula	< 24 hrs	40	25
Del Sette	> 24 hrs	75	12
Gucuyener	> 24 hrs	359	32
Koennecke	> 24 hrs	145	24
Lund	> 24 hrs	83	27
Poppert	> 24 hrs	653	6
Serena	> 24 hrs	182	9
Tong	> 24 hrs	38	11
Valton	> 24 hrs	73	21

Table 1. The prevalence of microemboli in various studies performed before and after 24 hours of stroke onset in various studies.

4.2 Prevalence in atherosclerotic carotid artery disease

The prevalence of microemboli is high in patients with large artery disease as in carotid artery stenosis. Table 2 shows a review of all studies in which prevalence of microemboli was assessed in symptomatic and asymptomatic carotid stenosis (Babikian, Hyde et al. 1994; Siebler, Kleinschmidt et al. 1994; Markus and Harrison 1995; Daffertshofer, Ries et al. 1996; Georgiadis, Lindner et al. 1997; Markus and MacKinnon 2005; Spence, Tamayo et al. 2005; Zuromskis, Wetterholm et al. 2008).

Author	n	Symptomatic(%)	Asymptomatic(%)
Zuromskis	197	32	4.5
Georgiadis	500	52	7
Siebler	89	82	
Babikian	75	28	
Daffertshofer	280	9	
Markus	38	34	3.5
Markus	230	48	
Spence	319		10

Table 2. Shows the prevalence of microemboli in symptomatic and asymptomatic carotid artery disease.

While the prevalence of microemboli in patients with carotid stenosis ranged from 20-90%, most of the studies showed a prevalence of more than 30% in symptomatic carotid stenosis (Markus and Harrison 1995). The large variation in the prevalence of microemboli in different studies may be attributed to differences in the timing of study, use of antiplatelet agents at the time of monitoring and the sample population itself. However the studies, which compared prevalence of microemboli in symptomatic and asymptomatic side, clearly shows a higher prevalence in the symptomatic side. A recent pooled analysis of microemboli in patients with symptomatic and asymptomatic carotid stenosis showed a prevalence of 42% and 8% respectively (Ritter, Dittrich et al. 2008).

4.3 Prevalence in intracranial stenosis

The prevalence microemboli in intracranial stenosis is less well studied compared to carotid stenosis. A review of those studies is given in table 3.

Author	n	Symptomatic	Asymptomatic
Wong	60	15	0
Nabavi	14	14	7
Gao	114	22	
Wong	30	33	
Droste	33	15	
Segura	29	36	

Table 3. Shows the prevalence of microemboli in the symptomatic and asymptomatic intracranial stenosis in various studies.

The available data shows that the prevalence of microemboli in intracranial stenosis to be between 7-33% (Nabavi, Georgiadis et al. 1996; Segura, Serena et al. 2001; Wong, Gao et al. 2001; Droste, Junker et al. 2002; Wong, Gao et al. 2002; Gao, Wong et al. 2004). The prevalence of microemboli in the largest of those studies (n=114) was 22%. The prevalence of microemboli in asymptomatic stenosis were between 0-7% (Nabavi, Georgiadis et al. 1996; Wong, Gao et al. 2001). A pooled analysis of patients with intracranial stenosis shows the prevalence of microemboli in the symptomatic and asymptomatic side to be 25% and 0% respectively (Ritter, Dittrich et al. 2008). Overall, the prevalence of microemboli in intracranial stenosis is lower compared to carotid artery stenosis. Lower prevalence of microemboli in intracranial stenosis may be because of the technical difficulty in performing microemboli monitoring in the presence of intracranial stenosis as well as the difference in plaque morphology.

4.4 Prevalence in various cardiac diseases

Microemboli from the heart originate either from the heart chambers itself or from prosthetic heart valves. Parallel to the known risk factors for cardioembolic stroke, microemboli are often observed in atrial fibrillation, prosthetic heart valves, patent foramen ovale, acute myocardial infarction and left ventricular dysfunction. The highest prevalence of microemboli is seen in patients with prosthetic heart valves, about 60% with mechanical prosthetic heart valves and about 10% with biological prosthetic heart valves (Eicke, Barth et al. 1996). In patients with atrial fibrillation, the prevalence of microemboli seems to be higher in symptomatic atrial fibrillation (29%) as opposed to asymptomatic atrial fibrillation (10%) (Kumral, Balkir et al. 2001). Similarly, there is a higher prevalence of microemboli in valvular atrial fibrillation as opposed to non-valvular atrial fibrillation corresponding to a higher risk for thromboembolic events (Kumral, Balkir et al. 2001). Except for mechanical prosthetic heart valves, the overall prevalence of microemboli in various heart conditions seems to be lesser than in carotid artery disease.

5. Application of microemboli monitoring

5.1 Application of microemboli monitoring in acute stroke

It is optimal to perform microemboli monitoring closer to the onset of symptoms because of the inverse relationship between timing of monitoring and the prevalence of microemboli

(Forteza, Babikian et al. 1996). The technical difficulty and the need for manpower make it difficult to perform monitoring within the first 24 hours after stroke onset. However, it may still be adequate to perform monitoring after the first 24 hours. Identification of microemboli will help us understand the etiology, predict outcome and assess the effectiveness of secondary prophylaxis.

5.1.1 Assessing the etiology of stroke

TOAST is one of the commonly used classifications to define stroke etiology. However, this classification fails to clearly define etiology in more than one third of the patients (Kolominsky-Rabas, Weber et al. 2001). More tools are needed to determine stroke etiology reliably. Microemboli are generally found in patients with embolic etiologies, both of arterial and of cardiac origin. A review of studies conducted in ischemic stroke patients shows that microemboli are mostly present when an embolic source is present (Del Sette, Angeli et al. 1997; Sliwka, Lingnau et al. 1997; Koennecke, Mast et al. 1998; Kaposzta, Young et al. 1999; Lund, Rygh et al. 2000; Serena, Segura et al. 2000; Poppert, Sadikovic et al. 2006; Iguchi, Kimura et al. 2008; Idicula, Naess et al. 2010). Some studies have, however, shown the presence of microemboli in lacunar stroke, even though less frequent than in other etiologies (Koennecke, Mast et al. 1998; Lund, Rygh et al. 2000; Iguchi, Kimura et al. 2008). Microemboli were absent in all lacunar stroke patients in most other studies including the largest of them (Poppert, Sadikovic et al. 2006). Even though the specificity of microemboli in determining an embolic etiology is not fully known, the presence of microemboli strongly suggests the possibility of an embolic source. Further differentiation between large-artery and cardioembolic stroke can also be made based on characteristics of microemboli. Bilateral microemboli may suggest microemboli from heart or arch of aorta (Kaposzta, Young et al. 1999), whereas unilateral microemboli suggest carotid artery stenosis or intracranial artery stenosis. This can especially be relevant when two potential embolic sources are simultaneously present as in carotid stenosis along with atrial fibrillation. Specificity of bilateral microemboli in determining cardiac source of embolism can further be improved by recording both the proximal carotid arteries and both middle cerebral arteries simultaneously.

5.1.2 Predicting outcome after stroke

The value of microemboli in predicting outcome and future vascular events following an ischemic stroke is known only to a limited extent due to the lack of sufficient studies. A review of all studies involving 602 patients reveals an interesting finding. All except one study showed that microemboli is an independent predictor of future vascular events with an odds ratio of 4 or above (Valton, Larrue et al. 1998; Censori, Partziguian et al. 2000; Gao, Wong et al. 2004; Markus and MacKinnon 2005; Iguchi, Kimura et al. 2008; Idicula, Naess et al. 2010). It infers that microemboli monitoring may be of value in predicting recurrence following acute ischemic stroke.

The functional outcome or disability after stroke is, however, less well predicted by the presence or absence of microemboli. Two studies in which data on functional outcome was available failed to observe any association between microemboli and functional outcome (Delcker, Schnell et al. 2000; Idicula, Naess et al. 2010). One of the studies showed a trend towards higher mortality among patients with microemboli, but the association was not significant after adjusting for confounding factors (Idicula, Naess et al. 2010). Thus, there is a paucity of evidence to suggest that microemboli predict poor functional outcome after ischemic stroke.

5.1.3 Assessing efficacy of secondary prophylaxis

Many platelet inhibitors are approved for secondary prophylaxis after ischemic stroke. It is difficult to predict which of the approved agents would be a better alternative in an individual patient. Microembolic mostly consist of platelet aggregates. Therefore, their measurement may be used as a surrogate marker for evaluating anti-platelet effect (Wong 2005). Glycoprotein IIb/IIIa receptor antagonist such as tirofiban infusion has shown to reduce the rate of microemboli and the effect was reversible with the cessation of infusion (Junghans and Siebler 2003). Administration of intravenous and oral acetylsalicyclic acid (ASA) has shown to reduce the frequency of microemboli rapidly (Goertler, Baeumer et al. 1999; Goertler, Blaser et al. 2001). Several small studies have shown that dual antiplatelet therapy might lead to rapid decline in microembolic frequency (Esagunde, Wong et al. 2006). The studies were not double blinded randomized studies. However, they showed that the frequency of microemboli was significantly reduced after administering antiplatelet agents. It indicates the potential of measuring microemboli as a surrogate marker of anti-platelet effect. This is particularly important in patients with recent symptomatic carotid stenosis.

In CARESS trial, a randomized double-blind study, patients with symptomatic carotid stenosis were randomized to either aspirin alone or aspirin and clopidogrel. Patients who received dual anti-platelet therapy with aspirin and clopidogrel had significantly lower microemboli compared to patients who received aspirin alone (Markus, Droste et al. 2005). Subsequently, fewer recurrent ischemic events were observed in patients who received dual antiplatelet therapy (Mackinnon, Aaslid et al. 2005). Dual antiplatelet therapy with aspirin and clopidogrel may be an optimal choice at least in a subgroup of high-risk stroke patients who can be identified with the help of microemboli monitoring. However, the long-term outcome or the optimal duration of dual antiplatelet therapy is not known yet. On the contrary, the effect of anticoagulation on microemboli is highly uncertain. Except for some anecdotal reports, there is no evidence that anticoagulation would abort microemboli (Poppert, Sadikovic et al. 2006).

5.2 Application of microemboli monitoring in carotid artery and intracranial artery stenosis

Microemboli from an unstable carotid plaque often represent inflammation within the plaque (Jander, Sitzer et al. 1998). Studies with FDG-PET in patients with carotid plaque have shown that patients with microemboli are more likely to have inflammation within the plaque (Moustafa, Izquierdo-Garcia et al. 2010). Plaque specimens in patients undergoing endarterectomy have shown that presence of microemboli is strongly associated with plaque fissuring and luminal thrombosis (Sitzer, Siebler et al. 1995). In patients with symptomatic carotid stenosis, microemboli is an indicator of plaque instability (Siebler, Kleinschmidt et al. 1994). Carotid endarterectomy results in drastic reduction or disappearance of microemboli (Orlandi, Parenti et al. 1997). Similarly, patients with asymptomatic carotid stenosis microemboli have proven to be a known marker of future vascular events as shown in several studies (Siebler, Nachtmann et al. 1995; Molloy and Markus 1999). Thus, the presence of microemboli might help choose the right therapeutic option including endarterectomy especially in patients with asymptomatic stenosis. Microemboli monitoring is also important in patients with intracranial artery disease as well. Even though there are technical difficulties in performing microemboli monitoring in the presence of intracranial stenosis, the presence of microemboli provides valuable information to choose appropriate management. The frequency of microemboli in the presence of intracranial artery stenosis has shown to be associated with the number of infarcts on imaging (Wong, Gao et al. 2002). In patients with frequent microemboli, dual antiplatelet agents has shown to reduce the frequency of microemboli from intracranial stenosis as in carotid artery stenosis (Sebastian, Derksen et al. 2011), arguing in favour of using it in those patients.

5.3 Application of microemboli monitoring in heart diseases

The clinical and prognostic significance of microemboli in patients with atrial fibrillation and prosthetic valves is unclear. Only few studies have shown that anticoagulation may reduce microembolic frequency in patients with atrial fibrillation (Tinkler, Cullinane et al. 2002). It is difficult to choose between anticoagulation versus anti-platelet agents based on the presence or absence of microemboli. However, the presence of microemboli may prompt the use either anticoagulation or anti-platelet agents in patients with atrial fibrillation regardless of any thromboembolic events.

5.4 Application of microemboli monitoring in special situations

5.4.1 Arterial dissection

As in embolic stroke, microemboli are often seen in patients with dissection. More microemboli are present in patients who present with stroke symptoms as opposed to local symptoms (Ritter, Dittrich et al. 2008). Presence of microemboli seems to be a predictor of stroke recurrence (Molina, Alvarez-Sabin et al. 2000). Microemboli are seen both in dissection of carotid and vertebral arteries, and possibly predict thromboembolic events (Droste, Junker et al. 2001). Presence of microemboli may be a determining factor in choosing the right medication, favoring anticoagulation over antiplatelet agents (Engelter, Brandt et al. 2007).

5.4.2 Monitoring during and after carotid endarterectomy

Presence of microemboli during carotid endarterectomy is an indicator of new ischemic events (Ackerstaff, Moons et al. 2000) (Ackerstaff, Jansen et al. 1995). Presence of microemboli should alert the physician to change the surgical technique. Ongoing microemboli after endarterectomy indicates other sources of emboli, which prompt reassessment of the operated carotid as well as searching for other sources.

6. Uncertainties and future directives

Microembolic signals have been identified in a number of clinical neurovascular settings with a variety of embolic sources, but predominantly in patients with large vessel atherosclerosis. In these patients microembolic signals may be an independent predictor of future stroke or TIA, but the association between microembolic signals and long-term clinical outcome has not always been found (Lund, Rygh et al. 2000; Abbott, Chambers et al. 2005). Research has mainly focused on quantity, i.e. presence or frequency of microemboli, but less on quality, i.e. size or constituents of microemboli due to technical limitations. After years of studies, the relevance of microemboli in the individual patient with acute stroke remains elusive and uncertainty prevails. There may be several reasons for this, of which the timing of assessment may be of great relevance. Studies have been performed within 24 hours, 48 hours, 72 hours, or even 7 days. The implications of microemboli in the early hours after stroke may be different from those at later stages. The number of microemboli seems to be inversely associated with the time from stroke onset. Early microemboli may reflect an ongoing acute vascular process, which might be satisfactorily controlled with adequate antithrombotic and statin treatment. Late microemboli persisting in spite of adequate treatment may reflect a true malignant vascular process with a high risk of future stroke. And in between, there is a transition time zone with microemboli of possibly varying long-term clinical relevance. Embolization is, however, not a continuous or a random process. Embolization occurs with temporal clustering and may occur outside the microemboli monitoring time window. Strength of TCD monitoring is it's time resolution. It is conceivable that repeated microemboli monitoring over time will yield more information than what a short glimpse at one single time-point does. The temporal variability of embolization underlines the need for repeated long-lasting microemboli monitoring to improve estimation of true embolic load and pattern of embolization (Mackinnon, Aaslid et al. 2005).

The size of an embolus is of obvious relevance. Although embolic signals become more intense with increasing thrombus size, there is currently no method for estimating size (Martin, Chung et al. 2009). Low-intensity signals are routinely rejected in standard monitoring set-up, but there may be many real microemboli among these low-intensity microemboli signals, and the presence of low-intensity microemboli signals significantly increases the chance of finding high-intensity microemboli signals (Telman, Sprecher et al. 2011). Therefore, low-intensity microemboli signals need increased attention as a possible marker of clinically significant embolization. Quality of microemboli may be further analyzed using transcranial power M-mode Doppler and an energy signature. This approach may define a subgroup of patients with malignant microemboli, who have larger baseline infarcts, and worse clinical outcome (Choi, Saqqur et al. 2010). In general, careful assessment of diffusion-weighted MRI may give indirect evidence of the size of microemboli (Droste, Knapp et al. 2007).

Microemboli are markers of disease activity, not the disease itself. Microemboli have been associated with carotid plaque inflammation (Moustafa, Izquierdo-Garcia et al. 2010), coagulopathies (Seok, Kim et al. 2010) and platelet activation markers (Ritter, Jurk et al. 2009). Adding information on basic disease mechanisms may improve our understanding of the complex pathophysiology of acute embolic stroke as defined by MES monitoring.

7. Conclusion

The assessment of microemboli in acute stroke needs to move from quantity to quality, taking into account the natural variability in embolization rates and the temporal clustering of embolization. There is need to establish optimal monitoring protocols with extensive time windows. The emboli as such need to be understood within the complex framework of acute stroke, including vessel wall or cardiac pathology, inflammation and coagulation, as well as end-organ damage. Multimodal approach, including transcranial microemboli monitoring, is a prerequisite for future advances in embolic stroke.

8. References

Abbott, A. L., B. R. Chambers, et al. (2005). "Embolic signals and prediction of ipsilateral stroke or transient ischemic attack in asymptomatic carotid stenosis: a multicenter prospective cohort study." *Stroke* 36(6): 1128-33.

Ackerstaff, R. G., C. Jansen, et al. (1995). "The significance of microemboli detection by means of transcranial Doppler ultrasonography monitoring in carotid endarterectomy." *J Vasc Surg* 21(6): 963-9.

Ackerstaff, R. G., K. G. Moons, et al. (2000). "Association of intraoperative transcranial doppler monitoring variables with stroke from carotid endarterectomy." *Stroke* 31(8): 1817-23.

Babikian, V. L., C. Hyde, et al. (1994). "Clinical correlates of high-intensity transient signals detected on transcranial Doppler sonography in patients with cerebrovascular disease." *Stroke* 25(8): 1570-3.

Brown, W. R., D. M. Moody, et al. (1996). "Histologic Studies of Brain Microemboli in Humans and Dogs After Cardiopulmonary Bypass." *Echocardiography* 13(5): 559-566.

Censori, B., T. Partziguian, et al. (2000). "Doppler microembolic signals predict ischemic recurrences in symptomatic carotid stenosis." *Acta Neurol Scand* 101(5): 327-31.

Choi, Y., M. Saqqur, et al. (2010). "Relative energy index of microembolic signal can predict malignant microemboli." *Stroke* 41(4): 700-6.

Daffertshofer, M., S. Ries, et al. (1996). "High-intensity transient signals in patients with cerebral ischemia." *Stroke* 27(10): 1844-9.

Del Sette, M., S. Angeli, et al. (1997). "Microembolic signals with serial transcranial Doppler monitoring in acute focal ischemic deficit. A local phenomenon?" *Stroke* 28(7): 1311-3.

Delcker, A., A. Schnell, et al. (2000). "Microembolic signals and clinical outcome in patients with acute stroke--a prospective study." *Eur Arch Psychiatry Clin Neurosci* 250(1): 1-5.

Dittrich, R., M. A. Ritter, et al. (2002). "Microembolus detection by transcranial doppler sonography." *Eur J Ultrasound* 16(1-2): 21-30.

Droste, D. W., K. Junker, et al. (2002). "Circulating microemboli in 33 patients with intracranial arterial stenosis." *Cerebrovasc Dis* 13(1): 26-30.

Droste, D. W., K. Junker, et al. (2001). "Clinically silent circulating microemboli in 20 patients with carotid or vertebral artery dissection." *Cerebrovasc Dis* 12(3): 181-5.

Droste, D. W., J. Knapp, et al. (2007). "Diffusion weighted MRI imaging and MES detection in the assessment of stroke origin." *Neurol Res* 29(5): 480-4.

Eicke, B. M., V. Barth, et al. (1996). "Cardiac microembolism: prevalence and clinical outcome." *J Neurol Sci* 136(1-2): 143-7.

Engelter, S. T., T. Brandt, et al. (2007). "Antiplatelets versus anticoagulation in cervical artery dissection." *Stroke* 38(9): 2605-11.

Esagunde, R. U., K. S. Wong, et al. (2006). "Efficacy of dual antiplatelet therapy in cerebrovascular disease as demonstrated by a decline in microembolic signals. A report of eight cases." *Cerebrovasc Dis* 21(4): 242-6.

Forteza, A. M., V. L. Babikian, et al. (1996). "Effect of time and cerebrovascular symptoms of the prevalence of microembolic signals in patients with cervical carotid stenosis." *Stroke* 27(4): 687-90.

Gao, S., K. S. Wong, et al. (2004). "Microembolic signal predicts recurrent cerebral ischemic events in acute stroke patients with middle cerebral artery stenosis." *Stroke* 35(12): 2832-6.

Georgiadis, D., A. Lindner, et al. (1997). "Intracranial microembolic signals in 500 patients with potential cardiac or carotid embolic source and in normal controls." *Stroke* 28(6): 1203-7.

Goertler, M., M. Baeumer, et al. (1999). "Rapid decline of cerebral microemboli of arterial origin after intravenous acetylsalicylic acid." *Stroke* 30(1): 66-9.

Goertler, M., T. Blaser, et al. (2001). "Acetylsalicylic acid and microembolic events detected by transcranial Doppler in symptomatic arterial stenoses." *Cerebrovasc Dis* 11(4): 324-9.

Gucuyener, D., N. Uzuner, et al. (2001). "Micro embolic signals in patients with cerebral ischaemic events." *Neurol India* 49(3): 225-30.

Idicula, T. T., H. Naess, et al. (2010). "Microemboli-monitoring during the acute phase of ischemic stroke: is it worth the time?" *BMC Neurol* 10: 79.

Iguchi, Y., K. Kimura, et al. (2008). "Microembolic signals at 48 hours after stroke onset contribute to new ischaemia within a week." *J Neurol Neurosurg Psychiatry* 79(3): 253-9.

Jander, S., M. Sitzer, et al. (1998). "Inflammation in high-grade carotid stenosis: a possible role for macrophages and T cells in plaque destabilization." *Stroke* 29(8): 1625-30.

Junghans, U. and M. Siebler (2003). "Cerebral microembolism is blocked by tirofiban, a selective nonpeptide platelet glycoprotein IIb/IIIa receptor antagonist." *Circulation* 107(21): 2717-21.

Kaposzta, Z., E. Young, et al. (1999). "Clinical application of asymptomatic embolic signal detection in acute stroke: a prospective study." *Stroke* 30(9): 1814-8.

Kaps, M., J. Hansen, et al. (1997). "Clinically silent microemboli in patients with artificial prosthetic aortic valves are predominantly gaseous and not solid." *Stroke* 28(2): 322-5.

Kessler, C. M. (1992). "Intracerebral platelet accumulation as evidence for embolization of carotid origin." *Clin Nucl Med* 17(9): 728-9.

Koennecke, H. C., H. Mast, et al. (1998). "Frequency and determinants of microembolic signals on transcranial Doppler in unselected patients with acute carotid territory ischemia. A prospective study." *Cerebrovasc Dis* 8(2): 107-12.

Kolominsky-Rabas, P. L., M. Weber, et al. (2001). "Epidemiology of ischemic stroke subtypes according to TOAST criteria: incidence, recurrence, and long-term survival in ischemic stroke subtypes: a population-based study." *Stroke* 32(12): 2735-40.

Kumral, E., K. Balkir, et al. (2001). "Microembolic signal detection in patients with symptomatic and asymptomatic lone atrial fibrillation." *Cerebrovasc Dis* 12(3): 192-6.

Lund, C., J. Rygh, et al. (2000). "Cerebral microembolus detection in an unselected acute ischemic stroke population." *Cerebrovasc Dis* 10(5): 403-8.

Mackinnon, A. D., R. Aaslid, et al. (2005). "Ambulatory transcranial Doppler cerebral embolic signal detection in symptomatic and asymptomatic carotid stenosis." *Stroke* 36(8): 1726-30.

Markus, H. S. and M. M. Brown (1993). "Differentiation between different pathological cerebral embolic materials using transcranial Doppler in an in vitro model." *Stroke* 24(1): 1-5.

Markus, H. S., D. W. Droste, et al. (2005). "Dual antiplatelet therapy with clopidogrel and aspirin in symptomatic carotid stenosis evaluated using doppler embolic signal detection: the Clopidogrel and Aspirin for Reduction of Emboli in Symptomatic Carotid Stenosis (CARESS) trial." *Circulation* 111(17): 2233-40.

Markus, H. S. and M. J. Harrison (1995). "Microembolic signal detection using ultrasound." *Stroke* 26(9): 1517-9.

Markus, H. S. and A. MacKinnon (2005). "Asymptomatic embolization detected by Doppler ultrasound predicts stroke risk in symptomatic carotid artery stenosis." *Stroke* 36(5): 971-5.

Martin, M. J., E. M. Chung, et al. (2009). "Thrombus size and Doppler embolic signal intensity." *Cerebrovasc Dis* 28(4): 397-405.

Molina, C. A., J. Alvarez-Sabin, et al. (2000). "Cerebral microembolism in acute spontaneous internal carotid artery dissection." *Neurology* 55(11): 1738-40.

Molloy, J. and H. S. Markus (1999). "Asymptomatic embolization predicts stroke and TIA risk in patients with carotid artery stenosis." *Stroke* 30(7): 1440-3.

Moustafa, R. R., D. Izquierdo-Garcia, et al. (2010). "Carotid plaque inflammation is associated with cerebral microembolism in patients with recent transient ischemic attack or stroke: a pilot study." *Circ Cardiovasc Imaging* 3(5): 536-41.

Nabavi, D. G., D. Georgiadis, et al. (1996). "Detection of microembolic signals in patients with middle cerebral artery stenosis by means of a bigate probe. A pilot study." *Stroke* 27(8): 1347-9.

Orlandi, G., G. Parenti, et al. (1997). "Silent cerebral microembolism in asymptomatic and symptomatic carotid artery stenoses of low and high degree." *Eur Neurol* 38(1): 39-43.

Poppert, H., S. Sadikovic, et al. (2006). "Embolic signals in unselected stroke patients: prevalence and diagnostic benefit." *Stroke* 37(8): 2039-43.

Ringelstein, E. B., D. W. Droste, et al. (1998). "Consensus on microembolus detection by TCD. International Consensus Group on Microembolus Detection." *Stroke* 29(3): 725-9.

Ritter, M. A., R. Dittrich, et al. (2008). "Prevalence and prognostic impact of microembolic signals in arterial sources of embolism. A systematic review of the literature." *J Neurol* 255(7): 953-61.

Ritter, M. A., K. Jurk, et al. (2009). "Microembolic signals on transcranial Doppler ultrasound are correlated with platelet activation markers, but not with platelet-leukocyte associates: a study in patients with acute stroke and in patients with asymptomatic carotid stenosis." *Neurol Res* 31(1): 11-6.

Russell, D., K. P. Madden, et al. (1991). "Detection of arterial emboli using Doppler ultrasound in rabbits." *Stroke* 22(2): 253-8.

Sebastian, J., C. Derksen, et al. (2011). "The role of transcranial Doppler embolic monitoring in the management of intracranial arterial stenosis." *J Neuroimaging* 21(2): e166-8.

Segura, T., J. Serena, et al. (2001). "Embolism in acute middle cerebral artery stenosis." *Neurology* 56(4): 497-501.

Seok, J. M., S. G. Kim, et al. (2010). "Coagulopathy and embolic signal in cancer patients with ischemic stroke." *Ann Neurol* 68(2): 213-9.

Serena, J., T. Segura, et al. (2000). "Microembolic signal monitoring in hemispheric acute ischaemic stroke: a prospective study." *Cerebrovasc Dis* 10(4): 278-82.

Siebler, M., A. Kleinschmidt, et al. (1994). "Cerebral microembolism in symptomatic and asymptomatic high-grade internal carotid artery stenosis.' *Neurology* 44(4): 615-8.

Siebler, M., A. Nachtmann, et al. (1995). "Cerebral microembolism and the risk of ischemia in asymptomatic high-grade internal carotid artery stenosis." *Stroke* 26(11): 2184-6.

Sitzer, M., M. Siebler, et al. (1995). "Cerebral microembolism in atherosclerotic carotid artery disease: facts and perspectives." *Funct Neurol* 10(6): 251-8.

Sliwka, U., A. Lingnau, et al. (1997). "Prevalence and time course of microembolic signals in patients with acute stroke. A prospective study." *Stroke* 28(2): 358-63.

Spence, J. D., A. Tamayo, et al. (2005). "Absence of microemboli on transcranial Doppler identifies low-risk patients with asymptomatic carotid stenosis." *Stroke* 36(11): 2373-8.

Spencer, M. P., G. H. Lawrence, et al. (1969). "The use of ultrasonics in the determination of arterial aeroembolism during open-heart surgery." *Ann Thorac Surg* 8(6): 489-97.

Telman, G., E. Sprecher, et al. (2011). "Potential relevance of low-intensity microembolic signals by TCD monitoring." *Neurol Sci* 32(1): 107-11.

Tinkler, K., M. Cullinane, et al. (2002). "Asymptomatic embolisation in non-valvular atrial fibrillation and its relationship to anticoagulation therapy." *Eur J Ultrasound* 15(1-2): 21-7.

Tong, D. C. and G. W. Albers (1995). "Transcranial Doppler-detected microemboli in patients with acute stroke." *Stroke* 26(9): 1588-92.

Valton, L., V. Larrue, et al. (1998). "Microembolic signals and risk of early recurrence in patients with stroke or transient ischemic attack." *Stroke* 29(10): 2125-8.

Wong, K. S. (2005). "Is the measurement of cerebral microembolic signals a good surrogate marker for evaluating the efficacy of antiplatelet agents in the prevention of stroke?" *Eur Neurol* 53(3): 132-9.

Wong, K. S., S. Gao, et al. (2002). "Mechanisms of acute cerebral infarctions in patients with middle cerebral artery stenosis: a diffusion-weighted imaging and microemboli monitoring study." *Ann Neurol* 52(1): 74-81.

Wong, K. S., S. Gao, et al. (2001). "A pilot study of microembolic signals in patients with middle cerebral artery stenosis." *J Neuroimaging* 11(2): 137-40.

Zuromskis, T., R. Wetterholm, et al. (2008). "Prevalence of micro-emboli in symptomatic high grade carotid artery disease: a transcranial Doppler study." *Eur J Vasc Endovasc Surg* 35(5): 534-40.

8

Intracranial Stenting for Acute Ischemic Stroke

Ahmad Khaldi and J. Mocco
University of Florida,
USA

1. Introduction

Stroke is the third major cause of death in the US. In the past decade there has been an exponential growth in modalities to treat acute stroke with acute recanalization therapies, including intravenous thrombolysis, intra-arterial chemical thrombolysis and mechanical thrombectomy, thromboaspiration, or angioplasty. While these new modalities of therapy have been promising, there remains a very real limitation to the overall rate of successful recanalization for current standard interventions. As a result, extrapolation from the cardiac literature has lead to early efforts using primary intracranial stenting to achieve safe recanalization. A major advantage of intracranial stenting is immediate flow restoration, as time to recanalization has repeatedly been shown to be a strong predictor of outcome in stroke. We will provide a cursory review each of the major established methods of acute stroke recanalization therapy, followed by a detailed review of intracranial stenting for acute stroke recanalization.

2. Intravenous tPA thrombolysis

Recombinant tissue-plasminogen activator (rt-PA) has been approved by the FDA for the use as a medical therapy in acute stroke. However, only 1% of acute stroke patients' patients in the US receive rt-PA (Barber 2001). The rate of recanalization using intravenous rt-PA is around 10%-30% when used within 3 hours of symptoms onset (Wolpert et al 2007). The rates of recanalization of large vessels are modest at best. Recanalization of a large internal carotid artery occlusion using intravenous rt-PA is around 10% and it can be as high as 30% of Middle Cerebral artery occlusion (Wolpert et al 2007) (Saqqur 2007). Recent studies, including European Cooperative Acute Stroke Study 3 (ECASS 3), have demonstrated that there may be a benefit in administrating intravenous rt-PA up to 4.5 hours from the time of onset (Hacke 2008).

3. Intraarterial tPA thrombolysis

Large proximal intracranial arteries can be recanalized more effectively with intra-arterial rt-PA than with intravenous rt-PA (Tomsick 2008). The Prolyse in Acute Cerebral Thromboembolism (PROACT) II trial revealed that intra-arterial proukinase within 6 hours of onset has 66% recanalization rate but with a higher intracranial hemorrhage 10% versus 2%. In other words, for every 7 patients that are treated with intraarterial rt-PA, 1 patient will benefit (Furlan Jama 1999). Following the IMS (Interventioanl Managmenet of Stroke) I and II pilot trials, where the combined intervention of both intravenous and intraarterial re-PA was more effective than the standard intravenous rt-PA alone for patients with NIH stroke scale of 10 or worse (IMS II 2007), the IMS III trial is currently underway. The aim of the IMS III trial is to enroll 900 patients with NIH stroke scale of 10 or higher and to randomize them to IV tPA therapy alone or IV tPA plus intra-arterial rt-PA infusion, MERCI thrombus-removal device (see below), Penumbra Aspiration Device (see below) or infusion of rt-PA with low intensity ultrasound at the site of the occlusion (Khatri 2008).

4. Mechanical thrombectomy

There are multiple mechanical thrombolysis techniques on the market today that treat acute stroke. They include Merci retriever (Concentric Medical, Mountain View, CA), snares and Alligator (EV3, Irvine, CA). Mechanical Embolus Removal in Cerebral Ischemia (MERCI) trial in 2004 revealed a recanalization rate of 64% within 6 hours of onset of stroke when used with or without intra-arterial rt-PA (Gobin 2004). Advancement in device design has lead to improved outcome with rate of recanalization exceeding 69% when using intra-arterial rt-PA as an adjunct to MERCI device (Smith 2008). The use of Snare (Medical Device Technologies, Gainesville, Fl) and alligator devices has been limited. Case report and small case series have been noted in the literature. For example, Hussain et al (Hussain 2009) describes a case series of 7 patients were alligator device was used to remove a clot in a straight segment vessels. Of the 7 patients, 5 attempts were successful in retrieving the clot with 1 complete recanalization and 4 with partial recanalization.

5. Thromboaspiration

Penumbra system (Penumbra, Alameda, CA) has shown to be very effective in acute stroke in early studies. One small series reported a revascularization rate of 100% in 21 vessels (20 patients) (TIMI 2 or 3) when using the Penumbra device (Bose 2008). At 30 days post-procedure, 45% of the patients had an improvement of 4 point or better on the NIH stroke scale with a modified Rankin scale of 2 or better. The mortality rate was high (45%) but was not unexpected as the initial NIH stroke scale had a mean of 21 (Bose 2008). Importantly, more comprehensive studies have revealed less successful revascularization rates of 81.6% and an increased rate of intracranial hemorrhage, 28% (Penumbra Pivotal Stroke Trial Investigators 2009). Additionally concerning was that only a modest number of patients did achieve independent outcome at 90 days. Of interest, there was a higher recanalization rate in both internal carotid artery (82.6%) and middle cerebral artery (83%) clots, which suggest that the penumbra device might be particularly useful for large vessel occlusions.

6. Angioplasty

Balloon angioplasty can augment thrombolysis especially in cases of proximal middle cerebral artery occlusion. There are two retrospective studies with 16 total patients revealing that the use angioplasty was successful in 10 patients when used followed failure of chemical thrombolytic agents (Mori 1999). Complications of angioplasty include arterial dissection and "snow plowing" effect (occlusion of vessel perforators at the ostium by plaque displacement) (Levy 2006). Inflating the balloon to 90% of the parent vessel diameter has been suggested as a angioplasty technique in order to reduce the potential risk the intracranial vessel walls (Levy 2007).

7. Intracranial stents

The use of intracranial stent provides a great benefit of restoring immediate flow to the effected area. The evolution of using intracranial stenting for recanalization is a concept that is adopted from the cardiac literature.

Early successful use of balloon-mounted coronary stents, in the setting of acute stroke, has advanced the field of intracranial stenting (Levy 2009). Self-expanding stents were first introduced in 2002 with a modification designed for intracranial atherosclerosis became available later in 2005. Until recently, intracranial stents have been viewed as a reasonable "last resort" technique in acute stroke revascularization, however increasing interest has developed around using stents as a first-line modality for stroke treatment.

Despite acute stentings origins being found in the cardiac literature, it is important to note that intracranial pathology differs from cardiac pathology in two major ways. First, cerebral arteries lack an extensive external elastic lamina and are relatively fixed in position because of small branching and perforating arteries (Lee 2009). Therefore, any technology used intracranially, must be appropriately navigable and atraumatic. Second, cerebral occlusion is often the result of emboli lodged in a healthy vessel, whereas coronary artery occlusion is more commonly a product of local vessel disease. This may mean that stenting is of less value in acute stroke; however, an alternative hypothesis is that stent placement allows the opening of a channel in an embolus while limiting distal emboli and perforator occlusion.

The first reports of using stents for acute stroke were retrospective series utilizing balloon-mounted cardiac stents. These achieved a high recanalization rate (79% had TIMI grade 2 or 3 flow) (Levy 2006). Of the 19 patients that were treated within 6.5 hours of the onset of symptoms, 6 died and 1 had asymptomatic intracranial hemorrhage. While these results were excellent, in general, balloon-mounted stents are relatively inflexible and are difficult to deploy in the anterior circulation.

The introduction of self-expanding stents has provided, at least a theoretical advantage, by decreasing the risk of vessel dissection or rupture and reducing the barotrauma to the parent's vessel (Levy 2006). Advantages of self-expanding stents include easier navigation to the target vessel, adaptation to the shape and anatomy of the affected vessel, and reduce rate of parent vessel rupture or dissection. The intracranial stents that are currently on the market in the US are Neuroform (Stryker Neurovascular, Freemont, CA), Wingspan (Stryker Neurovascular, Freemont, CA), and Enterprise (Codman, Raynham, MA). Only Wingspan is FDA-approved for the treatment of symptomatic intracranial stenosis, while others are indicated for coil assistant treatment. The Neuroform and the wingspan stents are open cell design while the Enterprise is a closed cell design.

Early case reports using the self expanding intracranial specific stents for arterial recanalization in 2 adults patients were first published in 2006 (Fitzsimmons 2006, Sauvageau 2006). This was followed by a multicenter, retrospective review of intracranial stenting for acute stroke in 2007 (Levy 2007) that demonstrated a successful recanalization rate of 79% (TIMI 2 or 3) in 18 patients (19 lesions). The use of self -expanding stents (Neuroform 16, wingspan 3) with a combination of thrombolysis and angioplasty, MERCI device, and/or glycoprotein IIb/IIIa inhibitor had no increased intraprocedural complication, however, there were 7 deaths with 4 due to progression of stroke, 2 from intracranial hemorrhage and an additional patient suffered respiratory failure. Of note, 7 patients had an improvement in their NIH scale within 24 hours from the procedure of 4 or greater points (Levy 2007).

A similar retrospective study of 9 patients who underwent placement of intracranial self-expanding stent intervention in the setting of acute stroke had recanalization rate of 89% (TIMI 2 or 3) (Zaidat 2008). The mean time to treatment was 5.1 hours with successful deployment of 9 stents (4 Neuroform, 5 Wingspan). Complications included 3 deaths, 1 intracrnial hemorrhage and 1 acute in-stent thrombosis that were treated with glycoprotein IIb/IIIa inhibitor. All the surviving patients had a good clinical outcome have modified Rakin Scale of 2 or better at 90 days follow-up appointment.

Brekenfeld et al., in a single center retrospective study of self-expanding stents for acute stroke achieved 92% recanalization (TIMI 2 or 3) in 12 patients (Brekenfeld 2009). Treatment also included the use of thrombolysis, thromboaspiration, thromboembolectomy, and angioplasty as well stent placement. Complications included 1 vessel dissection and 4 deaths but no intracranial hemorrhages. The overall outcome was good in 3 patients (modified Rankin Scale of 0-2) and moderate in 3 patients (modified Rankin Scale 3) and poor in 6 (modified Rankin Scale of 4-6) at 90 days follow-up.

Stent-Assisted Recanalization in Acute Ischemic Stroke (SARIS) trial was the first FDA approved prospective trial for the use of stenting in the treatment of acute stroke (Levy 2009 stroke). The patients that were included had poor NIH Stroke scale (mean 14) and were treated within 5.5 hours of onset of symptoms. Adjuvant therapy included angioplasty (8), intravenous rt-PA (2) and intra-arterial thrombolytics (10). There was 100% recanalization in 20 patients (Wingspan 17, Enterprise 2, No Deployment 1) and three intracranial hemorrhages occurring within 24 hours with one symptomatic hemorrhage. An improvement of 4 points or more on NIH stroke scale was achieved in 65% of the patients. Sub-acute outcomes demonstrated that 12 patients (60%) had a modified Rankin Scale of 3 or better at 30 days and additional 5 patients (25%) died of complications related to the stroke. More recently Mocco et al. revealed similar results in 20 patients with acute stroke were treated with Enterprise stent (Mocco 2010). Of the 20 patients, 10 had received intravenous rt-PA, which was unsuccessful. In addition, 12 patients had MERCI retrieval attempted, 7 had angioplasty, and 12 had administration of glycoprotein IIb-IIIa administration. Three patients had Wingspan stents deployed and one that had an Xpert Stent (Abbott, Abbott Park, and IL) deployed. Following the deployment of the Enterprise stent there was 100% recanalization with 75% of the patients having improved NIHSS (National Institute of Health Stroke Scale) > 4 points. There were 2 patients (10%) with symptomatic intracranial hemorrhage.

8. Intracranial stenting as a temporary measure:

The use of self-expanding stents as a temporary bypass, thereby allowing vessel recanalization while limiting the potential long-term complications that are associated with deploying a permanent stent such as in-stent stenosis or complications related to antiplatelet therapy. There are early case reports of using this technique in order to re-establish flow in a proximal Middle Cerebral artery occlusion despite failure of mechanical thrombolysis and chemical thrombolytics administration (Kelly 2008). The partial sheathing of an Enterprise stent allows for immediate revascularization of the artery without committing the patient for a permanent stent placement. After 20 minutes of blood flow, the stent was removed. The patient had a seven point's improvement to his NIH Stroke Scale following the procedure. A similar case was described using partially deployed Enterprise stent for a vertebrobasilar occlusion at 9 hours following onset. The patient did have 8 points improvement in their NIH stroke scale (Hauk 2009).

These early temporary deployment measures have led to further work in developing stent based thrombectomy tools, often referred to as "stent-on-a-stick". The most utilized of these rapidly expanding technology is the Solitaire device (EV3, Irvine, CA).
The Solitaire was first developed for assistance with wide-neck cerebral aneurysms (Lubicz 2010). Solitaire stent is a self-expanding stent that can be completely retrieved even when fully deployed (Lubicz 2010). A recent European study of 20 anterior circulation stroke patients treated within 8 hours of symptom onset with the Solitaire demonstrated a 90% revascularization rate, of which 16 had immediate restoration of flow following stent deployment (Castano 2010). Complications included 2 (10%) patients with intracranial hemorrhage, 4 (20%) died within 90 days. The 90 day follow up revealed that 45% of patients had a modified Rankin Scale score of 2 or better. There is also a recent randomized clinical trial of Solitaire Stent versus MERCI device, which has been completed, and the data is expected shortly. Additionally, there is an ongoing trial to evaluate a newer "stentriever" device called the Trevo (Concentric, Mountain View, CA). It is unknown, at this time, when this trial will be completed.

9. Conclusion

Acute stroke treatment has developed dramatically over the past decade and a half. Endovascular therapies have led to improved recanalization rates, while simultaneously extending the therapeutic time window. Recent publications suggest that intracranial stents effectively recanalize occluded cerebral blood vessels refractory to traditional techniques and, perhaps more excitingly, prospective data collected on the use of intracranial stents as a first line therapy have reported recanalization rates approaching 100%, and excellent clinical outcomes. While these data, from a highly selected series of patients, are certainly encouraging, significant concerns remain regarding the use of intracranial stents for acute stroke recanalization. These include the need for prolonged double antiplatelet therapy and continued limitations in the navigability of the current generation of intracranial stents. In the coming years we will doubtless see many further advances on the concepts of stent based acute stroke recanalization.

10. References

Barber, P. A., Zhang, J., Demchuk, A. M., Hill, M. D., & Buchan, A. M. (2001). Why are stroke patients excluded from TPA therapy? an analysis of patient eligibility. *Neurology, 56*(8), 1015-1020.

Bose, A., Henkes, H., Alfke, K., Reith, W., Mayer, T. E., Berlis, A., ... Penumbra Phase 1 Stroke Trial Investigators. (2008). The penumbra system: A mechanical device for the treatment of acute stroke due to thromboembolism. *AJNR.American Journal of Neuroradiology, 29*(7), 1409-1413. doi:10.3174/ajnr.A1110

Brekenfeld, C., Schroth, G., Mattle, H. P., Do, D. D., Remonda, L., Mordasini, P., . . . Gralla, J. (2009). Stent placement in acute cerebral artery occlusion: Use of a self-expandable intracranial stent for acute stroke treatment. *Stroke; a Journal of Cerebral Circulation, 40*(3), 847-852. doi:10.1161/STROKEAHA.108.533810

Castano, C., Dorado, L., Guerrero, C., Millan, M., Gomis, M., Perez de la Ossa, N., . . . Davalos, A. (2010). Mechanical thrombectomy with the solitaire AB device in large artery occlusions of the anterior circulation: A pilot study. *Stroke; a Journal of Cerebral Circulation, 41*(8), 1836-1840. doi:10.1161/STROKEAHA.110.584904

Fitzsimmons, B. F., Becske, T., & Nelson, P. K. (2006). Rapid stent-supported revascularization in acute ischemic stroke. *AJNR.American Journal of Neuroradiology, 27*(5), 1132-1134.

Furlan, A., Higashida, R., Wechsler, L., Gent, M., Rowley, H., Kase, C., . . . Rivera, F. (1999). Intra-arterial prourokinase for acute ischemic stroke. the PROACT II study: A randomized controlled trial. prolyse in acute cerebral thromboembolism. *JAMA : The Journal of the American Medical Association, 282*(21), 2003-2011.

Gobin, Y. P., Starkman, S., Duckwiler, G. R., Grobelny, T., Kidwell, C. S., Jahan, R., . . . Saver, J. L. (2004). MERCI 1: A phase 1 study of mechanical embolus removal in cerebral ischemia. *Stroke; a Journal of Cerebral Circulation, 35*(12), 2848-2854. doi:10.1161/01.STR.0000147718.12954.60

Hauck, E. F., Mocco, J., Snyder, K. V., & Levy, E. I. (2009). Temporary endovascular bypass: A novel treatment for acute stroke. *AJNR.American Journal of Neuroradiology, 30*(8), 1532-1533. doi:10.3174/ajnr.A1536

Hussain, M. S., Kelly, M. E., Moskowitz, S. I., Furlan, A. J., Turner, R. D.,4th, Gonugunta, V., . . . Fiorella, D. (2009). Mechanical thrombectomy for acute stroke with the alligator retrieval device. *Stroke; a Journal of Cerebral Circulation, 40*(12), 3784-3788. doi:10.1161/STROKEAHA.108.525618

IMS II Trial Investigators. (2007). The interventional management of stroke (IMS) II study. *Stroke; a Journal of Cerebral Circulation, 38*(7), 2127-2135. doi:10.1161/STROKEAHA.107.483131

Kelly, M. E., Furlan, A. J., & Fiorella, D. (2008). Recanalization of an acute middle cerebral artery occlusion using a self-expanding, reconstrainable, intracranial microstent as a temporary endovascular bypass. *Stroke; a Journal of Cerebral Circulation, 39*(6), 1770-1773. doi:10.1161/STROKEAHA.107.506212

Khatri, P., Hill, M. D., Palesch, Y. Y., Spilker, J., Jauch, E. C., Carrozzella, J. A., . . . Interventional Management of Stroke III Investigators. (2008). Methodology of the interventional management of stroke III trial. *International Journal of Stroke : Official Journal of the International Stroke Society, 3*(2), 130-137. doi:10.1111/j.1747-4949.2008.00151.x

Lee, V. H., Samuels, S., Herbst, T. J., Gallegos, M., Cochran, E. J., Chen, M., . . . Lopes, D. K. (2009). Histopathologic description of wingspan stent in acute ischemic stroke. *Neurocritical Care, 11*(3), 377-380. doi:10.1007/s12028-009-9258-0

Levy, E. I., & Chaturvedi, S. (2006). Perforator stroke following intracranial stenting: A sacrifice for the greater good? *Neurology, 66*(12), 1803-1804. doi:10.1212/01.wnl.0000227198.02597.15

Levy, E. I., Mehta, R., Gupta, R., Hanel, R. A., Chamczuk, A. J., Fiorella, D., . . . Hopkins, L. N. (2007). Self-expanding stents for recanalization of acute cerebrovascular occlusions. *AJNR.American Journal of Neuroradiology, 28*(5), 816-822.

Levy, E. I., Sauvageau, E., Hanel, R. A., Parikh, R., & Hopkins, L. N. (2006). Self-expanding versus balloon-mounted stents for vessel recanalization following embolic occlusion in the canine model: Technical feasibility study. *AJNR.American Journal of Neuroradiology, 27*(10), 2069-2072.

Levy, E. I., Siddiqui, A. H., Crumlish, A., Snyder, K. V., Hauck, E. F., Fiorella, D. J., . . . Mocco, J. (2009). First food and drug administration-approved prospective trial of primary intracranial stenting for acute stroke: SARIS (stent-assisted recanalization in acute ischemic stroke). *Stroke; a Journal of Cerebral Circulation, 40*(11), 3552-3556. doi:10.1161/STROKEAHA.109.561274

Lubicz, B., Collignon, L., Raphaeli, G., Bandeira, A., Bruneau, M., & De Witte, O. (2010). Solitaire stent for endovascular treatment of intracranial aneurysms: Immediate and mid-term results in 15 patients with 17 aneurysms. *Journal of Neuroradiology.Journal De Neuroradiologie, 37*(2), 83-88. doi:10.1016/j.neurad.2010.02.003

Mocco, J., Hanel, R. A., Sharma, J., Hauck, E. F., Snyder, K. V., Natarajan, S. K., . . . Levy, E. I. (2010). Use of a vascular reconstruction device to salvage acute ischemic occlusions refractory to traditional endovascular recanalization methods. *Journal of Neurosurgery, 112*(3), 557-562. doi:10.3171/2009.8.JNS09231

Mori, T., Kazita, K., Mima, T., & Mori, K. (1999). Balloon angioplasty for embolic total occlusion of the middle cerebral artery and ipsilateral carotid stenting in an acute stroke stage. *AJNR.American Journal of Neuroradiology, 20*(8), 1462-1464.

Penumbra Pivotal Stroke Trial Investigators. (2009). The penumbra pivotal stroke trial: Safety and effectiveness of a new generation of mechanical devices for clot removal in intracranial large vessel occlusive disease. *Stroke; a Journal of Cerebral Circulation, 40*(8), 2761-2768. doi:10.1161/STROKEAHA.108.544957

Saqqur, M., Uchino, K., Demchuk, A. M., Molina, C. A., Garami, Z., Calleja, S., ... Lotbust Investigators. (2007). Site of arterial occlusion identified by transcranial doppler predicts the response to intravenous thrombolysis for stroke. *Stroke; a Journal of Cerebral Circulation, 38*(3), 948-954. doi:10.1161/01.STR.0000257304.21967.ba

Sauvageau, E., & Levy, E. I. (2006). Self-expanding stent-assisted middle cerebral artery recanalization: Technical note. *Neuroradiology, 48*(6), 405-408. doi:10.1007/s00234-006-0077-0

Smith, W. S., Sung, G., Saver, J., Budzik, R., Duckwiler, G., Liebeskind, D. S., . . . Silverman, I. E. (2008). Mechanical thrombectomy for acute ischemic stroke: Final results of the multi MERCI trial. *Stroke; a Journal of Cerebral Circulation, 39*(4), 1205-1212. doi:10.1161/STROKEAHA.107.497115

Tissue plasminogen activator for acute ischemic stroke. the national institute of neurological disorders and stroke rt-PA stroke study group. (1995). *The New England Journal of Medicine, 333*(24), 1581-1587. doi:10.1056/NEJM199512143332401

Tomsick, T., Broderick, J., Carrozella, J., Khatri, P., Hill, M., Palesch, Y., . . . Interventional Management of Stroke II Investigators. (2008). Revascularization results in the interventional management of stroke II trial. *AJNR.American Journal of Neuroradiology, 29*(3), 582-587. doi:10.3174/ajnr.A0843

Wolpert, S. M., Bruckmann, H., Greenlee, R., Wechsler, L., Pessin, M. S., & del Zoppo, G. J. (1993). Neuroradiologic evaluation of patients with acute stroke treated with recombinant tissue plasminogen activator. the rt-PA acute stroke study group. *AJNR.American Journal of Neuroradiology, 14*(1), 3-13.

Zaidat, O. O., Wolfe, T., Hussain, S. I., Lynch, J. R., Gupta, R., Delap, J., . . . Fitzsimmons, B. F. (2008). Interventional acute ischemic stroke therapy with intracranial self-expanding stent. *Stroke; a Journal of Cerebral Circulation, 39*(8), 2392-2395. doi:10.1161/STROKEAHA.107.510966

9

Surgical Treatment of Patients with Ischemic Stroke Decompressive Craniectomy

Erion Musabelliu, Yoko Kato, Shuei Imizu, Junpei Oda and Hirotoshi Sano
Department of Neurosurgery, Fujita Health University, Toyoaka
Japan

1. Introduction

A number of patients with ischemic cerebrovascular stroke suffer a progressive deterioration secondary to massive cerebral ischemia, edema, and increased intracranial pressure (ICP). The evolution is often fatal. Stroke is the second - leading cause of death worldwide. Life-threatening, complete middle cerebral artery (MCA) infarction occurs in up to 10% of all stroke patients, and this may be characterized as massive hemispheric or malignant space - occupying supratentorial infarcts. Malignant, space - occupying supratentorial ischemic stroke is characterized by mortality up to 80%, several reports indicated a beneficial effect of hemicraniectomy in this situation, converting the closed, rigid cranial vault into a semi open.

The main cause of death encountered in these patients is severe postischemic brain edema leading to raised intracranial pressure, clinical deterioration, coma and death. The result is dramatic decrease in ICP and a reversal of the clinical and radiological signs of herniation. For these reasons, decompressive craniectomy has been increasingly proposed as a life-saving measure in patients with large, space-occupying hemispheric infarction. Recent successes with intra-venous and intra-arterial thrombolytic therapy have resulted in an increased awareness of stroke as a medical emergency. Thus, increasing numbers of patients are being evaluated in the early hours following the ictal event. In the process of gaining more experience in the early management of patients with acute ischemic stroke, it has become clear that in a number of these patients a progressive and often fatal deterioration secondary to mass effect from the edematous, infarcted tissue occurs. An increasing body of experimental and clinical evidence suggests that some of these patients may benefit from undergoing a decompressive craniectomy. But, the timing and indications for this potential lifesaving procedure are still debated.

The objectives of this chapter are;

- To help better define the selection criteria for performing the surgery in case of supratentorial infarctions,
- To assess the immediate outcome in terms of time conscious recovery and survival
- To assess long term outcome and quality of life, using standard and functional assessment scales

Complications have been reported in the literature when hemicraniectomy has been completed after cerebral infarction. Malignant cerebral ischemia occurs in a significant number of patients who undergo emergency evaluation for ischemic stroke. This patient

population can be identified by early clinical and neuroimaging characteristics. In some of these patients, Decompressive Craniectomy appears to be a life-saving procedure. If craniectomy is performed early, especially in young patients, a satisfactory functional outcome can be achieved in a significant proportion of cases. Clinical experience, however, demonstrates that even in such patients, an acceptable functional outcome can be achieved after surgery if some preservation of speech is present at the time of intervention.
Additional studies will have to be mounted to analyze in more detail these implications. Survival after Decompressive Craniectomy for MCA infarction is better than that reported after medical management alone. Early hemicraniectomy based on radiographic and clinical criteria, but before signs of brain stem herniation, has been proposed as a means of improving outcomes.

2. Historical background

Decompressive craniectomy procedures have been used to relieve increased ICP and cerebral oedema caused by a variety of pathological events. This technique (decompressive craniectomy) first applied in 1905. (10) In 1905, Cushing reported the use of this procedure to relieve the pressure caused by the growth of an intracranial tumour. (1, 39, 66) Since then, surgical decompression has been reported as a treatment option for traumatic head injury, (24, 26, 53, 42) subdural haematoma, (9, 56, 38) oedema resulting from vasospasm secondary to subarachnoid haemorrhage, (17) encephalitis, (39, 63) intracerebral haematoma, (13) cerebral venous and dural sinus thrombosis, (69) cerebellar infarction, (28, 31, 59) and supratentorial cerebral ischemia. (65, 45)
Non randomized and randomized control data published are reviewed and data are analyzed, enrolling result from recent and earlier studies.
In the 1950s and 60s, a number of reports were published in which the authors described cases of massive cerebral ischemia accompanied by acute and severe brain swelling. (1) These cases were often fatal, with the oedema caused by the infarct producing a "pseudotumour" increasing in pressure within the cranial vault. (44) In 1968, Greenwood used surgical intervention in the treatment of such cases, which decreased the mortality rate to below 50% as reported, (24) in his series of 9 patients with acute infarction involving the MCA or ICA, decompressive hemicraniectomy as well as resection of the necrotic parenchyma were performed. Six of these patients survived, although 3 suffered postoperatively from severe disability. In their report in 1971, Kjellberg and Prieto described a bifrontal decompressive craniectomy procedure for the treatment of a massive infarction; however, the patient did not survive. (41) In 1981, Rengachary and co-workers reported the first cases in which straightforward craniectomy were undertaken, without removal of necrotic brain tissue. (57) Since that study, more additional cases of hemicraniectomy and some with bilateral craniectomy have been reported in the treatment of massive cerebral ischemia. (50) Significant retrospective data support the hypothesis that decompressive hemicraniectomy decreases mortality rates due to this disease entity. Three randomized controlled studies shed light on these issues and enhance the quality of evidence revolving around this procedure.

3. "Malignant" cerebral infarction

Ischemic cerebral infarction is associated with a high rate of morbidity and mortality, which are highest when lesions involve the trunk of one or more of the main cerebral vessels. In fact, occlusion of either the distal Internal Carotid Artery (ICA) or proximal (MCA) trunk has been characterized as a "malignant" stroke in both clinical and animal studies, and these are the reason why we are considering this topic in relation with brain infarction in MCA territory. (15, 27) Of all cases with supratentorial infarctions in which an autopsy is performed, 13% are shown to suffer from severe brain swelling after an infarction involving the entire distribution of the ICA or MCA. (46, 49) Severe cerebral oedema can lead to herniation of cerebral structures through the tentorium or falx, as well as the brainstem structures through the foramen magnum. In fact, transtentorial herniation has been cited as the probable cause of death in many of these cases of malignant stroke. Bounds et al reviewed 100 autopsy cases of patients in whom an infarction involving the ICA distribution had been diagnosed. (5) Thirty-one patients died of tentorial herniation, which was the only neurological cause of death in all the cases reviewed.

The prognosis for patients who suffer a "malignant" cerebrovascular accident (CVA) is poor, with death occurring usually within the first 4 to 5 days. In this subset of patients, a mortality rate of 78% (estimated to be between 50% - 78%) was observed, (27) all deaths were attributed to transtentorial herniation, which occurred within 2 to 7 days (median 4 days). Similarly, in another set of data 81% of patients with malignant CVA died, and all deaths occurred within 5 days and were caused by herniation, (62, 64) given the poor prognosis in these patients, it is of critical importance to recognize imaging or clinical characteristics suggestive of such a progressive and rapid deterioration. In patients who suffer a malignant CVA the clinical course is generally predictable. The clinical course in these patients is uniform, with clinical deterioration developing within the first 2 to 3 days after stroke. Presenting symptoms may include the sudden onset of hemiplegia, homonymous hemianopsia, forced eye and head deviation toward the lesion side, and aphasia. Precipitous coma and papillary dilation usually occur together following the initial symptoms, (7, 12) in the absence of further intervention, death occurs.

To establish objective criteria for aggressive intervention, many investigators have measured intracranial pressure (ICP) once significant clinical deterioration is apparent. In an early study patients in whom ICP values were greater than 15 mm Hg did not survive the malignant infarct. (61) In subsequent studies other authors have shown that a fatal outcome occurred in most cases when the level was greater than 30 mm Hg. (7, 29, 51, 59, 74) In addition to clinical findings, neuroimaging criteria can help to identify those patients at particular risk for a malignant infarction in the early phase of their stroke. In patients with malignant CVA, a large area of parenchymal hypodensity in the MCA territory is often visualized on the admission CT scans (**Figure 1**). (59, 64, 74, 78)

With progressive clinical deterioration, CT-demonstrated signs may also include mass effect, effacement of the basal cisterns, compression of the ventricular system, a shift of midline structures, (78, 74) and herniation of tissue through the falx, foramen magnum, or tentorium. These patients present clinically with progressive deterioration of consciousness within the first 2 days. Thereafter, symptoms of transtentorial herniation occur within 2 to 4 days after onset of stroke. This clinical presentation is accompanied by early CT signs of major infarct during the first 12 hours after stroke, (74) as no model of medical treatment has been proven superior to the others, treatment options may vary, depending on each clinic protocol. The value of conventional therapies in this condition, as in others of raised ICP, consisting of artificial ventilation, osmotherapy, and barbiturate administration, has been a subject of debate.

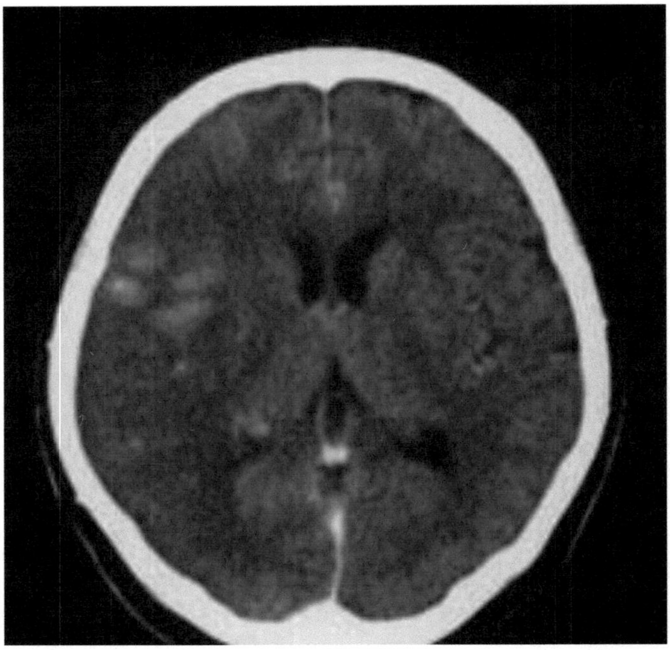

Fig. 1. CT scan demonstrating the R MCA territory infarction

4. Rationale for decompressive craniectomy and experimental studies

Cerebral ischemia results in oedema formation in and around the ischemic area, the larger the area of the infarction, the greater the extent of oedema. In the case of malignant CVA, the entire vascular distribution of the MCA, and possibly the anterior cerebral artery, is compromised. A severe oedematous response ensues throughout a large area. (61) Oedema is responsible for the parenchymal hypodensity that is demonstrated on CT scanning. (37, 56) One of the fundamental pathophysiological processes after cerebrovascular stroke is the development and propagation of an escalating cycle of brain swelling and an increase in ICP. The goals of the clinical management consist of interrupting this cycle by controlling ICP and maintaining cerebral perfusion pressure and cerebral blood flow to avoid brain ischemia. This management strategy has been developed as a result of reported strong correlations between uncontrollable high ICP and high rates of morbidity and mortality. The relationship between high ICP and poor outcome has been demonstrated consistently in both single-centre and multicenter studies and the ability to bring elevated ICP under control has long been considered a requirement for improving outcome of patients with severe head injuries. Progressive brain oedema and the exacerbating effect it has on increasing ICP can cause the area of damaged brain to extend. Within the confined cranial vault, the oedematous tissue places pressure against surrounding normal parenchyma. This is evidenced by the changes seen on CT scanning (**Figure 2**).

Intracranial hypertension results in decreased cerebral perfusion pressure and therefore decreasing blood supply throughout the cerebrum. Because of the increase in mechanical pressure and ICP, other major cerebral vessels may be compressed by the expanding tissue, against dural edges or against the skull. The result is secondary ischemia and a further expansion of the infracted area. (6)

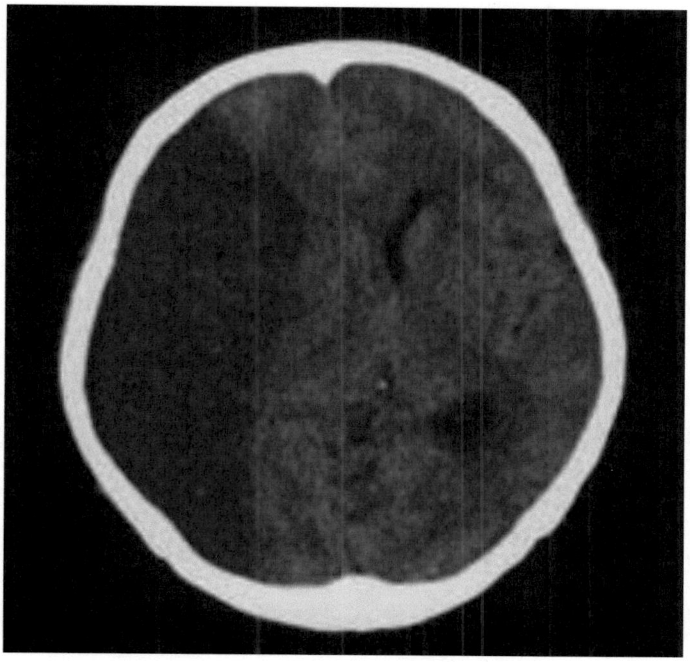

Fig. 2. CT scan on day one, demonstrating evolving R MCA infarction with mass effect and compression of the ventricular system. Clinical examination revealed right midriazis

Proposed as a life-saving procedure, increasing experimental and clinical evidence indicates that an early decompressive craniectomy can limit the extension of the infarcted area. From a mechanical perspective hemicraniectomy provides an immediate opening in the otherwise closed cranial vault. Therefore, compression of normal tissue is prevented or limited. The additional space created allows the tissue to expand through the bone defect, away from midline structures, so that CT-demonstrated changes normally observed when surgery is not performed like midline shift, decreased ventricular size, and herniation are minimized or completely resolved postoperatively. (37, 41, 61) As the cranial vault has essentially been expanded during surgery, there is an immediate decrease of ICP. The initial ICP values of 25 to 60 mm Hg decreased by 15% once the bone flap was removed, and by 70% once the dura was opened, resulting in the normalization of the ICP after surgery. (32) Similar findings were demonstrated when performed a bilateral craniectomy. (78, 80) In 2 patients with ischemic CVA whose initial ICP values were 54.8 mm Hg and 20 mm Hg, respectively, removal of the bone flap caused a decrease in ICP to 35.5 mm Hg and 10 mm Hg, and opening of the dura caused a reduction to 4.4 mm Hg and 3 mm Hg, respectively. In the immediate postoperative period, the ICP values were recorded as 4.4 mm Hg and 10.2 mm Hg. A decrease in ICP allows for an increase in cerebral perfusion pressure, aiding blood flow to the ischemic area, optimizing circulation to the damaged area through collateral vessels. Because hemicraniectomy alone may improve blood flow in the ischemic area, surgical resection of the infracted tissue should not be conducted in these patients. Although such resection or "strokectomy" has been associated with postoperative improvements in some cases, it is impossible in all the cases to differentiate at surgery between ischemic tissue and necrotic tissue. (34, 57) Being poorly delineated from necrotic tissue, the ischemic area may possibly be damaged or removed upon resection of the infarct.

5. Timing and indications of surgery

Hemicraniectomy has for a long time been used as a last resort to prevent impending death after all medical therapies have been attempted. The surgical procedure certainly preserves life, as evidenced by decreased mortality rates when compared with patients who undergo medical therapy alone. (61) In many of the reported cases, the symptoms of a severe herniation syndrome, fixed, dilated pupils, precipitous coma, cardiorespiratory difficulties and decerebrate posturing, were used to indicate the need for decompressive surgery. (37, 35, 40) Patients suffering malignant CVA receive antioedema medical treatment and hyperventilation or tissue plasminogen activator, (70) before considering a decompressive craniectomy. Usually, an initial reversal of symptoms, such as the degree of pupillary dilation, occurs with aggressive medical treatment. After its initial effectiveness, however, additional medical therapeutic efforts often fail to control or prevent herniation. In the case of massive cerebral ischemia, the effectiveness of such medical therapy is severely limited, at best, as evidenced by the high mortality rates observed in the absence of surgical intervention. In the case of stroke which is typically not treated surgically, physicians may wait too long to intervene surgically. Once the pupils are fixed and a deep coma has indicated an irreversible decline of cerebral function, surgery should not be performed. (57)

Parameter	Time of Surgery	Patient's outcomes. 1, 3, 6 months
Age	Mean ± SD	Survival after one month (in percentage - of enrolled patients)
Sex	Percentage	
Territory of infarction		Barthel Index
MCA	Number	NIHSS score
MCA/ ACA		MRS score
MCA/ PCA		
Hemisphere	Left / Right	
Pathological mechanism (if known)		Functionally independent
Emboli	Number	Mild to moderate disability
Dissection		Severely disabled
Other		
Other related disease/ conditions		
On admission		
Barthel Index Score	Mean ± SD	
SSS score		
GCS		
Time to surgery	Mean	
Imaging findings CT/ MRI		
Signs of herniation before surgery	Percentage	
Mortality rate (after surgery)	Percentage	
Time on NCU	Day	
Time of recovery		

NCU - Neurological Care Unit
ACA - Anterior Cerebral Artery
PCA - Posterior Cerebral Artery

Table 1. Clinical and instrumental criteria used in evaluation of the patient

Evaluation of experimental findings suggests that, early surgical decompressive surgery for the treatment of massive cerebral ischemia may limit the extension of the infarction and reduce morbidity. (14, 21) Craniectomy can decrease the infarct volume and improve neurological outcome in a rat model of MCA occlusion when surgery is completed early (1 hour postictus). (20) Similar results are found when surgery was completed 4 hours postictus. In the 4-hour treatment group, outcome and infarct volume were significantly better as compared with those observed in control animals and animals surgically treated at 12, 24 and 36 hours postictus. Animals treated at these later time periods improved, but no significant differences were reported among these three groups and the control group. (14) When patients who suffer malignant CVA were surgically treated on average 21 hours postictus, there was a greater decrease in mortality rate and length of stay in the intensive care unit as compared with patients who underwent surgery an average 39 hours postictus. There was also a trend of improved Barthel Index (BI) scores demonstrated at follow-up for patients in the earlier surgical group. Several factors need to be considered to optimize both the timing and the indication for decompressive craniectomy **(Table 1).** (26, 30, 32, 48, 71, 72)

6. Predictors of malignant cerebral edema

Severely compressive brain edema is associated with significant mortality and morbidity. From a pathophysiological view, early intervention could minimize secondary ischemia of viable tissue around the infarcted area and possibly prevent herniation. Optimal utility of this procedure would require identifying the population that is most likely to benefit in a way that meets patient's expectations as well as those of their families and caretakers.
By using diffusion weighted MR imaging, a stroke volume greater than 145 cm3 within 14 hours of onset of stroke symptoms has 100% sensitivity and 94% specificity for predicting the progression to malignant edema. (52) Additionally, in patients who suffered a massive MCA territory stroke, stroke volume greater than 50% of the MCA territory were identified, high white blood cell count, additional involvement of the anterior or posterior cerebral artery, systolic blood pressure higher than 180 mm Hg within 12 hours of stroke onset, and a history for the progression toward malignant edema. (36) Patients with an NIHSS score of 20 or greater on admission or who present with nausea or emesis are at high risk for developing malignant cerebral edema. (43) In addition to clinical and radiographic risk factors, serum levels of the astroglial protein S100B have been shown to be predictive of malignant cerebral edema with 94% sensitivity and 83% specificity (for a value of 1.03 mg/L at 24 hours from the ischemic event). (19) This may become a useful monitoring tool at crucial clinical time points at which the development of cerebral edema is believed to be an imminent possibility, once a commercially available bedside kit is available.

7. Time window for surgery

The question of the optimal time window for intervention has not yet been completely elucidated. (4, 26, 30, 32, 48, 71, 72) Although the pooled data from the European trials seem to show benefit from early surgery, only a small number of patients was included in the late group in the HAMLET, (30) and definite conclusions cannot be drawn at this time. Another sours of data, did not demonstrate a difference in outcome based on timing. (26) Clear definition of a time window for intervention will be essential to creating treatment guidelines. With that purpose in mind, 2 additional randomized control trials (RCTs), The

North American HeADDFIRST (Hemicraniectomy And Durotomy on Deterioration From Infarction Related Swelling Trial), aimed to evaluate patient outcome after hemicraniectomy within 96 hours from symptom onset, the HeMMI trial (Hemicraniectomy for Malignant Middle cerebral artery Infarcts) in the Philippines is studied patient morbidity and mortality after decompressive surgery within 72 hours from symptom onset.

8. Intracranial pressure monitoring

Intracranial pressure monitoring has been recommended as a guide to surgical timing. (81, 62) A measurement of greater than 25 mm Hg has been used despite attempts at medical therapy as an indicator for surgical intervention. (7, 59) Increased ICP measurements are preceded by the constellation of clinical signs and symptoms constituting the "malignant CVA syndrome;" thus, the usefulness of ICP monitoring in these cases has been questioned. But, brain tissue shifts rather than raised ICP are probably the most likely cause of the initial decrease in consciousness.

9. Neuroimaging studies

Extensive MCA infarction with oedema in greater than 50% of the MCA territory can be identified early after the ictal event on CT scans, and it is observed on the initial CT scan in approximately 69% of the reviewed cases by Hacke et al. (27) Parenchymal hypodensity in greater than 50% of the MCA territory is highly indicative of a progressive clinical course, leading to severe morbidity or death. With current, newer CT scanners, parenchymal hypodensity can be seen and followed soon after symptom onset **(Figure 3)**.

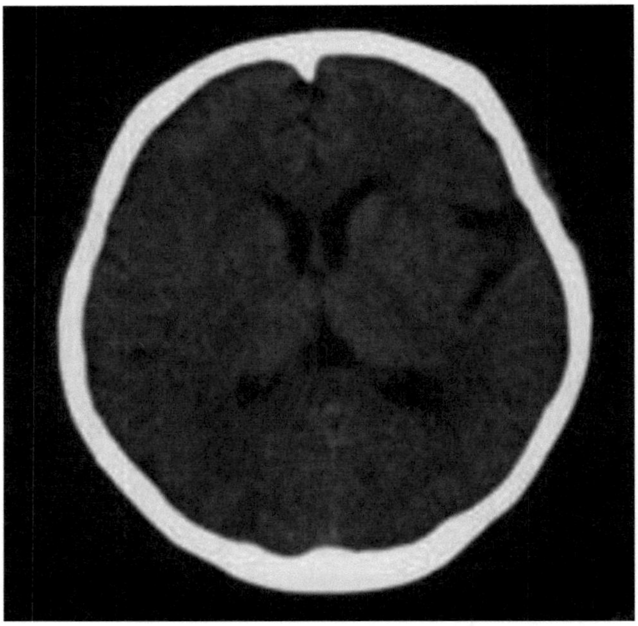

Fig. 3. CT scan demonstrating early CT findings of acute ischemic stroke (within 3 hours from onset) - slight changes, right sulci and Sylvian fissure effacement - effacement of R insular islands and structures of basal ganglia

In another set of data, most of the patients had at least two CT scans, one, within first 4 days after stroke and in some series within the first 12 hours after symptom onset, and the second one with the deterioration of symptoms and or after surgery **(Figures 4 and 5)**. (64, 65)

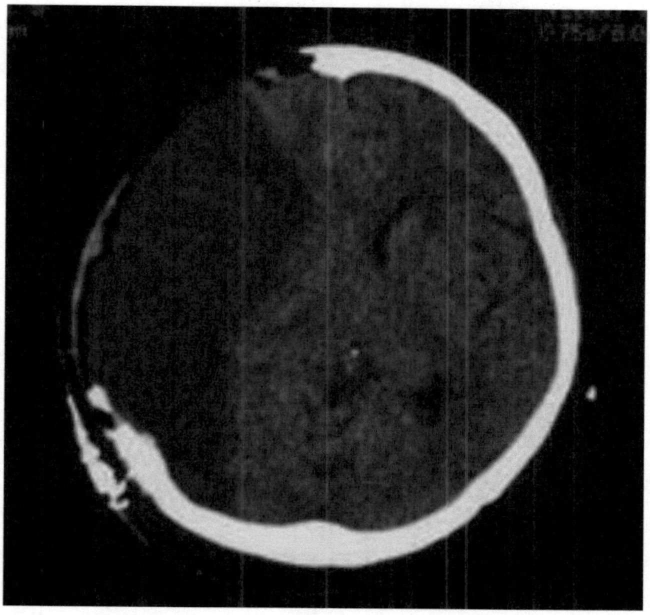

Fig. 4. CT scan, one day after hemicraniectomy (in which large frontoparieto-occipital bone was removed), revealing the resence of midline shift

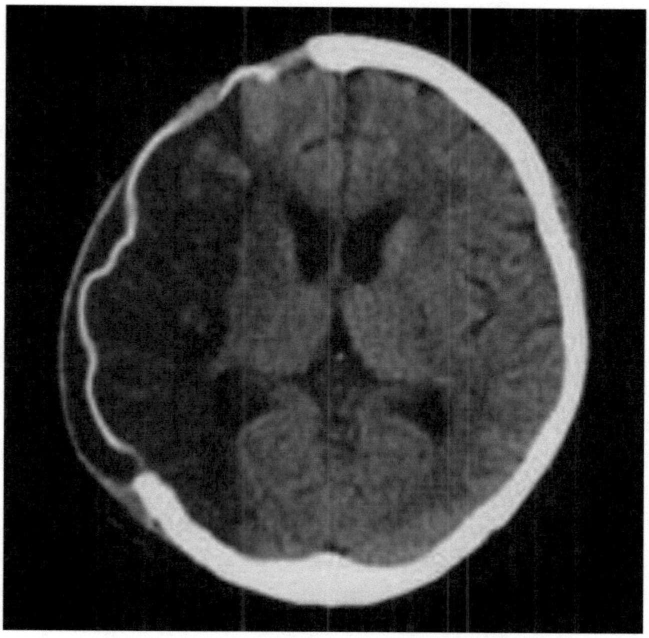

Fig. 5. CT scan, one month posthemicraniectomy, with resolution of previous midline shift

A midline shift of the cerebral structures is another phenomenon of increasing unilateral cerebral oedema that can be identified on CT scanning. The amount of midline shift was significantly different between survivors and nonsurvivors of malignant CVA. (59) In a study conducted to examine only the prognostic value of midline shift, it was suggested that at 32 hours after the occurrence of cerebral infarction, a shift of the third ventricle greater than 4 mm was indicative of a fatal outcome. (23) Regardless of its potential for prognostic significance however, midline shift is not visualized as early on CT scanning as is parenchymal hypodensity (**Figure 1**). Early changes demonstrated on CT scans are also an indicator of the viability of collateral circulation. Cerebral Angiography was performed (**Figure 6**) in patients in whom stroke was demonstrated early with CT scanning. (74)

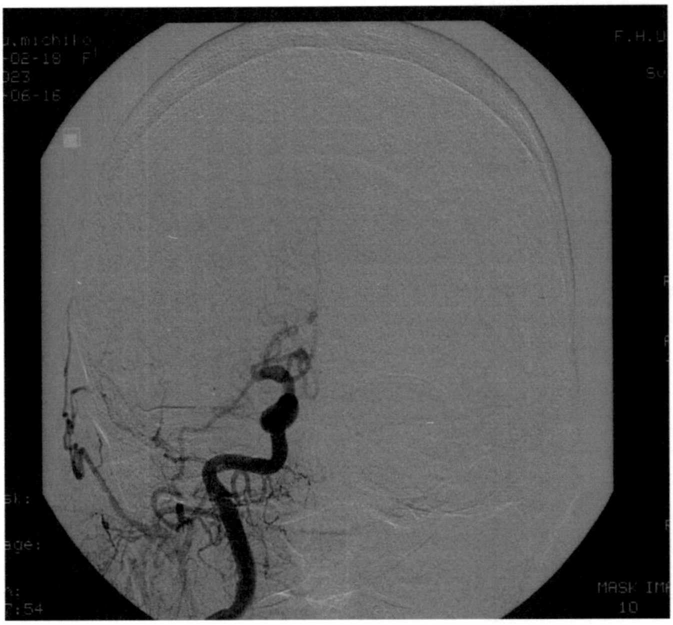

Fig. 6. R ICA AP angiogram reveals absence of R MCA - proximal occlusion

Comparing the angiographic findings with those obtained using CT scanning, the authors observed that parenchymal hypodensity in greater than 50% of the MCA territory was predictive of poor collateral circulation, as evidenced by the angiographic study. (74) These findings are important, because in patients with adequate collateral circulation, decompressive hemicraniectomy may not be necessary.

From neuroradiological studies it has been well recognized that "early visual radiolucency" in the CT examination is a negative outcome predictor. Continued refinements of newer imaging techniques such as diffusion / perfusion magnetic resonance will lead to an earlier identification of those patients more likely to benefit from early decompressive craniectomy. **(Figures 7 and 8)**

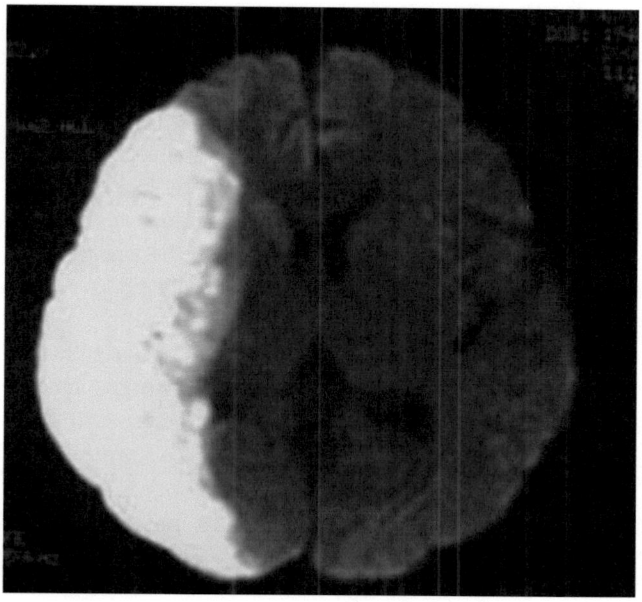

Fig. 7. MRI T2-weight diffusion, revealing R MCA territory infarction with early cytotoxic oedema

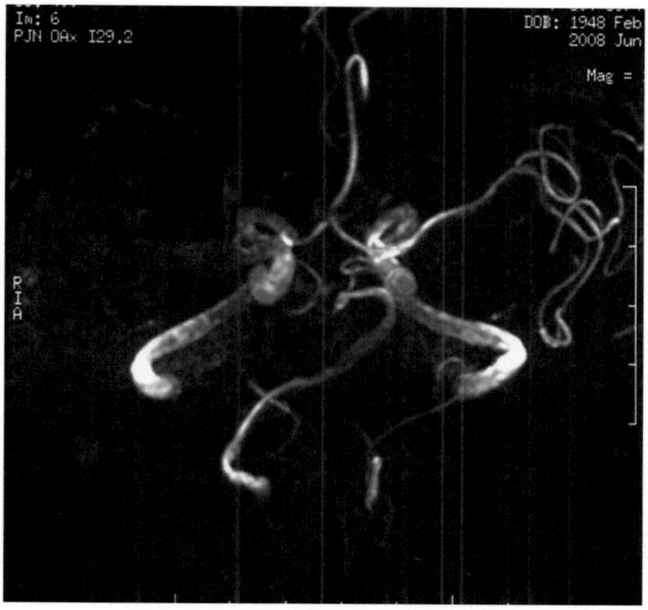

Fig. 8. MR angiography revealing the absence of flow - related enhancement in the R MCA. Confirming persistent proximal occlusion of R MCA.

10. Patient age and surgical age limit

The age of patients undergoing surgical intervention reported in the reviewed series ranged from 11 to 70 years of age. Based on data provided in the literature, it was impossible to determine if a certain age range of patients benefits more from surgical decompression. Most investigators, however, noted that they are more aggressive in performing hemicraniectomy in young patients in whom CVA has occurred and that the young seemed to benefit more from the procedure. By dividing patients by age in those younger than, and older than 50 years of age, it is found that patients under the age of 50 years made a good functional outcome (Barthel Index scores > 60 [100 = independent, 60-95 minimum assistance, and < 60 = dependent]), but not at all the patients over 50 years of age was this observed at follow-up examinations. (7) In theory and in practice, it would seem that younger patients with ischemic stroke would benefit from early decompressive surgery for the following reasons:

- Their brains are less atrophied, allowing less room for oedematous expansion within the cranial vault. Individuals aged 50 years and younger have been identified as benefiting more from bilateral decompressive craniectomy in cases of subarachnoid haemorrhage because of their unatrophied brains, as compared with those over 50 years of age.
- The ventricular system in younger persons is smaller than in older persons.
- It has been proposed that the oedematous response to ischemia is greater in younger individuals.

Randomized trials to date have focused on patients 60 years of age and younger, thus leaving us with very few data regarding patients older than 60 years of age. The HAMLET displayed conflicting results with previous review series (30) with a trend toward better outcome in the upper age categories (51–61 years). These results raised questions about the existence of an age limit for surgical benefit. The DESTINY RCT will shed more light on the impact of surgery in patients older than 60 years. (33) In patients older than 60 years of age, assessing outcome following decompressive craniectomy of malignant MCA infarction, mortality rate and functional outcome, as measured by Barthel Index (BI) and modified ranking scale (mRS), were significantly worse in patients older than 60 years of age following decompressive craniectomy. (3) Age is an important factor to consider in patient selection for surgery. However, cautious interpretation of the results is required because the outcome scores that were used only measure physical disability, whereas other factors, including psychosocial, financial, and caregiver burden, should be considered in addition to age alone.

11. Dominant hemisphere infarction

As a rule, investigators in the past did not undertake surgery in patients with dominant hemisphere infarctions. The loss of communicative abilities and a plegic dominant upper extremity were judged to be too damaging. Analysis of recent evidence suggests that considering a dominant hemisphere infarction to be a contraindication to surgery may be too harsh a criterion. (60, 65) Functionally, the patients with the dominant hemisphere infarct who underwent hemicraniectomy were not significantly different from those patients who underwent craniectomy after CVA in the nondominant hemisphere. Therefore, surgery can be considered in patients with dominant hemisphere infarction, especially if some residual language function is present at admission.

While the fear of complete aphasia was classically the reason behind the refusal to operate on large dominant hemispheric strokes, data have suggested that nondominant hemispheric injuries leading to serious depression and neglect can be as disabling as aphasia during the rehabilitation process. (76) Additionally a subset analysis in the DECIMAL trial showed no difference in the mRS scores of survivors with or without aphasia at 1 year; in addition, all surgical survivors agreed with the decisions to undergo surgery when asked retrospectively, including patients still experiencing aphasia. (72) Stroke laterality and its correlation with outcome (29, 30, 33, 34, 71) have also been the subject of subgroup analysis in other trials and controlled and uncontrolled studies have shown no predicative value for outcome related to laterality.

There has been interest in identifying which patients will develop malignant cerebral oedema after massive infarcts, patients at high risk (**Table 2**).

Inclusion criteria	Exclusion criteria
Age 18 - 60 years	Prestroke mRS score ≥ 2
NIHSS score nondominant hemisphere > 18 dominant hemisphere > 20	Prestroke score Barthel Index < 95
Imaging - documented unilateral infraction. MCA at least 2/3 of territory and at least part of basal ganglia. ± Additional infarctions in ACA or PCA territory. Ipsilateraly.	GCS < 6
Time – onset of symptoms	bilateral - pupils fixed and dilated Other brain related diseases Haemorrhagic transformation of the infarct Life expectancy < 3 years Other related disease/ conditions - affecting outcome. Especially coagulopathy/ systemic blooding disorders. Pregnancy. Contraindication for anaesthesia

Table 2. Criteria proposed to use for inclusion/ exclusion of patients and clinical outcome.

12. Surgical technique, results and limits

12.1 Operative technique

Hemicraniectomy for supratentorial infarction usually involves aggressive bone removal to alleviate better the symptoms of malignant cerebral oedema. The need for a radical approach, extension of bone removal, was recognized in the event of severe posttraumatic cerebral oedema, this was echoed in the case of massive cerebral ischemia when a few of initial surgically treated patients harboured a bone defect that was too small, not providing adequate space for decompression and resulting in brain herniation through the skull opening. (25, 60) Prolapsed of the oedematous brain through the edges of the craniectomy defect, with possible exacerbation of brain damage is one of the possible limitations of decompressive craniectomy. In the case of cerebral infarction, however, this phenomenon does not result in significant increased cerebral damage or venous stasis, because most likely the protruding tissue is already necrotic.

In the event of massive cerebral ischemia, the frontal, temporal, and parietal bones overlying the infracted hemisphere are removed. The dura is incised and reflected. A dural expansion graft of pericranium, lyophilized cadaver dura, homologous temporal fascia, or sintetic material is loosely sutured to the dura edges to prevent cortical adhesions. The dura is fixed to the craniectomy edges to prevent or limit epidural bleeding, and the temporal muscle and skin flap are reapproximated and sutured or stapled into place. The bone flap may be frozen and preserved or instead a fabricated artificial material can be used (e,g titanium), to close the bone defect, cranioplasty is then performed at a later date, when functional recovery has stabilized.

A technical note "In-window" craniotomy and "bridgelike" duraplasty as an alternative to decompressive hemicraniectomy has been lately introduced as an alternative, concluding that decompressive surgery, which uses an in-window craniotomy that gradually opens according to the intracranial pressure, is an alternative solution for deploying autologous material. The procedure has the advantage of obviating the need for a second surgical procedure to close the bone defect, and thus preventing the metabolic cerebral impairment associated with the absence of an overlying skull. (73)

By studying the impact of craniectomy size, shape, and location on parenchymal hemorrhagic and ischemic lesions, postoperative bleeding, and mortality, and interestingly found a 70% rate of hemicraniectomy-associated infarcts and hemorrhage. Bleeding was associated with a small craniectomy size and sharp bone defects. Parenchymal hemorrhage was the only factor that statistically affected mortality rate, with only 55% of patients surviving compared with 80% in the absence of hemorrhage, with a recommendation for craniectomy size in a diameter larger than 12 cm. This conclusion is validated by the fact that some studies suggest that doubling the diameter from 6 cm to 12 cm potentially increases the decompressive volume from 9 to 86 ml. (75, 79) Ideally, hemicraniectomy should be performed in the frontotemporoparietal region and reach the floor of the middle cranial fossa. The midline should be spared to avoid injury to the superior sagittal sinus.

12.2 Results of craniectomy

For more than 50 years, (1, 10, 39, 66) patients have been selected from case reports or series; range age 10 to 76 years, predominantly male patients, with a good outcome for up to 60% of the patients, several studies have shown that decompressive surgery is a possible treatment strategy for increased ICP after severe supratentorial stroke.

Although increasing numbers of studies have reported encouraging results after decompressive craniectomy for ischemic stroke, these studies are mostly limited to case series without a control group, a summery has is shown in a publication. (50) Study shows that mortality is lower in the surgically treated group compared with a higher mortality rate in the control group - medically treated, and with a better outcome in the surgically treated group. (60)

As decompressive craniectomy can be a life-saving procedure in patients who will most likely be left with a significant neurological deficit, the operation has important ethical and psychological implications. Because of their altered level of consciousness, patients cannot directly provide consent and in such cases, informed consent has to be obtained from the relatives. Psychological disturbances in this patient population were addressed, and mood disturbances were significant in patients who underwent decompressive craniectomy after right-sided hemisphere ischemic stroke, patients suffered severe depressive symptoms, and mild to moderate impairment was demonstrated. (7)

In deciding when surgery is indicated, it is important to know that in general, clinical signs precede critically raised ICP, drowsiness is one of the major clinical symptoms of developing brain oedema (61) thus, ICP monitoring of this condition might be helpful in guiding further therapy. However, elevated ICP is not a common cause of initial neurological deterioration from large hemispheric stroke. (21)

Even under full supportive therapy, the mortality rate is reported high (roughly 80%), and lately the effectiveness of many medical therapies such as chronic hyperventilation, osmotherapeutics, barbiturate therapy, has been challenged. (14, 20, 29, 34, 45) The clinical course of patients with severe supratentorial stroke is highly predictable, therefore, waiting for mesencephalic signs to occur potentially worsens prognosis. It was hypothesized that through decompressive surgery, the vicious circle of extensive oedema, which by elevation of ICP causes ischemia of neighbouring brain tissue and further infarction, may be interrupted. (14) This may then increase cerebral perfusion pressure and optimize retrograde perfusion of leptomeningeal collateral vessels, thus allowing functionally compromised but viable brain to survive. (21)

The timing of surgery, hemisphere infarcted, presence of signs of herniation before surgery, and involvement of other vascular territories may not significantly affect outcome, to identify the patients most likely to benefit from hemicraniectomy, age may be a crucial factor in predicting functional outcome after hemicraniectomy in patients with large MCA territory infarction, as from different review of data. (26, 33, 47, 60)

There are several limits to these reviews.

12.3 What limits?

These were data prior to RCTs but in the absence of randomized controlled data by that time, questions remained regarding optimal patient selection, timing of therapy, and prognosis.

Waiting for signs of herniation may worsen prognosis because of irreversible mesencephalic injury. Early decompressive surgery may further improve outcomes in these patients, considering for surgery nondominant hemisphere or incomplete aphasia before deterioration. For the patients, surgically treated before the occurrence of clinical signs of herniation, within the first 24 hours after stroke onset, hemicraniectomy is an effective therapy for the condition of malignant MCA infarction. Most related complications associated with the operation were epidural haematoma, subdural haematoma, and hygromas. However, whether and when decompressive surgery is indicated in these patients is still a matter of debate but, younger patients may have better functional outcome even if undergoing decompressive craniectomy of the dominant hemisphere. (65)

Given the unresolved questions regarding the role of decompressive craniectomy and appropriate patient selection, the following RCTs were conducted and designed, to investigate the efficiency of decompressive surgery: DECIMAL (Decompressive Craniectomy In MALignant middle cerebral artery infarcts) (72) DESTINY (DEcompressive Surgery for the Treatment of malignant INfarction of the middle cerebral arterY) (34, 71) and HAMLET (Hemicraniectomy After Middle cerebral artery infarction With Life-Threatening Edema Trial). (30) Not all the RCTs demonstrated statistical superiority of hemicraniectomy and failed to meet the primary end point. (71)

13. Surgery-related complications and the quality of life related surgery

Complications have been reported.
The outcomes of patients undergoing decompressive craniectomy may be impacted by the complications of the procedure, reported complications include inadequate decompression, infection, hemorrhage, and the development of contralateral fluid collections, postoperative epidural and subdural haemorrhage as well as hygromas has occurred. Furthermore, delayed sinking flap syndrome may result in headaches, seizure and focal neurological deficits and is typically cured by replacement of the bone flap. Similarly, hydrocephalus may develop in a delayed fashion. (7, 28, 29, 34, 45, 60, 65, 71, 77)
Available data are in agreement on a reduction of the mortality rate, but the reported functional outcome was highly variable. Older age, more severe neurological deficit on admission, and longer duration of intensive care treatment and mechanical ventilation were significantly associated with worse disability (BI < 50). The health-related quality of life (QOL) was considerably impaired in the subscales of mobility, household management, and body care. Decompressive hemicraniectomy improves survival in patients with malignant MCA infarction when compared with earlier reports of conservative treatment alone. Functional outcome and QOL remain markedly impaired, especially among elderly patients and in those with a severe neurological deficit at admission. (18) Early death is a result of transtentorial herniation while delayed death is typically due to the medical complications of prolonged hospitalization including pneumonia and pulmonary emboli. (67) Although the impact on mortality appeared unequivocal in most studies. Surgical age limit has not yet been fully defined very few data exist to support hemicraniectomy for patients older than 60 years. Data analysis, demonstrate significant mortality reduction in the surgically treated patients compared with those receiving medical treatment. Surgical decompression within 48 hours of stroke onset reduces the risk of death and the risk of significant morbidity and showed a statistically significant reduction in severely disabled, bedridden patients (mRS score > 4), effect on severe disability (mRS score 5) and effect on moderate disability (mRS score 4). (72, 34, 30)
Quality of life issues are difficult to put in proper perspective, studies help clarify some facets of this important subject. Future studies will need to focus more rigorously on the long-term quality of life in survivors and the neurological outcome. There exists a difficult balance between increasing survival and poor neurological outcome, which at the other end includes the subjective assessment of outcome and discussion with the patient and the family that should be held early, in the need for surgical decompression, while keeping in mind that RCTs reported a trend of reduced disability among survivors. (72, 34, 30, 55, 68)
Data refer that most patients remain in a vegetative state after this intervention, (11) however other data conclude that decompressive hemicraniectomy improves survival in patients with malignant MCA infarction when compared with earlier reports of conservative treatment alone. Functional outcome and QOL remain markedly impaired, especially among elderly patients and in those with a severe neurological deficit at admission. (3, 4, 8, 18, 33)

14. Conclusions

Malignant cerebral ischemia occurs in a significant number of patients who undergo emergency evaluation for ischemic stroke. The mortality rate in these patients is very high. Fatal outcome is usually related to progressive, severe cerebral oedema with brain herniation and compression of critical brainstem structures. This patient population can be identified by early clinical and neuroimaging characteristics. In some of these patients, decompressive craniectomy appears to be a life-saving procedure. If craniectomy is performed early, especially in young patients, a satisfactory functional outcome can be achieved in a significant proportion of cases. Questions persist regarding the indications for such a procedure in patients with dominant infarctions. Clinical experience, however, demonstrates that even in such patients, an acceptable functional outcome can be achieved after surgery if some preservation of speech is present at the time of intervention.

Best Medical Treatment or Optimal medical management for malignant edema due to stroke has not been standardized. Recommendations for medical management of stroke-related malignant edema included admission to the intensive care unit, osmotherapy with mannitol or glycerol, invasive monitoring of intracranial pressure, blood pressure control, elevation of the head to 30°, and maintenance of normothermia, normoglycemia, and normovolemia. Morbidity and mortality rates are high for this disease entity despite such aggressive measures. (30) Although decompressive craniectomy has been shown to significantly decrease mortality, high morbidity rates among survivors have tempered enthusiasm for this procedure. This reluctance has been most pronounced in elderly patients and those with dominant hemisphere infarcts. The span of the optimal operative time window when surgical decompression is superior to medical management alone is also subject to debate. (4)

We hope that our findings will add to existing information on decompressive hemicraniectomy and help until further data are available. However, there are some unanswered questions and questions persist regarding the age and the indications for such a procedure in patients with dominant infarctions:

- Which subset of patients will benefit maximally?
- Which patients will survive with an unacceptable degree of functional dependency?
- What is the optimal timing for surgery?

MCA infarction with malignant edema is a devastating disease for which hemicraniectomy can play a positive role.

Acknowledgement: To our patients, to whom we dedicate a very important part of our lives. To our professors who taught us how to treat our patients.

As disclosure, on behalf of the authors, I report no conflict of interest concerning the materials or methods used in our work or the findings specified.

15. References

[1] Adams JH, Graham DI: Twelve cases of fatal cerebral infarction due to arterial occlusion in the absence of atheromatous stenosis or embolism. J Neurol Neurosurg Psychiatry 1957, 30: 479-488

[2] Akins PT, Guppy KH: Sinking skin flaps, paradoxical herniation, and external brain tamponade: a review of decompressive craniectomy management. Neurocrit Care 2008, 9: 269–276

[3] Arac A, Blanchard V, Lee M, Steinberg GK: Assessment of outcome following decompressive craniectomy for malignant middle cerebral artery infarction in patients older than 60 years of age. Neurosurg. Focus. 2009, 26: E3 1-6

[4] Arnaout OM, Aoun SG, Batjer HH, Bendok BR: Decompressive hemicraniectomy after malignant middle cerebral artery infarction: rationale and controversies. Neurosurg Focus 2011, 30: E18 1-5
[5] Bounds JV, Wiebers DO, Whisnant JP, et al: Mechanism and timing of deaths from cerebral infarction. Stroke 1981, 12: 474-477
[6] Camarata PJ, Heros RC, Latchaw RE: "Brain attack": the rationale for treating stroke as a medical emergency. Neurosurg 1994, 34: 144-158
[7] Carter BS, Ogilvy CS, Candia GJ, et al: One-year outcome after decompressive surgery for nondominant hemispheric infarction. Neurosurg 1997, 40: 1168–1176
[8] Chang V, Hartzfeld P, Langlois M, Mahmood A, Seyfried D: Outcomes of cranial repair after craniectomy. J Neurosurg. 2010, 112: 1120–1124
[9] Cooper PR, Rovit RL, Ransohoff J: Hemicraniectomy in the treatment of acute subdural hematoma: a re-appraisal. Surg Neurol 1976, 5: 25-28
[10] Cushing H. The establishment of cerebral hernia as a decompressive measure for inaccessible brain tumors; with the description of intermuscular methods of making the bone defect in temporal and occipital regions. Surg Gynecol Obstet 1905, 1: 297-314
[11] Danish SF, Barone D, Lega BC, Stein SC: Quality of life after hemicraniectomy for traumatic brain injury in adults. A review of the literature. Neurosurg Focus 2009, 26: E2 1-5
[12] Delashaw JB, Broddaus WC, Kassell NF, et al: Treatment of right hemispheric cerebral infarction by hemicraniectomy. Stroke 1990, 21 :874-881
[13] Dierssen G, Carda R, Coca JM: The influence of large decompressive craniectomy on the outcome of surgical treatment in spontaneous intracranial hematomas. Acta Neurochir 1983, 69: 53-60
[14] Doerfler A, Forsting M, Reith W, Staff C, Heiland S, Scha¨bitz WR, von Kummer R, Hacke W, Sartor K: Decompressive craniectomy in a rat model of "malignant" cerebral hemispherical stroke: experimental support for an aggressive therapeutic approach. J Neurosurg 1996, 85: 853-859
[15] Engelhorn T, Doerfler A, Kastrup A, et al: Decompressive craniectomy, reperfusion, or a combination for early treatment of acute "malignant" cerebral hemispheric stroke in rats? Potential mechanisms studied by MRI. Stroke 1999, 30: 1456-1463
[16] Furlan A, Higashida RT, Wechsler L, et al: Intra-arterial prourokinase for acute ischemic stroke. The PROACT II study: a randomized controlled trial. JAMA 1999, 282: 2003-2011
[17] Fisher CM, Ojemann RG: Bilateral decompressive craniectomy for worsening coma in acute subarachnoid hemorrhage. Observations in support of the procedure. Surg Neurol 1994, 41: 65-74
[18] Foerch C, Lang JM., Krause J, Raabe A, Sitzer M, Seifert V, Steinmetz H, Kessler KR: Functional impairment, disability, and quality of life outcome after decompressive hemicraniectomy in malignant middle cerebral artery infarction. J Neurosurg 2004, 101: 248-54
[19] Foerch C, Otto B, Singer OC, Neumann-Haefelin T, Yan B, Berkefeld J, Steinmetz H, Sitzer M: Serum S100B predicts a malignant course of infarction in patients with acute middle cerebral artery occlusion. Stroke 2004, 35: 2160–2164

[20] Forsting M, Reith W, Schaebitz WR, et al: Decompressive craniectomy for cerebral infarction: an experimental study in rats. Stroke 1995, 26: 259-264

[21] Frank JI, Krieger D, Chyatte D: Hemicraniectomy and durotomy upon deterioration from massive hemispheric infarction: a proposed multicenter, prospective, randomized study. Stroke 1999, 30: 243

[22] Gerriets T, Stolz E, Modrau B, et al: Sonographic monitoring of midline shift in hemispheric infarctions. Neurol 1999, 52: 45-49

[23] Gower DJ, Lee KS, McWhorter JM: Role of subtemporal decompression in severe closed head injury. Neurosurg 1988, 23: 417-422

[24] Greenwood J Jr: Acute brain infarctions with high intracranial pressure: surgical indications. Johns Hopkins Med J 1968, 122: 254-260

[25] Guerra WKW, Gaab MR, Dietz H, et al: Surgical decompression for traumatic brain swelling: indications and results. J Neurosurg 1999, 90: 187–196

[26] Gupta R, Connolly ES, Mayer S, Elkind MS: Hemicraniectomy for massive middle cerebral artery territory infarction: a systematic review. Stroke 2004, 35: 539-543

[27] Hacke W, Schwab S, Horn M, Spranger M, De Georgia M, von Kummer R. Malignant middle cerebral artery territory infarction: clinical course and prognostic signs. Arch Neurol 1996, 53: 309-315

[28] Heros RC: Surgical treatment of cerebellar infarction. Stroke 1992, 23: 937-938

[29] Hofmeijer J, Amelink GJ, Algra A, van Gijn J, Macleod MR, Kappelle LJ, van der Worp HB: The HAMLET investigators. Hemicraniectomy after middle cerebral artery infarction with life-threatening edema trial (HAMLET): protocol for a randomised controlled trial of decompressive surgery in space-occupying hemispheric infarction. Trials 2006, 7: 29

[30] Hofmeijer J, Kappelle LJ, Algra A, Amelink GJ, van Gijn J, van der Worp HB: Surgical decompression for space-occupying cerebral infarction (the Hemicraniectomy After Middle Cerebral Artery infarction with Life-threatening Edema Trial [HAMLET]): a multicentre, open, randomised trial. Lancet Neurol. 2009 8: 326–333

[31] Ivamoto HS, Numoto M, Donaghy RMP: Surgical decompression for cerebral and cerebellar infarcts. Stroke 1974, 5: 365-370

[32] Jourdan C, Convert J, Mottolese C, et al: Evaluation of the clinical benefit of decompression hemicraniectomy in intracranial hypertension not controlled by medical treatment. Neurochirurgie 1993, 39: 304-310 (Fr)

[33] Jüttler E, Bösel J, Amiri H, Schiller P, Limprecht R, Hacke W, Unterberg A: DESTINY II: DEcompressive Surgery for the Treatment of malignant INfarction of the middle cerebral arterY II. Int J Stroke 2011, 6:79–86

[34] Jüttler E, Schwab S., Schmiedek P. et al., for the DESTINY Study Group. Decompressive Surgery for the Treatment of Malignant Infarction of the Middle Cerebral Artery (DESTINY) A Randomized, Controlled Trial Stroke 2007, 38: 2518-2525.

[35] Kalia KK, Yonas H: An aggressive approach to massive middle cerebral artery infarction. Arch Neurol 1993, 50: 1293-1297

[36] Kasner SE, Demchuk AM, Berrouschot J, Schmutzhard E, Harms L, Verro P, Chalela JA, Abbur R, McGrade H, Christou I, Krieger DW: Predictors of fatal brain edema in massive hemispheric ischemic stroke. Stroke 2001, 32: 2117–2123

[37] Kastrau F, Wolter M, et al: Recovery from aphasia after hemicraniectomy for infarction of the speech-dominant hemisphere. Stroke 2005, 36: 825

[38] Kilincer C, Simsek O, Hamamcioglu MK, Hicdonmez T, Cobanoglu S: Contralateral subdural effusion after aneurysm surgery and decompressive craniectomy: case report and review of the literature. Clin Neurol Neurosurg. 2005, 107: 412–416
[39] King AB: Massive cerebral infarction producing ventriculographic changes suggesting a brain tumor. J Neurosurg 1951, 8: 536-539
[40] Kirkham FJ, Neville BGR: Successful management of severe intracranial hypertension by surgical decompression. Dev Med Child Neurol 1986, 28:506-509
[41] Kjellberg RN, Prieto A Jr: Bifrontal decompressive craniotomy for massive cerebral edema. J Neurosurg 1971, 34: 488-493
[42] Kondziolka D, Fazl M: Functional recovery after decompressive craniectomy for cerebral infarction. Neurosurg 1988, 23: 143-147
[43] Krieger DW, Demchuk AM, Kasner SE, Jauss M, Hantson L: Early clinical and radiological predictors of fatal brain swelling in ischemic stroke. Stroke 1999, 30: 287–292
[44] Kunze E, Meixensberger J, Janka M, et al: Decompressive craniectomy in patients with uncontrollable intracranial hypertension. Acta Neurochir Suppl 1998, 71: 16-18
[45] Lanzino JD, Lanzino G: Decompressive caniectomy for space-occupying supratentorial infarction: rationale, indications, and outcome. Neurosurg. Focus 2000, 8: E3 1-7
[46] Major ongoing stroke trials. Stroke 2006, 37: E18-e26
[47] Mayer SA: Hemicraniectomy: a second chance on life for patients with space-occupying MCA infarction. Stroke 2007, 38: 2410–2412
[48] Mori K, Nakao Y, Yamamoto T, Maeda M: Early external decompressive craniectomy with duroplasty improves functional recovery in patients with massive hemispheric embolic infarction: timing and indication of decompressive surgery for malignant cerebral infarction. Surg Neurol. 2004, 62: 420–430
[49] Moulin DE, Lo R, Chiang J, Barnett HJM: Prognosis in middle cerebral artery occlusion. Stroke 1985, 16: 282-284
[50] Musabelliu E, Kato Y, Imizu S, Oda J, Hirotoshi S: Decompressive hemicraniectomy for malignant MCA territory infarction. Pan Arab Journal of Neurosurgery 2010, 591: 1-9
[51] Ng LKY, Nimmannitya J: Massive cerebral infarction with severe brain swelling: a clinicopathological study. Stroke 1970, 1: 158-163
[52] Oppenheim C, Samson Y, Manaï R, Lalam T, Vandamme X, Crozier S, Srour A, Cornu P, Dormont D, Rancurel G, Marsault C: Prediction of malignant middle cerebral artery infarction by diffusion-weighted imaging. Stroke 2000, 31: 2175–2181
[53] Pillai A, Menon SK, et al: Decompressive hemicraniectomy in malignant middle cerebral artery infarction: an analysis of long-term outcome and factors in patient selection. J Neurosurg 2007, 106: 59-65
[54] Polin RS, Shaffrey ME, Bogaev CA, et al: Decompressive bifrontal craniectomy in the treatment of severe refractory posttraumatic cerebral edema. Neurosurg 1997, 41: 84-94
[55] Puetz V, Campos CR, Eliasziw M, Hill MD, Demchuk AM: Assessing the benefits of hemicraniectomy: what is a favourable outcome? Lancet Neurol. 2007, 6: 580–581
[56] Ransohoff J, Benjamin MV, Gage EL Jr, et al: Hemicraniectomy in the management of acute subdural hematoma. J Neurosurg 1971, 34: 70-76

[57] Rengachary SS, Batnitzky S, Moranz RA, et al: Hemicraniectomy for acute massive cerebral infarction. Neurosurg 1981, 8: 321-328
[58] Rengachary SS: Surgery for acute brain infarction with mass effect. In: Wilkins RH, Rengachary SS (eds): Neurosurgery. New York: McGraw-Hill, 1985, Vol 2, pp 1267-1271
[59] Rieke K, Krieger D, Adams HP, et al: Therapeutic strategies in space-occupying cerebellar infarction based on clinical, neuroradiological and neurophysiological data. Cerebrovasc Dis 1993, 3: 45-55.
[60] Rieke K, Schwab S, Krieger D, et al: Decompressive surgery in space-occupying hemispheric infarction: results of an open prospective trial. Crit Care Med 1995, 23: 1576-1578
[61] Ropper AH, Shafran B: Brain edema after stroke: clinical syndrome and intracranial pressure. Arch Neurol 1984, 41: 26-29
[62] Schwab S, Aschoff A, Spranger, et al: The value of ICP monitoring in acute hemispheric stroke. Neurol 1996, 47: 393-398
[63] Schwab S, Junger E, Spranger M, et al: Craniectomy: an aggressive approach in severe encephalitis. Neurol 1997, 48: 412-417
[64] Schwab S, Rieke K, Aschoff A, et al: Hemicraniectomy in space-occupying hemispheric infarction: useful intervention or desperate activism? Cerebrovasc Dis 1996, 6: 325-329
[65] Schwab S, Steiner T, Aschoff A, et al: Early hemicraniectomy in patients with complete middle cerebral artery infarction. Stroke 1998, 29: 1888-1893
[66] Shaw CM, Alvord EC Jr, Berry RG: Swelling of the brain following ischemic infarction with arterial occlusion. Arch Neurol 1959, 1: 161-177
[67] Silver FL, Norris JW, Lewis AJ, Hachinski VC: Early mortality following stroke: a prospective review. Stroke 1984, 15: 492- 496
[68] Staykov D, Gupta R: Hemicraniectomy in malignant middle cerebral artery infarction. Stroke 2011, 42: 513–516
[69] Stefini R, Latronico N, Cornali C, et al: Emergent decompressive craniectomy in patients with fixed dilated pupils due to cerebral venous and dural sinus thrombosis: report of three cases. Neurosurg 1999, 45: 626-630
[70] The National Institute of Neurological Disorders and Stroke rt-PA Stroke Study Group: Tissue plasminogen activator for acute ischemic stroke. N Engl J Med 1995, 333: 1581-1587
[71] Vahedi K, Hofmeijer J, Juettler E, Vicaut E, George B, Algra A, Amelink GJ, Schmiedek P, Schwab S, Rothwell PM, Bousser MG, van der Worp HB, Hacke W: The DECIMAL, DESTINY, and HAMLET investigators. Early decompressive surgery in malignant middle cerebral artery infarction: pooled analysis of three randomized controlled trials. Lancet Neurol 2007, 6: 215-222
[72] Vahedi K, Vicaut E, Mateo J, Kurtz A, Orabi M, Guichard JP, Boutron C, Couvreur G, Rouanet F, Touzé E, Guillon B, Carpentier A, Yelnik A, George B, Payen D, Bousser MG: Sequential-design, multicenter, randomized, controlled trial of early decompressive craniectomy in malignant middle cerebral artery infarction (DECIMAL Trial). Stroke 2007, 38: 2506–2517

[73] Valença MM, Martins C, da Silca JC: "In-window" craniotomy and "bridgelike" duraplasty: an alternative to decompressive hemicraniectomy: Technical note. J Neurosurg 2010, 113: 982-9
[74] Von Kummer R, Meyding-Lamade´ U, Forsting M, Rosin L, Rieke K, Sartor K, Hacke W: Sensitivity and prognostic value of early computed tomography in middle cerebral artery trunk occlusion. Am J Neuroradiol 1994, 15: 9 -15
[75] Wagner S, Schnippering H, Aschoff A, Koziol JA, Schwab S, Steiner T: Suboptimum hemicraniectomy as a cause of additional cerebral lesions in patients with malignant infarction of the middle cerebral artery. J Neurosurg. 2001, 94: 693–696
[76] Walz B, Zimmermann C, Böttger S, Haberl RL: Prognosis of patients after hemicraniectomy in malignant middle cerebral artery infarction. J Neurol. 2002, 249: 1183–1190
[77] Waziri A, Fusco D, Mayer SA, McKhann GM II, Connolly ES Jr: Postoperative hydrocephalus in patients undergoing decompressive hemicraniectomy for ischemic or hemorrhagic stroke. Neurosurgery 2007, 61: 489–494
[78] Wijdicks EFM, Schievink WI, McGough PF: Dramatic reversal of the uncal syndrome and brain edema from infarction in the middle cerebral artery territory. Cerebrovasc Dis 1997, ;7: 349-352
[79] Wirtz CR, Steiner T, Aschoff A, Schwab S, Schnippering H, Steiner HH, Hacke W, Kunze S: Hemicraniectomy with dural augmentation in medically uncontrollable hemispheric infarction. Neurosurg. Focus 1997, 2: E3 1-9
[80] Yoo DS, Kim DS, Cho KS, et al: Ventricular pressure monitoring during bilateral decompression with dural expansion. J Neurosurg 1999, 91: 953-959
[81] Young PH, Smith KR, Dunn RC: Surgical decompression after cerebral hemispheric stroke: indications and patient selection. South Med J 1982, 75: 473-474

10

Understanding and Augmenting Collateral Blood Flow During Ischemic Stroke

Gomathi Ramakrishnan, Glenn A. Armitage and Ian R. Winship
Centre for Neuroscience and Department of Psychiatry, University of Alberta, Canada

1. Introduction

Stroke refers to brain damage and dysfunction that occurs due to the obstruction of blood flow to brain tissue. Stroke is one of the leading causes of death and disability worldwide, accounting for 10% of all deaths (Grysiewicz et al., 2008; Donnan et al., 2008). Risk of stroke is affected by a number of modifiable and non-modifiable risk factors. Age is the primary non-modifiable risk factor, while modifiable risk factors include chronic hypertension, diabetes, smoking, cholesterol and lack of exercise (Simons et al., 1998; Knuiman & Vu, 1996; Iso et al., 1989; Wadley et al., 2007).

Ischemic stroke, the rapid development of a neurological deficit due to the disruption of blood supply to a specific region of the brain, is the most common cause of stroke. Usually caused by the blockage of an artery or vein by an embolus or blood clot, an ischemic stroke is a major cerebrovascular trauma with a mortality rate of 25% after one month (Donnan et al., 2008; Hossmann, 2006). Ischemic strokes are differentiated from transient ischemic attacks by neurological symptoms lasting for more than 24 hours (Albers et al., 2002). Death and extent of disability due to ischemic stroke is largely defined by location of the occlusion and corresponding size and location of the infarct.

Brain injury following ischemic stroke results from an "ischemic cascade" of pathological events triggered by reduced blood flow. Disturbed ion homeostasis, excitotoxity, elevation of intracellular calcium concentrations, peri-infarct depolarisations, free radical generation, lipid peroxidation and protein synthesis dysfunction are all triggered by reduced blood flow and contribute to necrotic and apoptotic processes in ischemic tissue and expansion of the infarct (Dirnagl et al., 1999 and Hossmann et al., 2006). Notably, necrotic cell death tends to be fast and irreversible in the core or infarct of the stroke area, where blood flow falls below ~20% of baseline perfusion and results in energy failure in resident neurons (Hossman, 2006). However, in "penumbral" regions surrounding the core, partial blood flow is maintained and tissue is considered functionally silent but structurally intact. Importantly, damage in the penumbra is reversible, though this reversibility is time-limited (Hakim, 1987). Because pathophysiology in the penumbra evolves over hours and days after ischemic onset, it is believed that early treatments that restore blood flow or reduce brain damage can reduce damage and improve outcome (Green, 2008). Although hundreds to thousands of prospective treatments to salvage ischemic tissue or halt the pathological ischemic cascade have been identified, few have successfully been translated to clinical practice (Ginsberg , 2008; Wahlgren & Ahmed, 2005). In fact, only thrombolytic drugs have thus far produced significant positive results for stroke patients in clinical trials. Of the thrombolytic drugs, intravenous recombinant tissue plasminogen activator (rtPA) has proved effective in reducing mortality and disability associated with ischemic stroke (Wardlaw et al., 2000). When it is administered in selected patients with acute ischemic stroke within 4.5 h of symptom onset, rtPA is highly effective in reducing death and disability (Buchan & Kennedy, 2007; Toni et al., 2005 and Lansberg et al., 2009; Clark et al., 1999). Clinically, relatively few patients are treated with rtPA, primarily because the therapeutic window is prohibitively short compared to the usual delays in stroke recognition and patient transport, triaging and neuroimaging (Kwan et al., 2004). Moreover, 40% of patients with early treatment and indications of salvageable tissue still do not respond to rtPA (Kaur et al., 2004). For middle cerebral artery occlusion (MCAo)—the most common cause of focal ischemic stroke—rtPA treatment restores blood flow in only 25–30% of patients (Kaur et al., 2004).

2. Collateral blood flow and collateral therapeutics

With a paucity of effective treatments for acute stroke, new approaches to neuroprotection or reperfusion are needed. One strategy currently under investigation to improve post-stroke outcome is to increase blood supply to ischemic tissue via intracerebral collateral circulation. The collateral circulatory system is defined as the vascular network through which blood flow can be partially maintained after the primary vascular routes are blocked (Liebeskind, 2003). "Collateral therapeutics" attempt to harness these endogenous vascular redundancies to improve blood flow to at-risk tissue.

Cerebral collaterals can be classified as veinous, primary or secondary. The venous collateral circulation is highly variable, and augments drainage of cerebral blood flow during primary venous occlusion (Liebeskind, 2003). Primary collaterals refer to short arterial segments in the Circle of Willis, while the secondary collaterals refer to the ophthalmic and leptomeningeal collaterals (Liebeskind, 2003). The Circle of Willis is a circular vascular structure situated on the base of the brain that creates redundancy in cerebral blood flow between the internal carotid arteries and vertebrobasilar system (Hendrikse et al., 2005). In the case of occlusion or stenosis in these feeding arteries, blood can flow through the Circle of Willis and maintain blood flow in regions downstream of the narrowing or occlusion (Cieślicki et al., 1997). Similarly, collateral flow through the ophthalmic artery can partially restore blood flow to the distal carotid in the case of severe internal carotid artery occlusion or stenosis (Henderson et al., 2000; Reynolds et al., 2002). Leptomeningeal collaterals (or pial collaterals) are anastomatic connections between distal branches of the cerebral arteries found along the surface of the brain that permit blood flow from the territory of an unobstructed artery into the territory of an occluded artery(Liebeskind, 2005).

In this chapter, we will review methods for imaging cerebral blood flow relevant to investigations of stroke collaterals and illustrate the important link between stroke outcome and collateral circulation. Our review will focus primarily on the leptomeningeal collaterals and will incorporate both clinical and pre-clincial studies exploring the relevance of collateral blood flow for stroke prognosis and the potential benefits of collateral therapeutics.

3. Imaging collateral blood flow in clinical and pre-clinical settings

In this section, we will briefly outline some of the methods used to image blood flow in the clinical and pre-clinical setting. To image collateral vessels, single vessel resolution is required. While no ideal strategy to image collateral blood flow has been identified, a number of techniques have been employed in the clinic and in animal research to image cerebral collateral circulation and begin to define the anatomy, physiology, and significance of collateral circulation in stroke. Collateral circulation is an important predictor of infarct size (Angermaier et al., 2011; Bang et al., 2008 and Zhang et al., 2010), and accurate imaging approaches are essential to optimize its predictive value and to properly evaluate the benefits and mechanisms of collateral therapeutics.

3.1 Collateral blood flow imaging in humans

A number of direct and indirect methods can be used to image cerebral blood flow in the clinical setting. Indirect measurements of cerebral blood flow during stroke allow inferences about collateral perfusion of ischemic tissue. Techniques such as magnetic resonance (MR) perfusion imaging, computed tomography (CT) perfusion, xenon-enhanced CT, single-photon emission CT, and positron-enhanced tomography can be used to measure cerebral blood flow and assess the collateral status (Liebeskind, 2003). However, the utility of these methods is somewhat limited since only indirect information about collaterals blood flow is attained (Liebeskind, 2003). Single vessel resolution permits a more direct assessment of collateral blood flow in stroke patients. Direct visualization of collateral vessels can be obtained using cerebral digital angiography, CT angiography, MR angiography, and transcranial Doppler sonography (TCD) (Liebeskind, 2003). Below we will briefly discuss these direct imaging techniques for collateral blood flow during stroke.

3.1.1 Cerebral angiography

Cerebral digital angiography involves injection of a contrast dye (typically via the femoral artery) during X-ray imaging. A series of radiographs are collected as the contrast agent spreads through the cerebral vasculature, yielding high-resolution images of cerebral blood flow. Digital subtraction angiography improves resolution of vasculature in bony structures such as the cranium by subtracting a "mask" image acquired without contrast.

Conventional angiography is the "gold standard" for observing cerebral blood vessels and angiography during stroke has confirmed the importance of collateral blood flow in determining tissue fate (Bang et al., 2008). However, the various methods used to quantify cerebral collaterals have not been well validated. Moreover, conventional angiography involves radiation exposure and is relatively invasive with a risk of complications including embolism, dissection, hematoma, allergic reaction to contrast dye, and nephropathy (Barlinn & Alexandrov, 2011; Hankey et al., 1990). Such complications are more common in older patients with atherosclerosis, a particularly relevant contraindication in the stroke population where both age and high cholesterol represent significant risk factors (Barlinn & Alexandrov, 2011, Simons et al., 1998; Knuiman & Vu, 1996; Iso et al., 1989).

3.1.2 Magnetic resonance angiography

Magnetic resonance angiography (MRA) uses MR imaging approaches to map blood vessels in the brain (Hartung et al., 2011). While there are several MRA variants, time-of-flight (TOF) MRA and contrast-enhanced (CE) MRA are most frequently used to image cerebral blood flow in patients with cerebrovascular disease (Barlinn & Alexandrov, 2011). Both techniques allow either 2-dimensional (2D) or 3-dimensional (3D) volume acquisition and are capable of detecting aneurysms, occlusions or stenosis in cerebral vasculature, with the major differences being the requirement for a bolus injection of a contrast medium (gadolinium) for CE-MRA. Additionally, TOF-MRA permits higher-resolution images while CE-MRA allows faster collection over a larger anatomical volume, and reduced artefacts due to blood flow and vascular pulsation (Barlinn & Alexandrov, 2011; Hartung et al., 2011). Notably, MRA does not use ionization radiation, does not require an invasive catheter, and the "low-dose" contrast agent used with CE-MRA is considered less toxic than contrast media associated with conventional angiography. In fact, MRA techniques are considered the most powerful non-invasive methods to examine collateral circulation and hemodynamically relevant anatomical variations in Circle of Willis (Fürst et al., 1993). Still, MRA is not without limitations. Gadolinium based contrast agents have generally excellent safety profiles, but recent reports suggest a link to nephrogenic systemic fibrosis in patients with impaired kidney function (Weinreb & Abu-Alfa, 2009). Moreover, some stroke patients cannot tolerate or cooperate with the requirements for MRA, leading to movement artefacts, and MR cannot be used in patients with pacemakers or other magnetic appliances (Barlinn & Alexandrov, 2011).

3.1.3 Computed tomography angiography

Because it is widely available and well-tolerated by most stroke patients (Barlinn & Alexandrov, 2011), computed tomography angiography (CTA) is the most commonly used tool for diagnostic vascular imaging in the clinical stroke setting (Schellinger, 2005). A single bolus of iodine injected intravenously permits fast acquisition of high-resolution, thin slice CT images of cerebral vasculature. With proper post-acquisition processing, CTA images are comparable to DSA and allow 3D resolution of brain vasculature. With respect to stroke, CTA is very effective in detecting proximal arterial occlusions, allowing for differentiation between complete and near-occlusions, and stenoses, and provides information to predict functional outcome and response to thrombolysis. While CTA results in fewer motion artefacts than MRA, it requires radiation exposure and the toxicity and dose-size of the iodine used as a contrast agent is greater than that of the gadolinium. Moreover, risk of radio-contrast nephropathy after CTA is a serious concern, particularly in patients with kidney disease or diabetes (Barlinn & Alexandrov, 2011). Such concerns are particularly important with multiple examinations that lead to larger cumulative doses of radiation and iodine.

3.1.4 Transcranial Doppler sonography

Transcranial Doppler ultrasonography (TCD) can be used to measure the velocity of blood flow and waveforms in intracranial blood vessels through spectral Doppler sampling over particular cerebral blood vessels. TCD is relatively quick, non-invasive and inexpensive method to measure blood flow in the brain that offers information complementary to MRA and CTA. By analysing frequency shifts caused by the velocity of moving particles in the cerebral blood vessels, TCD provides real-time information on cerebral blood flow and hemodynamics and can be used to monitor blood flow without exposing patients to repeated doses of radiation or contrast agents. TCD is limited in that it does not allow for 2D or 3D reconstruction of vascular networks in the brain, and is highly dependent on the experience and aptitude of the sonographer (Barlinn & Alexandrov, 2011). While it is primarily used in human patients, a recent study using TCD in a rat model of middle cerebral artery occlusion identified a redistribution of blood flow after stroke (Li et al., 2010).

3.2 Imaging collateral blood flow in laboratory animals

Due to the heterogeneity of the clinical population and differences in delay from onset, the availability of diagnostic imaging, and the varying treatment options in human stroke patients, interpretation of data on collateral blood flow from clinical imaging can be difficult. Recent advances in blood flow imaging in animal models of stroke provide new opportunities to study the dynamics, persistence, and importance of collateral blood flow and the mechanisms and efficacy of collateral therapeutics in pre-clinical studies. Below we will discuss two methods for imaging single-vessel blood flow in animal models of stroke: laser speckle contrast imaging and two-photon laser scanning microscopy.

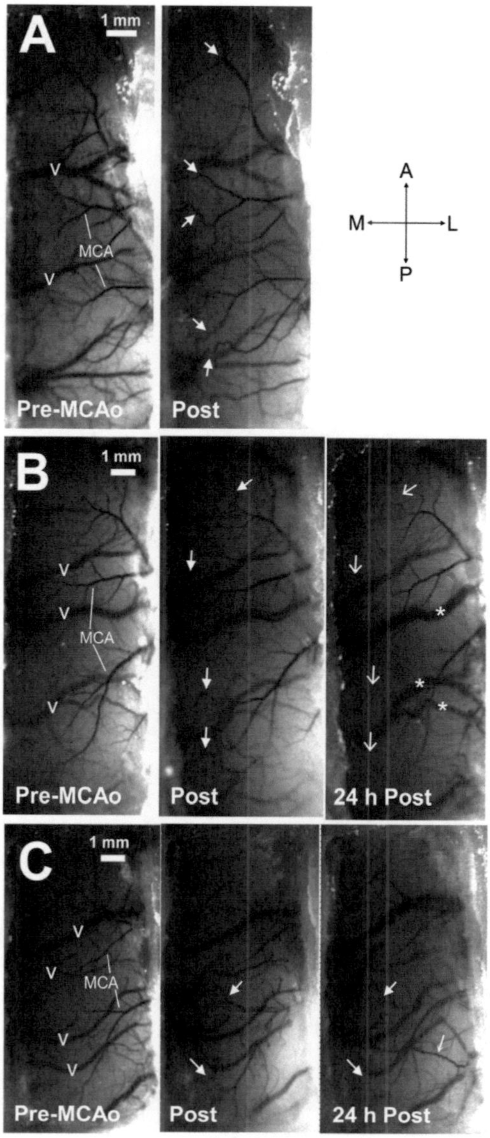

Fig. 1. LSCI of dynamic leptomeningeal collaterals during acute stroke. A, LSCI image showing blood flow in the surface veins (V) and branches of the middle cerebral artery

(MCA) over the hindlimb and forelimb sensorimotor cortex. Note the blood flow through anastomatic connections between the distal segments of the ACA and MCA immediately after MCAo (arrows). B, Left and middle panels show blood flow prior to and immediately after MCAo mapped with LSCI, while the right panel shows blood flow 24 hours after stroke. Spontaneous reperfusion occurred between imaging sessions and blood flow through anastomatic connections ceased by 24 h (large arrows). Darker veins indicative of increased veinous blood flow from the territory of the MCA were observed after reperfusion (asterisks). C, Left, midle and right panels show LSCI blood flow maps before, after, and 24 hours after MCAo. Arrows indicate new patterns of collateral flow through anastomatic connections between the ACA and MCA that were apparent soon after MCAo and persisted at 24 h after onset. The small arrow identifies an anastamose with blood flow 24 h after MCAo that was not apparent immediately after onset. A, anterior; P, posterior; M, medial; L, lateral. Figure from Armitage et al., 2010 (used with perimission).

3.2.1 Laser speckle contrast imaging (LSCI)

LSCI is a technique that allows high spatial and temporal resolution during full-field imaging of changes in blood flow on the surface of the brain. Requiring only inexpensive instrumentation and simple analysis, LSCI provides resolution to individual blood vessels and is extremely effective in mapping changes in collateral blood flow during stroke (Armitage et al., 2010). LSCI maps of blood flow are based on blurring of the characteristic laser speckle pattern produced by illumination of the brain surface (or skull) with coherent laser light. Importantly, the speckle pattern is dynamic and blurred by moving particles (such as blood cells) on or below the illuminated surface. By analyzing fluctuations in the speckle pattern in a particular image, speckle contrast values that provide a measure of relative changes in blood flow can be calculated. The speckle contrast factor (K) is a measure of the local spatial contrast of the laser speckle pattern and is defined as the ratio of the standard deviation to the mean intensity ($K = \sigma s/I$) in a small region of the speckle image (typically 5× 5 or 7 x 7 pixels). Speckle contrast and motion of the scattering particles are inversely related. K values ranges from 0 to 1, with values near 1 suggesting no blood flow in that vessel and values closer to zero reflect greater blood flow. By plotting K values, LSCI allows for maps of blood flow and can reveal changes in the pattern of blood flow after focal ischemia, including enhanced collateral perfusion or spontaneous reperfusion. LSCI has been used in animal models after middle cerebral artery occlusion (MCAo) to measure cerebral blood flow changes after stroke (Figure 1, Armitage et al., 2010; Dunn et al., 2001; Shin et al., 2008; Strong et al., 2008).

While LSCI permits sensitive mapping of blood flow in surface vessels, the exact quantitative relationship between speckle contrast and blood flow velocity remains undefined (Duncan & Kirkpatrick, 2008). LSCI is susceptible to experimental artifacts that can vary between animals and imaging sessions (Parthasarathy et al., 2008; Ayata et al., 2004) and is best restricted to describing relative changes in the pattern of blood flow rather than quantifying blood flow velocity (Parthasarathy et al., 2008; Ayata et al., 2004).

3.2.2 Two photon laser scanning microscopy (TPLSM)

TPLSM permits visualization of fluorescent molecules up to 1 mm below the surface in opaque tissues such as brain. During single photon fluorescence microscopy, short excitation wavelengths prevent deep penetration into tissues and increase light scattering and phototoxicity (Helmchen & Denk, 2005; Svoboda & Yasuda, 2006 and Mulligan & MacVicar, 2007). Because it uses "pulse lasers" that facilitate multiphoton excitation of fluorophores, TPLSM allows the use of longer excitation wavelengths. In addition to improving penetration into the tissue, these wavelengths have lower phototoxicity. Moreover, multiphoton excitation will only occur in the focal volume of the objective, meaning that all fluorescence collected arises from fluorophores in the focal plane, allowing for optical sectioning and 3D reconstructions of flourophore distribution. TPLSM has previously been used to demonstrate that stroke induces a rapid loss of this dendritic microstructure in individual neurons (Zhang et al., 2005; Zhang & Murphy, 2007). Importantly, synapses can be restored even after delayed reperfusion (Li & Murphy, 2008) and long-term recovery is associated with enhanced synaptogenesis beside the stroke core (Brown & Murphy, 2008; Brown et al., 2007; Brown et al., 2009), suggesting that methods to facilitate synapse preservation during acute stroke or spine formation during recovery may be of functional benefit. In vivo calcium imaging using TPLSM also demonstrated functional rewiring of sensorimotor neurons as new regions of the cortex adopt the function of tissue lost to stroke (Winship & Murphy, 2008; Winship & Murphy, 2009).

TPLSM has been important in defining the rules governing cerebral blood flow (Zhang & Murphy 2007; Shih et al., 2009; Takano et al., 2006; Nishimura et al., 2010; Mulligan & MacVicar, 2004). Cortical microcirculation can be precisely measured in vivo during TPLSM after blood plasma is labelled with a fluorescent-conjugated dextran (Figure 2). This technique permits resolution of blood flow in veins and arteries on the brain surface as well as arterioles and capillaries in the microvascular bed below the surface of the cortex. Moreover, it allows for precise quantification of the direction and speed of motion of blood cells in these vessels, something that is not possible with LSCI. After stroke, TPLSM can identify vessels at the capillary level that were not previously carrying blood (Schaffer et al., 2006 and Shih et al., 2009). Red blood cell velocity can then be precisely measured in individual arterioles, veins, and capillaries in the penumbral cortex and three-dimensional reconstructions of the microvascular architecture and diameter of these vessels can be created.

4. Collaterals and ischemia

As noted previously, the collateral circulation is divided into three distinct pathways. Primary collateral circulation is particularly important after occlusion or stenosis of the brains major feeding arteries, the ICAs and the vertibrobasalar system. In patients with severe stenosis of the ICA, collateral flow through anterior and posterior communicating arteries and retrograde filling through the ophthalmic artery correlate with patient survival rate. Moreover, collateral flow is correlated with a lower risk of hemispheric stroke and transient ischemic attack (Henderson et al., 2000). After severe stenosis of the ICA, enhanced collateral flow through anterior Circle of Willis is observed and the diameter of the communicating arteries is increased (Hartkamp, 1999). Similarly, patients with bilateral ICA occusion exhibit significant collateral flow through the posterior Circle of Willis and increased posterior communicating artery diameters (Hartkamp, 1999). In fact, in patients with ICA occlusion, blood flow in the territory of the MCA ipsilateral to the occluded ICA is derived primarily from the vertebrobasilar arteries while ACA flow is mainly supplied by the contralateral ICA (Van Laar et al., 2007).

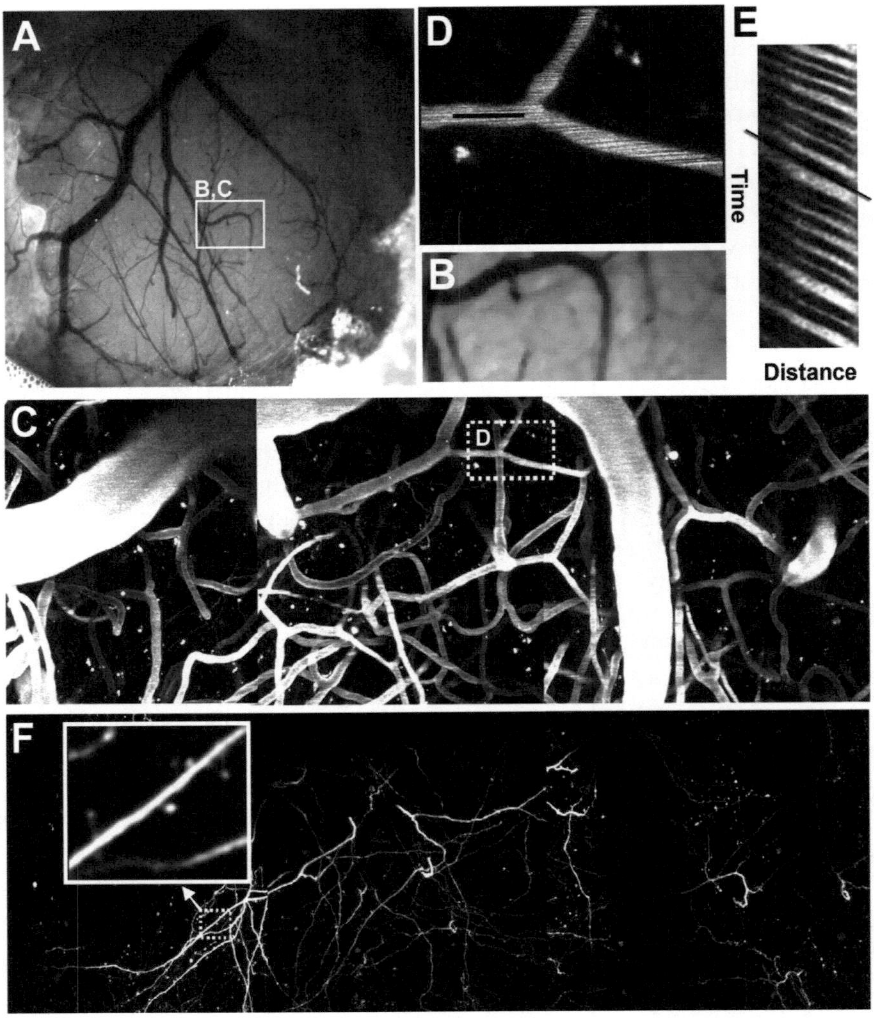

Fig. 2. Quantitative measurement of cerebral blood flow and vascular anatomy. A, B Photomicrographs of the surface of the mouse sensorimotor cortex. C, TPLSM of vasculature loaded with rhodamine dextran, showing surface arterioles and microvascular bed below the cortical surface. D, E, Quantitative measurement of blood cell velocity using line scans was made in the region denoted by the line in D. Resulting line scans are compiled in E, and by calculating the slope (time/ distance), a quantitative measure of blood flow velocity can be calculated. Using two channel imaging in mice expressing green fluorescent protein in subset of neurons, neuronal microstructure can be imaged simultaneously with cerebral blood flow (F). Images complements of Dr. Craig E. Brown, University of Victoria.

4.1 Leptomeningeal collateral vasculature

First described by Heubner in 1874, a leptomeningeal artery is described as a pial artery that connects two major cerebral arteries supplying distinct areas of the cerebral cortex (Heubner 1874; Brozici et al., 2003). Similar to the primary collateral vascular system, it is thought that augmentation of the leptomeningeal collateral vascular system, by flow diversion from the primary circulation, could lead to increased cerebral blood flow and decreased infarct volume after a focal ischemic stroke.

During middle cerebral artery occlusion (MCAo), high-velocity blood flow in the anterior cerebral artery (ACA) or posterior cerebral artery (PCA) are indicative of flow diversion. In turn, increased blood flow in the ACA and PCA is a potential source of blood flow to leptomeningeal arteries and may improve perfusion in ischemic tissue downstream of the MCAo. Kim et al (2009) used transcranial doppler ultrasonography, in combination with angiography, to measure flow diversion and collateral flow in 51 patients suffering from middle cerebral artery stenosis. Dividing the patients into three groups based on severity of stenosis, they found that patients with less severe stenosis had lower amounts of leptomeningeal collateral circulation, while more severe stenosis correlated with increased leptomeningeal blood flow. These results correlated with flow diversion in the ACA and PCA that was identified in 47% of individuals and increased with the severity of stenosis.

A recent mathematical model of post-stroke blood flow suggests that the leptomeningeal collateral vascular system can maintain approximately 15% of the normal cerebral blood flow during MCAo (Ursino & Gianessi, 2010). Although blood flow at 15% of normal is well below the limit to preserve cellular function, this same study suggests that over time, collaterals may be able to increase their luminal diameter by 50%, thereby preserving normal cellular function until full blood flow can be restored (Ursino & Gianessi, 2010).

4.2 Clinical importance of leptomeningeal collaterals

While CT, positron emission tomography, MR perfusion and TCD have all been used to assess leptomeningeal collateral blood flow in a variety of different disorders, the most effective single method to visualize leptomeningeal collateral blood flow in humans remains through angiographic assessment (Mori et al., 2009; Derdeyn et al., 1999; Thurley et al., 2009; Wu et al., 2008). However, a combination of multiple imaging modalities is ideal to gain a greater understanding of blood flow in the ischemic cortex (Bang et al., 2008; Wu et al., 2008; Kim et al., 2009). By combining these imaging approaches, leptomeningeal collaterals have been linked to positive outcome after stoke including decreased infarct volumes and decreased National Institute of Health Stroke Scale (NIHSS) scores (Christaforidis et al., 2005; Miteff et al., 2009; Lima et al., 2010).

While leptomeningeal collaterals are seen as a positive indicator of post stroke outcome, it is interesting to note that the presence of leptomeningeal collaterals in humans can indicate cerebrovascular impairment, the presence of vascular occlusive diseases, and are predictive of stoke in certain individuals. For example, Moyamoya disease is a chronic cerebrovascular disorder caused by progressive stenosis or occlusion of the internal carotid artery, leading to headaches, transient ischemic attacks and stroke (Robertson et al., 1997). Due to the long-term occlusive nature of this disease, leptomeningeal arteries become highly developed and have been shown to be a positive indicator of severity of ischemic symptoms (Mori et al., 2009), and are associated with engorged pial networks and slow blood flow (Chung & Park, 2009).

Yamauchi et al (2004) investigated the link between the patterns of collateral circulation and the types of infarcts. This study investigated 42 patients with symptomatic ICA occlusion using four-vessel angiography to assess Willsonian, ophthalmic, and leptomeningeal collaterals and MR imaging to measure infarct type and location. The study showed that the oxygen extraction fraction (a measure of the relative concentration of oxyhemoglobin and deoxyhemoglobin that can be an indicator of a chronic ischemic condition) was significantly higher in patients with well developed ophthalmic or leptomeningeal collaterals and associated with the presence of striaocapsular infarcts, indicating that those with leptomeningeal and opthalmic collaterals were suffering from chronic cerebrovascular impairment.

Although the presence of leptomeningeal collaterals are a positive indicator for future stroke risk, they are also associated with positive outcomes after stoke. For instance, in a retrospective angiographic study on collateral blood flow and clinical outcome after thromboembolic stroke, Christoforidis et al (2005), found that infarct volume and modified Rankin scale scores at discharge were significantly lower for patients with better angiographically-assessed lepotmeningeal collateral scores. This same study also found that, NIHSS score was significantly higher for patients with lower collateral scores. Similarly, Bang et al (2008) used MRI diffusion and perfusion in combination with angiographic assessment to measure collaterals in patients receiving recanalization therapy for acute cerebral ischemia. While this study found that diffusion-perfusion mismatch (a measure of penumbral or salvageable brain tissue) did not correlate with either good or poor collaterals, it showed that patients with good collaterals had larger areas with only mild hypoperfusion and infarct growth within the penumbra was smaller in these patients. Moreover, the study showed that patients with good pre-treatment collaterals more frequently had good recanalization and less infarct growth. Later studies confirmed that recanalization rate is heavily influenced by the collateral grade in patients undergoing endovascular revascularization therapy (Bang et al., 2011).

Another study using angiographic assessment of collateral status in acute ischemic stroke demonstrated that major reperfusion was associated with good collateral status, and that good collateral status was significantly associated with reduced infarct expansion and more favorable outcomes (Miteff et al., 2009). Similar findings were also reported in a prospective cohort study by Lima et al (2010), which investigated patterns of leptomeningeal collateral blood flow by CTA and evaluated patient outcome after stroke. Lima et al. (2010) studied 196 patients and found that a favourable pattern of leptomeningeal collaterals, along with younger age, lower baseline NIHSS, absence of diabetes and administration of rtPA, predicted improved outcomes 6 months after stroke. Additionally, Chistaforidis et al (2009) demonstrated that good collateral blood flow is linked to lower rates of hemorrhagic transformation. Of 104 patients who underwent intra-arterial thrombolysis, 25% of patients with poor leptomeningeal collaterals suffered significant hemorrhage, while only 2.78% of those with good collaterals suffered significant hemorrhage. Interestingly, this study also found that low platelet counts were predictive of significant hemorrhage, indicating that the administration of platelets after intra-arterial therapy may be beneficial.

One explanation for improved patient outcome with increased leptomeningeal collateral circulation in stroke patients is due to the potential facilitation of recanalization and reperfusion. Currently, thrombolysis with rtPA is the most effective therapy for acute ischemic stroke. However, rtPA is ineffective in many patients who receive treatment within its short therapeutic window, particularly in the case of MCAo (Kaur et al., 2004). Part of this low success rate can be attributed to futile recanalization, defined as the lack of clinical benefit due to endovascular treatment of acute ischemic stroke even when recanalization is successful. Futile recanalization may be due to re-occlusion of the artery after initial thrombolysis or due to leptomeningeal collaterals that are insufficient to sustain tissue viability until recanalization occurs (Hussein et al., 2010; Liebeskind et al., 2008).

Good collateral status may also augment the effectiveness of neuroprotective drug therapies by providing increased routes for pharmacological agents such as rtPA to reach the ischemic penumbra and aid in recanalization.

4.3 Animal models and leptomeningeal collaterals

Clinical evidence strongly suggests that increased leptomeningeal collateral blood flow is a positive indicator for post stroke outcome. Moreover, it is thought that augmenting collateral blood flow via the leptomeningeal arteries by pharmacological or mechanical means may maintain blood supply in the ischemic penumbra and reduce cell death in this at-risk tissue. However, much about the dynamics of collateral blood flow during ischemic stroke remains unknown. As noted, clinical studies are limited by the access to imaging modalities and heterogeneity in treatment options and patient demographics. Animal models offer greater experimental control and facilitate an understanding of collateral vascular dynamics.

When assessing collateral dynamics and therapeutics in animal models, it is important to consider strain differences in the number of collaterals before stroke. While animal studies have shown that collateral growth is enhanced in the weeks after stroke, and highly developed collateral blood flow prior to stroke is associated with decreased infarct size, estimation of the leptomeningeal collateral network size, a number that varies from birth, is difficult (Wei et al., 2001; Lin et al., 2002; Chalothorn et al., 2007; Zhang et al., 2010). In fact, Zhang et al (2010) investigated 16 different mouse strains to determine numbers of native collaterals. This study found statistically significant variation in collateral length, numbers of penetrating arterioles and infarct volume after middle cerebral artery occlusion. As expected, infarct volume correlated inversely with collateral number, diameter and number of penetrating arterioles (Zhang et al., 2010). As in human patients, the number and quality of collateral connections can vary greatly between individuals or animal strains, and is a predictor of stroke outcome. However, by examining collateral dynamics and the mechanisms and efficacy of collateral therapeutics in animal models with different collateral networks, inferences into the importance of leptomeningeal collateral blood flow after stroke can be made regardless of collateral density.

Early studies in animal models focused on the regulation of leptomeningeal collateral blood flow. These studies showed that the pryriform branch of the MCA has collateral communication with the ACA, and that the parietal and temporal branches collateralize with the posterior cerebral artery after MCAo in Sprague-Dawley (SD) rats (Menzies et al., 1993). After a MCAo or common carotid artery occlusion, leptomeningeal arterial blood pressure correlates with blood flow in ischemic areas and these arteries can further dilate to increase blood flow to the brain after stroke (Shima et al., 1983; Morita et al., 1997). Using laser doppler flowmetry in SD rats, Morita et al (1997) showed that pial arteries took ~12 s to become maximally dilated and around 131 seconds to become stable after common carotid artery occlusion. Although this rapid response is promising, it has been suggested that leptomeningeal collateral blood flow does not provide enough blood flow to maintain normal blood flow over a long time period (Derdeyn et al., 1998).

In a recent study, LSCI was used to assess the dynamics and persistence of leptomeningeal collateral blood flow to ischemic territories over the 24 hours following thromboembolic MCAo in SD rats (Armitage et al., 2010). As shown in Figure 1, maps of blood flow revealed several (~ 3 - 6) anastomatic connections between the ACA and MCA that developed soon after vessel occlusion. Notably, these anastomoses were both persistent and dynamic: Blood flow through approximately 75% of these anastomoses persisted for at least 24 hours. The anastomoses were dynamic during the imaging period: Blood flow through these collateral connections ceased after spontaneous reperfusion and, in some animals, collateral connections that were not apparent immediately after stroke were visible 24 hours post-stroke. Importantly, in this study LSCI confirmed the persistence of blood flow though ACA-MCA anastomoses up to 24 hours after MCAo. However, more quantitative methods (such as TPLSM) will be necessary to better address the persistence of leptomeningeal collateral blood flow velocity as it relates to tissue viability.

Changes in collateral flow in the first hours after stroke, including measures below the cortical surface, have been quantified using TPLSM. Importantly, TPLSM has confirmed flow reversal in distal sections of the MCA downstream from anastomoses with the ACA in a mouse model of transient MCAo (Murphy & Li, 2008). Overall, red blood cell velocity in arterioles downstream MCAo are reduced to 30% of baseline, and lumen diameters in small (< 23 μm diameter) surface arterioles and penetrating arterioles increased by approximately 20% (Shih et al., 2009) during acute ischemia. Importantly, this vasodilation persisted over 90 minutes of MCAo. Schaffer et al (2006) quantified blood flow reversals downstream of the occlusion and showed that approximately half of the arterioles downstream of the MCAo showed flow reversal, as would result from retrograde flow from the ACA into the territory of the MCA, within the two hours after occlusion. More recent studies suggest that these flow reversals are restricted to surface arterioles and do not persist to penetrating arterioles (Shih et al., 2009). Targeted occlusions of penetrating arterioles in the cortex have demonstrated that compensation is somewhat limited in penetrating vessels, as occlusion-induced dilations were restricted to vessels downstream of the occlusion and that neighbouring penetrating arterioles do not dilate to enhance collateral compensation (Nishimura et al., 2010).

In addition to acute changes in collateral circulation, changes in leptomeningeal collaterals are observed after long-term recovery from MCAo. Coyle & Heistad (1987) demonstrated that normotensive Wistar Kyoto rats exhibited extreme collateralization (~27 anastamoses between the ACA and MCA) and little infarct one month after chronic MCAo. In fact, collateral vessels supplying blood to the MCA territory were able to restore blood flow to near baseline levels in the territory of the MCA one month after stroke. Contrasting this, stroke prone hypertensive rats (derived from a WKY background) exhibited the same number of anastomoses one month after stroke, but these connections were significantly narrower than WKY rats and hypertensive rats had significant infarction due to MCAo.

5. Augmenting collateral blood flow during stroke

Animal models and clinical data have clearly demonstrated the importance of collateral circulation during acute ischemic stroke in determining stroke prognosis and response to recanalization therapy. Based on these subsidiary vascular networks, it has also been suggested that enhancing collateral blood flow may reduce ischemia without targeting the clot. While therapies to enhance collateral flow such as adjusting head position, intravenous fluid support, and pressure augmentation have been suggested as neuroprotective strategies, collateral therapeutics remain a relatively unexploited neuroprotective strategy (Liebeskind 2003, 2005). In this section, we will explore different means of collateral blood flow augmentation and their efficacy in the treatment of acute ischemic stroke.

5.1 Angiogenesis and collaterals

A number of studies have highlighted the importance of angiogenesis in the development of collateral channels throughout the vascular system and their role in ischemia. Angiogenesis is mediated by a number of angiogenic factors including vascular endothelial growth factor (VEGF), fibroblast growth factor (FGF), granulocyte colony stimulating factor (G-CSF) and angiopoietin (among others) and can be induced by circulating inflammatory cells during atherosclerosis (accounting for the increased collateral vasculature seen with chronic cerebrovascular insufficiencies) (Schirmer et al., 2009; Deb, 2010). After portal vein ligation, VEGF expression and collateral angiogenesis is upregulated, and inhibition of VEGF receptor-2 via a monoclonal antibody (DC101) or autophosphorylation (by SU5416) can decreases portal-systemic collateral density by up to 68% or 52%, respectively (Frenandez et al., 2004). In fact, VEGF expression appears to be critical for the formation of the collateral vasculature in many models of ischemia. In a mouse model of altered lipid metabolism, ApoE-/- deficient mice have reduced expression of VEGF and decreased hind limb vascular collateral development (Couffinhal et al., 1999). Strain differences in the expression of the vegfa gene account for a 54% difference in collateral remodelling after hind limb ischemia between BALB/C and C57BL/6 mice, as well as reduced collateral density in the intestine and cerebral cortex of BALB/C mice when compared to C57BL/6 mice. The influence of VEGF-A on collateral density has been directly related to models of cerebral ischemia, where it has been shown that transgenic mice that express low levels of VEGF form fewer leptomeningeal collaterals during the perinatal period and have increased infarct volume after MCAo when compared to mice expressing high levels of VEGF (Clayton et al., 2008).

Hepatocyte growth factor (HGF) is another angiogenic growth factor which promotes the growth of endothelial cells. HGF has been shown to efficiently increase the number of collateral vessels and improved the blood flow after hindlimb ischemia in rabbits (Pyun et al., 2010).

Perhaps the most promising data relating angiogenic compounds to improved stroke outcome relates to G-CSF and granulocyte monocyte colony stimulating factor (GM-CSF). GM-CSF stimulates angiogenesis by releasing growth factors from mobilised monocytes and macrophages. The importance of G-CSF and GM-CSF was first reported in heart and cerebral artery disease and they were more recently shown effective for treating cerebral ischemia (Buschmann et al., 2003). In fact, a number of groups have identified a neuroprotective role for G-CSF and GM-CSF administered before or after ischemia in rodent models (Todo et al., 2008; Nakagawa et al., 2006; Schäbitz et al., 2008), likely in part due to its upregulation of the formation of collateral vascular channels. Prophylactic injection of GM-CSF in rats for 6 weeks prior to bilateral common carotid artery occlusion has been shown to attenuate functional impairment of cerebrovascular reserve capacity and increase leptomeningeal collateral density (Schneider et al., 2007). A recent study demonstrated that five days of daily GM-CSF or G-CSF administered to C57/BL6 mice after unilateral occlusion of the common carotid artery also promoted leptomeningeal collateral growth and decreased infarct volume (Sugiyama et al., 2011). A subset of these animals received MCAo seven days after common carotid occlusion. Of this subset, animals that were treated with G-CSF or GM-CSF had smaller infarcts and greater cerebral perfusion than untreated animals. Although promising, the feasibility of GM-CSF injection has yet to be tested in humans.

5.2 Vasodilation and collateral flow

For the most part, attempts to improve cerebral blood flow during stroke using vasodilatory compounds have not been neuroprotective. This may be because ischemic vasculature is already fully dilated during stroke, and therefore only non-ischemic vasculature dilates, resulting in vascular stealing that is deleterious to ischemic tissue (Bremer et al., 1980 and

Kuwabara et al., 1995). Bath application of N-Methyl-D-aspartate (NMDA) has been shown to enhance blood flow to collateral dependent tissue in a canine model of MCAo independent of neuronal nitric oxide production (Robertson & Loftus 1998). As such, collateral vessels appear to be under additional vasodilatory influences that are yet to be determined. Defining these mechanisms may aid the development of therapies directed at augmenting flow through collateral vessels to reduce infarct size.

5.3 Augmenting cerebral blood flow by inducing mild hypertension

Perhaps the most obvious way to increase collateral blood flow is by inducing systemic hypertension through pharmacological agents or volume expansion. As cerebral autoregulation is impaired during stroke, changes in mean arterial blood pressure have a linear effect of cerebral blood flow. Similarly, decreasing the blood pressure in ischemic patients during acute stroke can exacerbate neurological deficits (Oliveira-Filho et al., 2003; Ahmed et al., 2000; Vlcek et al., 2003). Therefore, it is thought that by artificially inducing hypertension, global cerebral blood flow can be increased, enhancing flow through leptomeningeal collaterals and thereby preserving blood supply to the ischemic penumbra and protecting neuronal function therein (Wityk, 2007; Bogoslovsky et al., 2006). A neuroprotective role for mild induced hypertension has been confirmed in animal models. Shin et al (2008) used intravenous phenylepherine to increase blood pressure after MCAo. The mild hypertension induced by phenylephrine increased blood pressure and cerebral blood flow when injected either 10 or 60 minutes after occlusion (Shin et al., 2008). Treated rats displayed decreased infarct volume after stoke, and the authors hypothesized that this was due to increased perfusion of ischemic territories via leptomenigneal anastomoses between the posterior cerebral artery, ACA, and MCA (Shin et al., 2008). Similarly, hypertensive treatment with phenylephrine that increased blood pressure by 65mm Hg reduced infarct volume by 97% in rabbits after one hour of MCAo and 45% in rabbits subjected to two hours of MCAo (Smrcka et al., 1998). Increasing blood pressure through angiotensin was also demonstrated to increase the mean arterial pressure by 40-60% and reduce infarct volume after transient MCAo in rats (Chileuitt et al., 1996). While mild induced hypertension may be neuroprotective, it is important to note that chronic hypertension worsens stroke outcome (Aslanyan et al., 2003; Geeganage et al., 2011; Toyoda et al., 2009), possibly due to inhibition of collateral blood flow. In spontaneously hypertensive rats, compensatory growth of leptomeningeal collaterals in response to chronic cerebral hypoperfusion is impaired relative to normotensive rats, though this compensatory growth is restored by anti-hypertensive therapies (Omura-Matsuoka et al., 2011).

Clinically, blood pressure is often elevated during MCAo and clinical trials have not demonstrated unequivocal beneficial results in neurological outcome after stroke (Liebeskind, 2003). Moreover, the risks of elevated blood pressure in stroke patients are not well defined, and hypertensive treatments may increase the risk of intracerebral hemorrhage, reflex bradycardia and possibly even ischemic bowel disease (Wityk, 2007).

Still, preliminary data suggest some benefit. An increase in mean arterial pressure of at least 10mm Hg (induced by norephenephrine administration) improved perfusion pressure in patients with MCAo with only a small increase in intracranial pressure (Schwarz et al., 2002). Additionally, several preliminary studies have suggested that inducing mild hypertension may have functional benefits as measured by NIHSS scores and volume of hypoperfused tissue (Hillis et al., 2003; Rordorf et al., 2001). Induced hypertension may be particularly useful for patients ineligible for thrombolysis. In these patients, mild hypertension induced via pheynylephrine increased mean arterial pressure by 20% resulted in a three point reduction on the NIHSS scale and moderate functional improvement on follow up measured using the Rankin scale (Bogoslovsky et al., 2006).

5.4 Augmenting cerebral blood flow using partial aortic occlusion

Another approach to facilitating reperfusion of ischemic territories is to increases global cerebral blood flow via temporary partial occlusion of the descending aorta. Using a catheter and balloon introduced via the femoral artery and inflated to occlude 70% of the suprarenal descending aorta, it is hoped that global cerebral perfusion and perfusion of ischemic territories by collateral pathways can be enhanced. Partial aortic occlusion has previously been shown to improve cerebral perfusion and neurological deficits in symptomatic vasospasm after subarachnoid hemorrhage (Lylyk et al., 2005), but its efficacy in ischemic stroke is unproven. Because many focal strokes are resistant to rtPA—particularly MCAo—pilot studies are ongoing to assess the safety and efficacy of aortic occlusion treatment in animal models and stroke patients (Noor et al., 2009 and Shuaib et al., 2011). In a non-ischemic porcine model, it was shown that partial occlusion of descending suprarenal aorta increased cerebral blood flow by 35-52% and that global cerebral perfusion remained elevated for 90 min after deflation (Hammer et al., 2009). Exciting preclinical data in a rat model of thromboembolic stroke supported a neuroprotective role for partial aortic occlusion, and demonstrated that aortic occlusion significantly reduces infarct volume at 24 hours post-occlusion without increasing the risk of hemorrhagic transformation. Notably, treatment in combination with rtPA further reduced the infarct volume (Noor et al., 2009), suggesting a synergistic relationship between aortic occlusion and thrombolysis.

Recently, the safety and efficacy of partial aortic occlusion was tested in patients up to 14 hours after ischemic onset in the Safety and Efficacy of NeuroFlo in Acute Ischemic Stroke (SENTIS) trial (Shuaib et al., 2011). Importantly, the treatment appeared safe with no significant increase in adverse events as compared to standard stroke treatments. While overall efficacy was unclear, preliminary results suggest that aortic occlusion was effective in patients treated within 5 hours of onset, older than 70 years or age, and with moderate stroke severity. Moreover, partial aortic occlusion as an adjunct to thrombolysis appears safe, suggesting that studies of combination therapy are warranted (Emery et al., 2011).

5.5 Augmenting cerebral blood flow with sphenopalatine and cervical spinal stimulation

While partial aortic occlusion attempts to improve cerebral blood flow and reperfusion of ischemic territories by physically diverting blood from the periphery, other approaches attempt to manipulate the neurovascular interface to improve cerebral blood flow during stroke. One approach involves selective electrical stimulation of the parasympathetic nerves in the sphenopalatine ganglion. These fibres provide parasympathetic innervation of the anterior cerebral circulation, and a number of studies in animal models suggest that sphenopalatine stimulation elicits significant increases in cerebral blood flow (Ayajiki et al., 2005; Suzuki et al., 1990; Yarnitsky et al., 2005). Recently, MR imaging and behavioural assessment was used to assess tissue characteristics and stroke recovery in MCAo rats after sphenopalatine ganglion stimulation treatment that began 18 hours after ischemic onset (Bar-Shir et al., 2010). Notably, n-acetyl-aspartate (NAA) levels (a marker of neuronal density and viability) were significantly greater in treated rats, and measures of neurological impairment at 8 and 28 days after stroke suggested a benefit of sphenopalatine ganglion stimulation. Conversely, cutting the nerves eminating from the sphenopalatine ganglion increases infarct volume after MCAo (Diansan et al., 2010). Based on preliminary data, the safety of sphenopalatine ganglion stimulation is currently being evaluated in human stroke patients (Khurana et al., 2009).

Spinal cord stimulation has been found effective in treating a number of disorders related to low cerebral blood flow (Robaina & Clavo, 2007). While it has not yet been tested in stroke patients, spinal cord stimulation in non-stroke patients significantly enhances blood flow in the common carotid and MCA (Robaina & Clavo, 2007). In rats, electrical stimulation of the cervical spinal cord increases cerebral blood flow (measured via laser Doppler flowmetry) by over 50% in control rats (Sagher et al., 2003). When initiated 20 minutes after MCAo, cervical spinal stimulation also improved blood flow in ischemic territories by over 30% (~64% reduction in blood flow prior to stimulation and ~30% below baseline after stimulation) and profoundly reduced infarct volume measured six hours after ischemic onset (Sagher et al., 2003). Similarly, cervical spinal stimulation in cats significantly reduced infarct size 24 hours after stroke and mortality due to MCAo (Matsui & Hosobuchi, 1989). Based on these preliminary data, further studies in animal models and human patients are warranted.

5.6 Augmenting cerebral blood flow using head positioning

Cerebral blood flow to the brain can be augmented by supine positioning of head that results in increased arterial flow due to gravity. Importantly, this treatment can be applied as soon as an ischemic stroke patient is diagnosed. When head position is reduced from 30° to 0° elevation during the first 24 hours after ischemic onset, the mean flow velocity of MCA (measured using Transcranial Doppler) is increased by 20%, resulting in functional improvement in 15% of patients (NIHSS) (Wojner-Alexander, 2005). Conversely, a decrease in cerebral blood flow was observed by increasing the head position from 0° to 30° or 45° (Schwarz et al., 2002; Moraine et al., 2000), with cerebral blood flow determined according to the arteriovenous pressure gradient (Moraine et al., 2000). Applying a supine head positioning procedure may increase the intracranial pressure of some patients, and is therefore advisable when a higher perfusion rate is required even at the risk of increased intracranial pressure (Schwarz et al., 2002). More research is required, however, since it is not clear to what extent head position augments collateral blood flow, nor is it known how delay and duration of head positioning influence outcome.

6. Summary

Collateral circulation refers to subsidiary vascular networks in the brain whose pathophysiological recruitment can partially maintain blood flow when primary vascular routes are blocked. With respect to MCAo, clinical imaging suggests that blood flow through the leptomeningeal collaterals, anastomoses connecting the distal segments of the MCA to distal branches of the ACA, can partially restore blood flow to ischemic territories. Based on these subsidiary vascular networks, it has been suggested that enhancing collateral blood flow may reduce ischemia without targeting the clot. While therapies to enhance collateral flow remain relatively unexploited neuroprotective strategies, promising data from animal models and clinical evaluation suggest that collateral therapeutics offer a legitimate alternative and/or adjuvant to thrombolytic therapies. By furthering our understanding of the dynamics, persistence, and regulation of collateral blood flow and expanding on studies evaluating the mechanisms and efficacy of collateral therapeutics, improved strategies for stroke care can be developed.

7. References

Ahmed N, Näsman P, Wahlgren NG. (2000). Effect of intravenous nimodipine on blood pressure and outcome after acute stroke. *Stroke.* Vol.31, No.6, pp.1250-1255, ISSN 1524-4628

Albers GW, Caplan LR, Easton JD, Fayad PB, Mohr JP, Saver JL, et al.(2002).Transient ischemic attack—proposal for a new definition. *N Engl J Med.* Vol.347, No.21, pp. 1713–1716, ISSN 1533-4406

Armitage GA, Todd KG, Shuaib A, Winship IR. (2010). Laser speckle contrast imaging of collateral blood flow during acute ischemic stroke. *J Cereb Blood Flow Metab.* Vol.30, No.8, pp. 1432-1436, ISSN 1559-7016

Aslanyan S, Fazekas F, Weir CJ, Horner S, Lees KR; GAIN International Steering Committee and Investigators.(2003). Effect of blood pressure during the acute period of ischemic stroke on stroke outcome: a tertiary analysis of the GAIN International Trial. *Stroke.* Vol.34, No.10, pp.2420-2425, ISSN 1524-4628

Ayajiki K, Fujioka H, Shinozaki K, Okamura T(2005). Effects of capsaicin and nitric oxide synthase inhibitor on increase in cerebral blood flow induced by sensory and parasympathetic nerve stimulation in the rat. *J Appl Physiol.* Vol.98, No.5, pp.1792-1798, ISSN 1522-1601

Ayata C, Shin HK, Salomone S, Ozdemir-Gursoy Y, Boas DA, Dunn AK, Moskowitz MA.(2004). Pronounced hypoperfusion during spreading depression in mouse cortex. *J Cereb Blood Flow Metab.* Vol. 24,No.10, pp.1172-1182, ISSN 1559-7016

Bang OY, Saver JL, Buck BH, Alger JR, Starkman S, Ovbiagele B, Kim D, Jahan R, Duckwiler GR, Yoon SR, Viñuela F, Liebeskind DS. (2008). Impact of collateral flow on tissue fate in acute ischaemic stroke. *J Neurol Neurosurg Psychiatr,* Vol.79, No.6, pp. 625-9, ISSN 1468-330X.

Bang OY, Saver JL, Kim SJ, Kim GM, Chung CS, Ovbiagele B, Lee KH, Liebeskind DS. (2011).Collateral flow predicts response to endovascular therapy for acute ischemic stroke. *Stroke.* Vol.42, No.3, pp. 693-699, ISSN 1524-4628

Barlinn K, Alexandrov AV. (2011). Vascular Imaging in Stroke: Comparative Analysis. *Neurotherapeutics.* Vol.NA, No.NA, pp.NA, ISSN 1878-7479

Bar-Shir A, Shemesh N, Nossin-Manor R, Cohen Y.(2010).Late stimulation of the sphenopalatine-ganglion in ischemic rats: improvement in N-acetyl-aspartate levels and diffusion weighted imaging characteristics as seen by MR. *J Magn Reson Imaging.*Vol. 31, No.6, pp.1355-1363,ISSN 1522-2586

Bogoslovsky T, Häppölä O, Salonen O, Lindsberg PJ. (2006). Induced hypertension for the treatment of acute MCA occlusion beyond the thrombolysis window: case report. *BMC Neurol.* Vol.19, No.6,pp.46-51 ISSN 1471-2377

Bremer AM, Yamada K, West CR. (1980). Ischemic cerebral edema in primates: effects of acetazolamide, phenytoin, sorbitol, dexamethasone, and methylprednisolone on brain water and electrolytes. *Neurosurgery.* Vol.6, No.2, pp.149-154, ISSN 1524-4040

Brown CE, Aminoltejari K, Erb H, Winship IR, Murphy TH. (2009). In vivo voltage-sensitive dye imaging in adult mice reveals that somatosensory maps lost to stroke are replaced over weeks by new structural and functional circuits with prolonged modes of activation within both the peri-infarct zone and distant sites. *J Neurosci.*Vol.29,No.6, pp.1719-1734,ISSN 1529-2401

Brown CE, Li P, Boyd JD, Delaney KR, Murphy TH.(2007). Extensive turnover of dendritic spines and vascular remodeling in cortical tissues recovering from stroke. *J Neurosci.* Vol.27,No.15,pp.4101-4109, ISSN 1529-2401

Brown CE, Murphy TH. (2008).Livin' on the edge: imaging dendritic spine turnover in the peri-infarct zone during ischemic stroke and recovery. *Neuroscientist.* Vol.14,No.2,pp.139-146. ISSN 1089-4098

Brozici M, van der Zwan A, Hillen B. (2003). Anatomy and Functionality of Leptomeningeal Anastomoses: A Review. *Stroke.* Vol.34, No.11, pp. 2750-2762, ISSN 1524-4628

Buchan AM, Kennedy J. (2007). Strategies for therapy in acute ischemic stroke. *Nat Clin Pract Neurol.*Vol. 3, No.1,pp.2–3,ISSN 1745-8358

Buschmann IR, Busch HJ, Mies G, Hossmann KA. (2003). Therapeutic induction of arteriogenesis in hypoperfused rat brain via granulocyte–macrophage colony-stimulating factor. *Circulation.* Vol.108, No.5, pp. 610–615, ISSN 1524-4539

Chalothorn D, Clayton JA, Zhang H, Pomp D, Faber JE. (2007). Collateral density, remodeling, and VEGF-A expression differ widely between mouse strains. *Physiol Genomics.* Vol.30, No.2, pp.179-191, ISSN 1531-2267.

Chileuitt L, Leber K, McCalden T, Weinstein PR. (1996). Induced hypertension during ischemia reduces infarct area after temporary middle cerebral artery occlusion in rats. *Surg Neurol.* Vol.46, No.3, pp. 229-234, ISSN 1879-3339

Christoforidis GA, Mohammad Y, Kehagias D, Avutu B, Slivka AP. (2005). Angiographic assessment of pial collaterals as a prognostic indicator following intra-arterial thrombolysis for acute ischemic stroke. *AJNR Am J Neuroradiol,* Vol.26, No.7, pp. 1789–1797, ISSN 1936-959X

Christoforidis GA, Karakasis C, Mohammad Y, Caragine LP, Yang M, Slivka AP. (2009). Predictors of hemorrhage following intra-arterial thrombolysis for acute ischemic stroke: the role of pial collateral formation. *AJNR Am J Neuroradiol.* Vol.30, No.1, pp. 165-70, ISSN 1936-959X

Chung P-W, Park K-Y. (2009). Leptomeningeal enhancement in petients with moyamoya disease: correlation with perfusion imaging. *Neurology.Vol.* 72, No.21, pp. 1872-1873, ISSN 1526-632X

Cieślicki K, Gielecki J, Wilczak T. (1997). Redundancy of the main cerebral arteries in morphological variations of the Willis circle. *Neurol Neurochir Pol.* Vol. 31,No.3, pp.463-474, ISSN 0028-3843

Clark WM, Wissman S, Albers GW, Jhamandas JH, Madden KP, Hamilton S. (1999) . Recombinant tissue-type plasminogen activator (Alteplase) for ischemic stroke 3 to 5 hours after symptom onset. The ATLANTIS Study: a randomized controlled trial. Alteplase Thrombolysis for Acute Noninterventional Therapy in Ischemic Stroke. *JAMA.* Vol.282, No.21, pp. 2019-2026, ISSN 1538-3598

Clayton JA, Chalothorn D, Faber JE. (2008). Vascular endothelial growth factor-A specifies formation of native collaterals and regulates collateral growth in ischemia. *Circ Res. Vol.*103, No.9, pp.1027-1036, ISSN 1524-4571

Couffinhal T, Silver M, Kearney M, Sullivan A, Witzenbichler B, Magner M, Annex B, Peters K, Isner JM. (1999).Impaired collateral vessel development associated with reduced expression of vascular endothelial growth factor in ApoE-/- mice. *Circulation.* Vol.99 , No.24, pp. 3188-3198 , ISSN 1524-4539

Coyle P, Heistad DD. (1987). Blood flow through cerebral collateral vessels one month after middle cerebral artery occlusion. *Stroke.* Vol.18, No.2, pp. 407-411, ISSN 1524-4628

Deb P, Sharma S, Hassan KM. (2010). Pathophysiologic mechanisms of acute ischemic stroke: An overview with emphasis on therapeutic significance beyond thrombolysis. *Pathophysiology.* Vol.17, No.3, pp. 197-218, ISSN 0928-4680.

Derdeyn CP, Powers WJ, Grubb RL. (1998). Hemodynamic effects of middle cerebral artery stenosis and occlusion. *AJNR Am J Neuroradiol.* Vol.19 , No.8, pp. 463-469, ISSN 1936-959X

Derdeyn CP, Shaibani A, Moran CJ, Cross DT, Grubb Jr RL, Powers WJ. (1999). Lack of Correlation Between Pattern of Collateralization and Misery Perfusion in Patients With Carotid Occlusion. *Stroke.* Vol.30, No.5, pp. 1025-1032, ISSN 1524-4628

Diansan S, Shifen Z, Zhen G, Heming W, Xiangrui W.(2010). Resection of the nerves bundle from the sphenopalatine ganglia tend to increase the infarction volume following middle cerebral arteryocclusion. *Neurol Sci.* Vol.31, No.4, pp.431-435. ISSN 1590-3478

Dirnagl U, Iadecola C, Moskowitz MA. (1999). Pathobiology of ischaemic stroke: an integrated view.*Trends Neurosci.* Vol. 22, No.9,pp.391-397, ISSN 1878-108X

Donnan GA, Fisher M, Macleod M, Davis SM. (2008). Stroke. *Lancet,* Vol. 371, No. 9624, pp. 1612-23, ISSN 1474-547X

Duncan DD, Kirkpatrick SJ. (2008). Can laser speckle flowmetry be made a quantitative tool? J Opt Soc Am A Opt Image Sci Vis. Vol.25, No.8, pp.2088-2094, ISSN 1520-8532

Dunn AK, Bolay H, Moskowitz MA, Boas DA. (2001). Dynamic imaging of cerebral blood flow using laser speckle. *J Cereb Blood Flow Metab.* Vol.21, No.3, pp. 195-201, ISSN 1559-7016

Emery DJ, Schellinger PD, Selchen D, Douen AG, Chan R, Shuaib A, Butcher KS. (2011) . Safety and feasibility of collateral blood flow augmentation after intravenous thrombolysis. *Stroke. Vol.*42, No.4, pp. 1135-1137, ISSN 1524-4628

Fernandez M, Vizzutti F, Garcia-Pagan JC, Rodes J, Bosch J. (2004).Anti-VEGF receptor-2 monoclonal antibody prevents portal-systemic collateral vessel formation in portal hypertensive mice. *Gastroenterology.* Vol.126, No.3, pp. 886-94, ISSN 1528-0012

Fürst G, Steinmetz H, Fischer H, Skutta B, Sitzer M, Aulich A, Kahn T, Mödder U. (1993). Selective MR angiography and intracranial collateral blood flow. *J Comput Assist Tomogr.* Vol.17, No.2, pp. 178-183, ISSN 1532-3145

Geeganage C, Tracy M, England T, Sare G, Moulin T, Woimant F, Christensen H, De Deyn PP, Leys D, O'Neill D, Ringelstein EB, Bath PM; for TAIST Investigators. (2011). Relationship between baseline blood pressure parameters (including mean pressure, pulse pressure, and variability) and early outcomeafter stroke: data from the Tinzaparin in Acute Ischaemic Stroke Trial (TAIST). *Stroke.*Vol.42, No.2, pp.491-493.ISSN 1524-4628

Ginsberg MD. (2008). Neuroprotection for ischemic stroke: past, present and future. *Neuropharmacology.*Vol.55, No.3, pp.363-389. ISSN 1873-7064

Green AR. (2008). Pharmacological approaches to acute ischaemic stroke : reperfusion certainly, neuroprotection possibly. *Br J Pharmacol.* Vol.153, No.S1,pp.325-38, ISSN 1476-5381

Grysiewicz RA, Thomas K, Pandey DK. (2008). Epidemiology of ischemic and hemorrhagic stroke: incidence, prevalence, mortality, and risk factors. *Neurol Clin.* Vol.26, No.4, pp. 871-95, ISSN 1557-9875

Hakim AM. (1987). The cerebral ischemic penumbra.*Can J Neurol Sci.Vol.* 14,No.4, pp.557-559, ISSN 0317-1671

Hammer M, Jovin T, Wahr JA, Heiss WD. (2009). Partial occlusion of the descending aorta increases cerebral blood flow in a nonstroke porcine model. *Cerebrovasc Dis.* Vol.28, No.4, pp. 406-410, ISSN 1421-9786

Hankey GJ, Warlow CP, Molyneux AJ. Complications of cerebral angiography for patients with mild carotid territory ischaemia being considered for carotid endarterectomy. *J Neurol Neurosurg Psychiatry.* 1990 Jul;53(7):542-8.

Hartkamp MJ, van Der Grond J, van Everdingen KJ, Hillen B, Mali WP. (1999). Circle of Willis collateral flow investigated by magnetic resonance angiography. *Stroke.* Vol.30, No.12, pp. 2671-2678, ISSN 1524-4628

Hartung MP, Grist TM, François CJ. (2011). Magnetic resonance angiography : current status and future directions.*J Cardiovasc Magn Reson.* Vol.13, No.19, pp.NA, ISSN 1532-429X

Helmchen F, Denk W. (2006). Deep tissue two-photon microscopy. *Nat Methods.* Vol. 2, No.12, pp.932-940. *Nat Methods.* ISSN 1548-7105

Henderson RD, Eliasziw M, Fox AJ, Rothwell PM, Barnett HJ. (2000). Angiographically defined collateral circulation and risk of stroke in patients with severe carotid artery stenosis. North American Symptomatic Carotid endarterectomy Trial (NASCET) Group.*Stroke.* Vol.31, No.1, pp. 128-132, ISSN 524-4628

Hendrikse J, van Raamt AF, van der Graaf Y, Mali WP, van der Grond J.(2005). Distribution of cerebral blood flow in the circle of Willis. *Radiology.* Vol.235, No.1, pp.184-189.ISSN 1527-1315

Heubner O. (1874). Die luetischen Erkrankungen der Hirnarterien. Leipzig, Germany: FC Vogel. Vol.NA, No.NA, pp.170–214.

Hillis AE, Ulatowski JA, Barker PB, Torbey M, Ziai W, Beauchamp NJ, Oh S, Wityk RJ. (2003). A pilot randomized trial of induced blood pressure elevation: effects on function and focal perfusion in acute and subacute stroke. *Cerebrovasc Dis.* Vol.16, No.3, pp. 236-246, ISSN 1421-9786

Hossmann K-A. (2006). Pathophysiology and therapy of experimental stroke. *Cell Mol Neurobiol.* Vol.26, No.7-8, pp. 1057-1083, ISSN 1573-6830

Hussein HM, Georgiadis AL, Vazquez G, Miley JT, Memon MZ, Mohammad YM, Christoforidis GA, Tariq N, Qureshi, AI. (2010). Occurrence and Predictors of Futile Recanalization following Endovascular Treatment among Patients with Acute Ischemic Stroke: A Multicenter Study. *AJNR Am J Neuroradiol.* Vol.31, No.3, pp. 454–458, ISSN 1936-959X

Iso H, Jacobs DR Jr, Wentworth D, Neaton JD, Cohen JD. 1989. Serum cholesterol levels and six-year mortality from stroke in 350,977 men screened for the multiple risk factor intervention trial. *N Engl J Med.* Vol.320,No.14 ,pp.904-910, ISSN 1533-4406

Kaur J, Zhao Z, Klein GM, Lo EH, Buchan AM. (2004). The neurotoxicity of tissue plasminogen activator? *J Cereb Blood Flow Metab.* Vol.24, No.9, pp. 945-963, ISSN 1559-7016

Kim Y, Sin D-S, Park H-Y, Park M-S, Cho, K-H. (2009). Relationship between Flow Diversion on Transcranial Doppler Sonography and Leptomeningeal Collateral Circulation in Patients with Middle Cerebral Artery Occlusive Disorder. *Journal of Neuroimaging.* Vol.19, No.1, pp. 23-26, ISSN 1552-6569

Khurana D, Kaul S, Bornstein NM. (2009). ImpACT-1 Study Group. Implant for augmentation of cerebral blood flow trial 1: a pilot study evaluating the safety and effectiveness of the Ischaemic StrokeSystem for treatment of acute ischaemic stroke. *Int J Stroke.*Vol.4, No.6, pp.480-485, ISSN 1747-4949

Knuiman MW, Vu HT. (1996). Risk factors for stroke mortality in men and women: The Busselton Study.*J Cardiovasc Risk.* Vol. 3,No.5, pp.447-452. ISSN 1350-6277

Kuwabara Y, Ichiya Y, Sasaki M, Yoshida T, Masuda K.(1995).Time dependency of the acetazolamide effect on cerebral hemodynamics in patients with chronic occlusive cerebral arteries. Early steal phenomenon demonstrated by [15O] H2O positron emission tomography. *Stroke.* Vol.26, No.10, pp.1825-1829, ISSN 1524-4628

Kwan J, Hand P, Sandercock P.(2004).A systematic review of barriers to delivery of thrombolysis for acute stroke. *Age Ageing.* Vol.33,No.2,pp.116–121,ISSN1468-2834

Lansberg MG, Bluhmki E, Thijs VN.(2009). Efficacy and safety of tissue plasminogen activator 3 to 4.5 hours after acute ischemic stroke: a metaanalysis. Stroke. Vol.40, No.7, 2438-2441,ISSN 1524-4628

Lee JY, Lee KY, Suh SH. (2010). Different meaning of vessel signs in acute cerebral infarction. Neurology. Vol.75, No.7, pp. 11970-11979, ISSN 1529-2401

Li L, Ke Z, Tong KY, Ying M. (2010). Evaluation of cerebral blood flow changes in focal cerebral ischemia rats by using transcranial Doppler ultrasonography. *Ultrasound Med Biol.* Vol.36, No.4, Different meaning of vessel signs in acute cerebral infarction. *Neurology.* Vol.75, No.7, pp. 595-603, ISSN 1879-291X

Li P, Murphy TH. (2008). Two-photon imaging during prolonged middle cerebral artery occlusion in mice reveals recovery of dendritic structure after reperfusion. *J Neurosci.* Vol.28, No.46

Liebeskind DS , MD. (2003).Collateral Circulation .*Stroke.* Vol.34, No.9, 2279-2284, 1524-4628

Liebeskind DS, Kim D, Starkman S, Changizi K, Ohanian AG, Jahan R, Viñuela F. (2008). Collateral Failure? Late Mechanical Thrombectomy after Failed Intravenous Thrombolysis. *J Neuroimaging.* Vol.20 , No.1, pp. 78-82, ISSN 1552-6569

Liebeskind DS. (2005) .Neuroprotection from the collateral perspective. *IDrugs.* Vol.8,No.3,pp.222-228, ISSN 2040-3410

Liebeskind DS. (2005). Collaterals in acute stroke: beyond the clot. *Neuroimaging Clin N Am.* Vol.15, No.3, pp.553-573,ISSN 1557-9867

Liebeskind DS.(2004). Collateral therapeutics for cerebral ischemia. *Expert Rev Neurother.*Vol.4,No.2,255- 265,ISSN 1744-8360

Lima FO, Furie KL, Silva GS, Lev MH, Camargo ECS, Singhal AB, Harris GJ, Halpern EF, Koroshetz WJ, Smith WS, Yoo AJ, Nogueira RG. (2010). The Pattern of Leptomeningeal Collaterals on CT Angiography Is a Strong Predictor of Long-Term Functional Outcome in Stroke Patients With Large Vessel Intracranial Occlusion. *Stroke.* Vol.41, No.10, pp. 2316-2322, ISSN 1524-4628

Lin T-N, Sun S-W, Cheung W-M, Li F, Chang C. (2002).Dynamic Changes in Cerebral Blood Flow and Angiogenesis After Transient Focal Cerebral Ischemia in Rats: Evaluation

With Serial Magnetic Resonance Imaging. *Stroke*. Vol.33, No.12, pp. 2985-2991, ISSN 1524-4628

Lylyk P, Vila JF, Miranda C, Ferrario A, Romero R, Cohen JE. (2005). Partial aortic obstruction improves cerebral perfusion and clinical symptoms in patients with symptomatic vasospasm. *Neurol Res*. Vol.27, No.NA, pp.129-135, ISSN 1743-1328

Matsui T, Hosobuchi Y.(1989).The effects of cervical spinal cord stimulation (cSCS) on experimental stroke. *Pacing Clin Electrophysiol*. Vol.12, No.4.2, pp.726-732,ISSN 1540-8159

Menzies SA, Hoff JT, Betz AL. (1992) .Middle cerebral artery occlusion in rats: a neurological and pathological evaluation of a reproducible model. *Neurosurgery*. Vol.31, No.1, pp. 100-106, ISSN 1524-4040

Miteff F, Levi CR, Bateman GA, Spratt N, McElduff P,Parsons MW. (2009). The independent predictive utility of computed tomography angiographic collateral status in acute ischaemic stroke. *Brain*.Vol.132, No.pt.8, pp. 2231–2238, ISSN 1460-2156

Moraine JJ, Berré J, Mélot C.(2000). Is cerebral perfusion pressure a major determinant of cerebral blood flow during head elevation in comatose patients with severe intracranial lesions? *J Neurosurg*. Vol.92, No.4, pp.606-614, ISSN 1933-0693

Mori N, Mugikura S, Higano S, Kaneta T, Fujimura M, Umetsu A, Murata T, Takahashi S. 2009. The Leptomeningeal "Ivy Sign" on Fluid- Attenuated Inversion Recovery MR Imaging in Moyamoya Disease: A Sign of Decreased Cerebral Vascular Reserve? *AJNR*. Vol.30, No.5, pp. 930-935, ISSN 1936-959X

Mulligan SJ, MacVicar BA. (2007). Two-Photon Fluorescence Microscopy: Basic Principles, Advantages and Risks. Modern Research and Educational Topics in Microscopy, ISBN 13: 978-84-611-9418-6, Spain.

Mulligan SJ, MacVicar BA.(2004). Calcium transients in astrocyte endfeet cause cerebrovascular constrictions. *Nature*. Vol.431, No.7005, pp.195-199, ISSN 1476-4687

Nakagawa T, Suga S, Kawase T, Toda M. (2006). Intracarotid injection of granulocyte-macrophage colony-stimulating factor induces neuroprotection in a rat transient middle cerebral artery occlusion model. *Brain Res*. Vol.1089, No.1, pp. 179-185, ISSN 1872-6240

Nishimura N, Rosidi NL, Iadecola C, Schaffer CB.(2010). Limitations of collateral flow after occlusion of a single cortical penetrating arteriole. *J Cereb Blood Flow Metab*. Vol.30,No.12, pp.1914-1927,ISSN 1559-7016

Noor R, Wang CX, Todd K, Elliott C, Wahr J, Shuaib A. (2010). Partial intra-aortic occlusion improves perfusion deficits and infarct size following focal cerebral ischemia. *J Neuroimaging*. Vol.20, No.3, pp. 272-276, ISSN 1552-6569

Oliveira-Filho J, Silva SC, Trabuco CC, Pedreira BB, Sousa EU, Bacellar A. (2003). Detrimental effect of blood pressure reduction in the first 24 hours of acute stroke onset. *Neurology*. Vol.61, No.8, pp. 1047-1051, ISSN 1526-632X

Omura-Matsuoka E, Yagita Y, Sasaki T, Terasaki Y, Oyama N, Sugiyama Y, Todo K, Sakoda S, Kitagawa K. (2010).Hypertension impairs leptomeningeal collateral growth after common carotid artery occlusion: Restoration by antihypertensive treatment. *J Neurosci Res*. Vol. 89, No.1, pp. 108-116, ISSN 1097-4547

Parthasarathy AB, Tom WJ, Gopal A, Zhang X, Dunn AK.(2008). Robust flow measurement with multi-exposure speckle imaging. *Opt Express*. Vol.16, No.3, pp.1975-1989, ISSN 1094-4087

Pyun WB, Hahn W, Kim DS, Yoo WS, Lee SD, Won JH, Rho BS, Park ZY, Kim JM, Kim S. (2010). Naked DNA expressing two isoforms of hepatocyte growth factor induces collateral artery augmentation in a rabbit model of limb ischemia. *Gene Ther.* Vol.17, No.12, pp. 1442-1452, ISSN 1476-5462

Robertson RL, Burrows PE, Barnes PD, Robson CD, Poussaint TY, Scott RM. (1997). Angiographic changes after pial synangiosis in childhood moyamoya disease. *AJNR Am J Neuroradiol.* Vol.18, No.5, pp. 837-845, ISSN 1936-959X

Robertson SC, Loftus CM. (1998) . Effect of N-methyl-D-aspartate and inhibition of neuronal nitric oxide on collateral cerebral blood flow after middle cerebral artery occlusion. *Neurosurgery. Vol.*42, No.1, pp. 117-123, ISSN 1524-4040

Robaina F, Clavo B. (2007). Spinal cord stimulation in the treatment of post-stroke patients: current state and future directions. *Acta Neurochir Suppl.* Vol.97, No.1, pp.277-282, ISSN 0065-1419

Reynolds PS, Greenberg JP, Lien LM, Meads DC, Myers LG, Tegeler CH.(2002).Ophthalmic artery flow direction on color flow duplex imaging is highly specific for severe carotid stenosis. *J Neuroimaging.* Vol.12, No.1, pp.5-8, ISSN 1552-6569

Rordorf G, Koroshetz WJ, Ezzeddine MA, Segal AZ, Buonanno FS. (2001). A pilot study of drug-induced hypertension for treatment of acute stroke. *Neurology.* Vol.56, No.9, pp.1210-1213, ISSN 1526-632X

Sagher O, Huang DL, Keep RF. (2003). Spinal cord stimulation reducing infarct volume in a model of focal cerebral ischemia in rats. *J Neurosurg.*Vol.99, No.1, pp.131-137, ISSN 1933-0693

Schäbitz WR, Krüger C, Pitzer C, Weber D, Laage R, Gassler N, Aronowski J, Mier W, Kirsch F, Dittgen T, Bach A, Sommer C, Schneider A.(2008). A neuroprotective function for the hematopoietic protein granulocyte-macrophage colony stimulating factor (GM-CSF).J Cereb Blood Flow Metab.Vol. 28, No.1, pp.29-43, ISSN 1559-7016

Schaffer CB, Friedman B, Nishimura N, Schroeder LF, Tsai PS, Ebner FF, Lyden PD, Kleinfeld D. (2006) .Two-photon imaging of cortical surface microvessels reveals a robust redistribution in blood flow after vascular occlusion. *PLoS Biol.* Vol.4, No.2, pp. 0258-0270, ISSN 1545-7885

Schellinger PD.(2005).The evolving role of advanced MR imaging as a management tool for adult ischemic stroke: a Western-European perspective. Neuroimaging Clin N Am. Vol.15, No.2, pp.245-58, ISSN 1557-9867

Schirmer SH, van Nooijen FC, Piek JJ, van Royen N. (2009). Stimulation of collateral artery growth: travelling further down the road to clinical application. *Heart.* Vol.95, No.3, pp. 191-197, ISSN 1468-201X

Schneider UC, Schilling L, Schroeck H, Nebe CT, Vajkoczy P, Woitzik J. 2007. Granulocyte-Macrophage Colony-Stimulating Factor-Induced Vessel Growth Restores Cerebral Blood Supply After Bilateral Carotid Artery Occlusion. *Stroke.* Vol.38, No.4, pp. 1320-1328, ISSN 1524-4628

Schwarz S, Georgiadis D, Aschoff A, Schwab S. (2002). Effects of body position on intracranial pressure and cerebral perfusion in patients with large hemispheric stroke. Stroke Vol.33, No.2, pp.497-501, ISSN 1524-4628

Schwarz S, Georgiadis D, Aschoff A, Schwab S. (2002). Effects of induced hypertension on intracranial pressure and flow velocities of the middle cerebral arteries in patients with large hemispheric stroke. *Stroke.* Vol.33, No.4, pp. 998-1004, ISSN 1524-4628

Shin HK, Nishimura M, Jones PB, Ay H, Boas DA, Moskowitz MA, Ayata C. (2008).Mild Induced Hypertension Improves Blood Flow and Oxygen Metabolism in Transient Focal Cerebral Ischemia. *Stroke.* Vol.39, No.5, pp. 1548-1555, ISSN 1524-4628

Shih AY, Friedman B, Drew PJ, Tsai PS, Lyden PD, Kleinfeld D.(2009). Active dilation of penetrating arterioles restores red blood cell flux to penumbral neocortex after focal stroke.*J Cereb Blood Flow Metab.* Vol.29,No.4, pp.738-51,ISSN 1559-7016

Shuaib A, Bornstein NM, Diener HC, Dillon W, Fisher M, Hammer MD, Molina CA, Rutledge JN, Saver JL, Schellinger PD, Shownkeen H; for the SENTIS Trial Investigators. (2011). Partial Aortic Occlusion for Cerebral Perfusion Augmentation: Safety and Efficacy of NeuroFlo in Acute Ischemic Stroke Trial. *Stroke.* Vol.42, No.6, pp. 1680-1690, ISSN 1524-4628

Simons LA, McCallum J, Friedlander Y, Simons J.(1998). Risk factors for ischemic stroke: Dubbo Study of the elderly. *Stroke.* Vol.29,No.7,pp.1341-1346 ,ISSN 1524-4628

Smrcka M, Ogilvy CS, Crow RJ, Maynard KI, Kawamata T, Ames A 3rd. (1998). Induced hypertension improves regional blood flow and protects against infarction during focal ischemia: time course of changes in blood flow measured by laser Doppler imaging. *Neurosurgery.* Vol.42, No.3, pp. 617-624; ISSN 1524-4040

Strong AJ, Bezzina EL, Anderson PJ, Boutelle MG, Hopwood SE, Dunn AK.(2006). Evaluation of laser speckle flowmetry for imaging cortical perfusion in experimental stroke studies: quantitation of perfusion and detection of peri-infarct depolarisations. *J Cereb Blood Flow Metab.* Vol.26,No.5, pp.645-653,ISSN 1559-7016

Sugiyama Y, Yagita Y, Oyama N, Terasaki Y, Omura-Matsuoka E, Sasaki T, Kitagawa K. (2011). Granulocyte colony-stimulating factor enhances arteriogenesis and ameliorates cerebral damage in a mouse model of ischemic stroke. *Stroke.* Vol.42, No.3, 770-775, ISSN 1524-4628

Suzuki N, Hardebo JE, Kåhrström J, Owman C. (1990). Selective electrical stimulation of postganglionic cerebrovascular parasympathetic nerve fibers originating from the sphenopalatineganglion enhances cortical blood flow in the rat.*J Cereb Blood Flow Metab.* Vol.10, No.3,pp.383-391, ISSN 1559-7016

Svoboda K, Yasuda R. (2006). Principles of two-photon excitation microscopy and its applications to neuroscience.*Neuron. Vol.*50,No.6, pp.823-39, ISSN 1097-4199

Thurley PD, Altaf N, Dineen R, MacSweeney S, Auer DP. (2009). Pial vasodilation and moderate hyperaemia following carotid endarterectomy: new MRI diagnostic signs in hyperperfusion/reperfusion syndrome? *Neuroradiology.* Vol.51, No.6, pp. 427-428, ISSN 1432-1920

Todo K, Kitagawa K, Sasaki T, Omura-Matsuoka E, Terasaki Y, Oyama N, Yagita Y, Hori M. (2008). Granulocyte-Macrophage Colony-Stimulating Factor Enhances Leptomeningeal Collateral Growth Induced by Common Carotid Artery Occlusion. *Stroke.* Vol.39, No. 6, pp. 1875-1882, ISSN 1524-4628

Toni D, Lorenzano S, Sacchetti ML, Fiorelli M, De Michele M, Principe M.(2005). Specific therapies for ischaemic stroke: rTPA and others. *Neurol Sci.*Vol. *26,* No.*NA,* pp.S26–S28, ISSN1590-3478

Toyoda K, Fujimoto S, Kamouchi M, Iida M, Okada Y.(2009). Acute blood pressure levels and neurological deterioration in different subtypes of ischemic stroke.*Stroke.* Vol. 40, No.7, pp.2585-2588. ISSN 1524-4628

Ursino M, Giannessi M. (2010). A Model of Cerebrovascular Reactivity Including the Circle of Willis and Cortical Anastomoses. *Annals of biomedical engineering.*Vol.38, No.3, pp.975-994, ISSN 1521-6047

Wadley VG, McClure LA, Howard VJ, Unverzagt FW, Go RC, Moy CS, Crowther MR, Gomez CR, Howard G. (2007). Cognitive status, stroke symptom reports, and modifiable riskfactors among individuals withno diagnosis of stroke or transientischemicattack inthe REasons for Geographic and Racial Differences in Stroke (REGARDS) Study. *Stroke.* Vol. 38, No.4, pp.1143-1147. ISSN 1524-4628

Wahlgren NG, Ahmed N.(2004). Neuroprotection in cerebral ischaemia: facts and fancies--the need for new approaches. *Cerebrovasc Dis.* Vol.17, No.NA, pp.153-166, ISSN 1421-9786

Wardlaw JM, del Zoppo G, Yamaguchi T.(2000). Thrombolysis for acute ischaemic stroke. *Cochrane Database Syst Rev.*Vol.NA, No.2, pp.NA, ISSN 1469-493X

Wei L, Erinjeri JP, Rovainen CM, Woolsey TA. (2001). Collateral Growth and Angiogenesis Around Cortical Stroke. *Stroke.* Vol.32, No.9, pp. 2179-2184, ISSN 1524-4628

Weinreb JC, Abu-Alfa AK.(2009). Gadolinium-based contrast agents and nephrogenic systemic fibrosis: why did it happen and what have we learned? *J Magn Reson Imaging.* Vol.30, No.6, pp.1236-1239, ISSN 1522-2586

Wityk RJ. Blood pressure augmentation in acute ischemic stroke. (2007). *J Neurol Sci.* Vol.261, No.1-2, pp. 63-73, ISSN 1878-5883

Wojner-Alexander AW, Garami Z, Chernyshev OY, Alexandrov AV. (2005). Heads down: flat positioning improves blood flow velocity in acute ischemic stroke. Neurology. Vol.64, No.8, pp.1354-1357, ISSN1526-632X

World health organisation. May, 2011. Available from <http://www.strokecenter.org/patients/stats.htm>

Wu B, Wang X, Guo J, Xie S, Wong EC, Zhang J, Jiang X, Fang J. (2008). Collateral circulation imaging: MR perfusion territory arterial spin-labeling at 3T. *AJNR Am J Neuroradiol.* Vol. 29, No.10, pp. 1855-1860, ISSN 1936-959X

Van Laar PJ, Hendrikse J, Klijn CJ, Kappelle LJ, van Osch MJ, van der Grond J. (2007). Symptomatic carotid artery occlusion: flow territories of major brain-feeding arteries. *Radiology.* Vol.242, No.2, pp. 526-534, ISSN 1527-1315

Vlcek M, Schillinger M, Lang W, Lalouschek W, Bur A, Hirschl MM. (2003). Association between course of blood pressure within the first 24 hours and functional recovery after acute ischemic stroke. *Ann Emerg Med.* Vol.42, No.5, pp. 619-626, ISSN 1097-6760

Yamauchi H, Kudoh T, Sugimoto K, Takahashi M, Kishibe Y, Okazawa H. (2004).Pattern of collaterals, type of infarcts, and haemodynamic impairment in carotid artery occlusion. *J Neurol Neurosurg Psychiatr.* Vol.75, No.12, pp. 1697-1701, ISSN 1468-330X

Yarnitsky D, Lorian A, Shalev A, Zhang ZD, Takahashi M, Agbaje-Williams M, Macdonald RL. (2005). Reversal of cerebral vasospasm by sphenopalatine ganglion stimulation in a dog model of subarachnoid hemorrhage.*Surg Neurol.*Vol.64, No.1, pp.5-11, ISSN 1879-3339

Zhang H, Prabhakar P, Sealock R, Faber JE. (2010). Wide genetic variation in the native pial collateral circulation is a major determinant of variation in severity of stroke. *J Cereb Blood Flow Metab.* Vol.30, No.5, pp. 923-934, ISSN 1559-7016

Zhang S, Boyd J, Delaney K, Murphy TH.(2005). Rapid reversible changes in dentritic spine structure in vivo gated by the degree of ischemia. *J Neurosci.*Vol.25, No.22, pp.5333-5338, ISSN 1529-2401

Zhang S, Murphy TH. (2007). Imaging the impact of cortical microcirculation on synaptic structures and sensory-evoked hemodynamic responses in vivo. *PLoS Biol.* Vol.5, No.5,pp.1152-1167,ISSN1545-7885

11

Does Small Size Vertebral or Vertebrobasilar Artery Matter in Ischemic Stroke?

Jong-Ho Park
Department of Neurology, Stroke Center,
Myongji Hospital, Kwandong University College of Medicine,
South Korea

1. Introduction

The vertebral arteries (VAs) are originated from the subclavian arteries and are major arteries for posterior circulation. The left and right VAs are typically described as having 4 segments each (V_1 through V_4), the first 3 of which are extracranial [1]: the V_1 segments extend cephalad and posteriorly from the origin of the vertebral arteries between the longus colli and scalenus anterior muscles to the level of the transverse foramina, typically adjacent to the sixth cervical vertebra. The V_2 segments extend cephalad from the point at which the arteries enter the most inferior transverse portion of the foramina to their exits from the transverse foramina at the level of the second cervical vertebra. These segments of the left and right VAs therefore have an alternating intraosseous and interosseous course, a unique anatomic environment that exposes the V_2 segments to the possibility of extrinsic compression from spondylotic exostosis of the spine. Small branches from the V_2 segments supply the vertebrae and adjacent musculature and, most importantly, may anastomose with the spinal arteries. The V_3 segments extend laterally from the points at which the arteries exit the C_2 transverse foramina, cephalad and posterior to the superior articular process of C_2, cephalad and medially across the posterior arch of C_1, and then continue into the foramen magnum. Branches of the V_3 segments typically anastomose with branches of the occipital artery at the levels of the first and second cervical vertebrae. The V_4 segments of each vertebral artery extend from the point at which the arteries enter the dura to the termination of these arteries at the vertebrobasilar junction. Important branches of the V_4 segments include the anterior and posterior spinal arteries, the posterior meningeal artery, small medullary branches, and the posterior inferior cerebellar artery (PICA) [1].

2. Significance of hypoplastic vertebral artery on ischemic stroke

Congenital variations in the arrangement and size of the cerebral arteries are frequently recognized [2], ranging from asymmetry or hypoplasia of VA on cerebral angiography. The term, hypoplasia was defined as a lumen diameter of ≤2 mm in a pathoanatomical study [3]. Up to 10 or 15% of the healthy population have one hypoplastic VA (HVA) and makes little contribution to basilar artery (BA) flow [4, 5]. The left VA is dominant in approximately 50%; the right in 25% and only in the remaining quarter of cases are the two VAs of similar caliber [4].

The usual absence of vertebrobasilar insufficiency symptoms among people with HVA has led to an underestimation of clinical significance of HVA. However, ipsilateral HVA is commonly noted in patients with PICA infarction (Fig. 1-A and 1-B) or lateral medullary infarction (LMI, Fig. 2-A and 2-B), suggesting that HVA confers an increased probability of ischemic stroke [6].

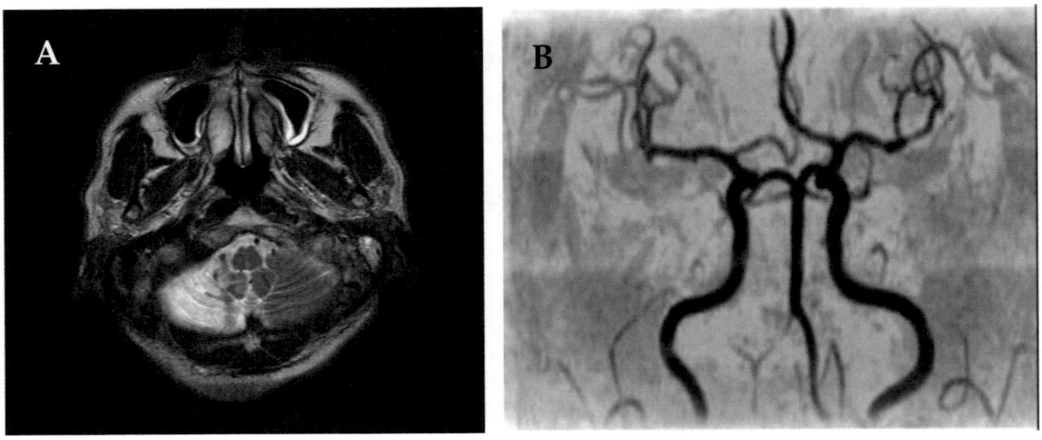

PICAI, posterior inferior cerebellar artery infarction; VA, vertebral artery

Fig. 1. A case of right PICAI with the responsible VA showing hypoplasia.

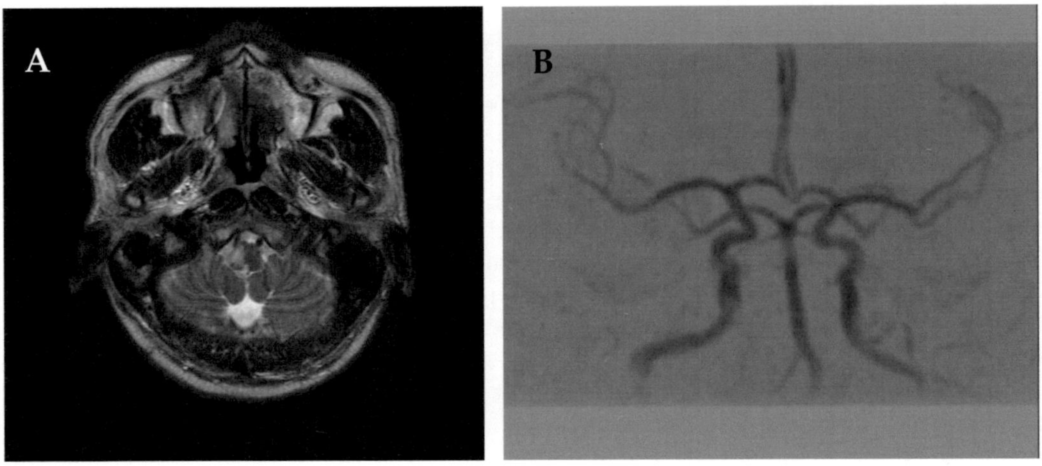

LMI, lateral medullary infarction; VA, vertebral artery

Fig. 2. A case of LMI with the responsible VA showing hypoplasia

Although the HVA is observed in up to 10 or 15% of normal populations [4, 5], there may be many patients with HVA who suffered from posterior circulation stroke (PCS). A Taiwan study [7] examined 191 acute ischemic stroke patients (age 55.8 ± 14.0 years) using a cervical magnetic resonance angiogram (MRA) and a duplex ultrasonography on bilateral VA (V_2 segment level) with flow velocities and vessel diameter within 72 h after stroke onset. The overall incidence of a unilateral congenital HVA was higher especially in cases of brainstem/cerebellar infarction (P=0.022). Subjects with HVA had a preponderance of the large-artery atherosclerosis subtype and a topographic preponderance of ipsilateral PCS.

They suggested HVA seemed a contributing factor of acute ischemic stroke, especially in PCS territories. Perren et al [8] investigated 725 first-ever stroke patients, using color-coded duplex flow imaging of the V_2 segment, and showed that HVA (diameter ≤2.5 mm) was more frequent in PCS (mostly brainstem and cerebellum) than in strokes in other territories (13% vs. 4.6%, $P<0.001$), whereas distribution of all other risk factors (e.g. hypertension, hyperlipidemia, diabetes, smoking) were comparable ($P>0.05$). They concluded that HVA may be predisposed to PCS.

Park et al [6] investigated the frequency and clinical relevance of HVA in 529 stroke patients [303 anterior (ACS) and 226 PCS] and in 306 normal healthy people. When classified by stroke location, patients with PCS (45.6%) showed more significant frequency of HVA than those with ACS (27.1%) and normal healthy people (26.5%, $P<0.001$ for all). Out of 226 patients with PCS, ischemic lesion distribution of VA territory stroke (PICA or LMI) in 102 PCS patients was examined by the group of VA (hypoplastic, dominant, and symmetric). HVA was defined as a VA with a diameter of ≤2 mm, and the larger (contralateral) one was defined as a dominant VA. The VA symmetry was defined when both VAs have a diameter >2 mm. Cardioembolic stroke was more prevalent in the symmetric group ($P<0.05$). In terms of demographic features, risk factors, and laboratory findings, there were no significant differences. Acute ischemic lesions of the VA territory stroke were present mostly in the PICA territory and then lateral medulla, PICA territory + lateral medulla, PICA territory + BA territory or more. It is because the HVA may terminate in the PICA or extends beyond the PICA to the BA, contributing little to BA blood flow [1].

Ischemic lesion distributions in the VA feature groups are displayed in Fig. 3 [6]. LMI and PICAI were dominant in the HVA group. Multiple infarctions, such as LMI + PICAI, and PICAI + ≥BA territory infarction were also more prominent in the HVA group than in the symmetric group. In the dominant VA group, the lesions were present dominantly in the PICA territory, and then in the lateral medulla. Ipsilateral HVA tended to predict the involvement of multiple and extensive lesions, and a higher incidence of steno-occlusion.

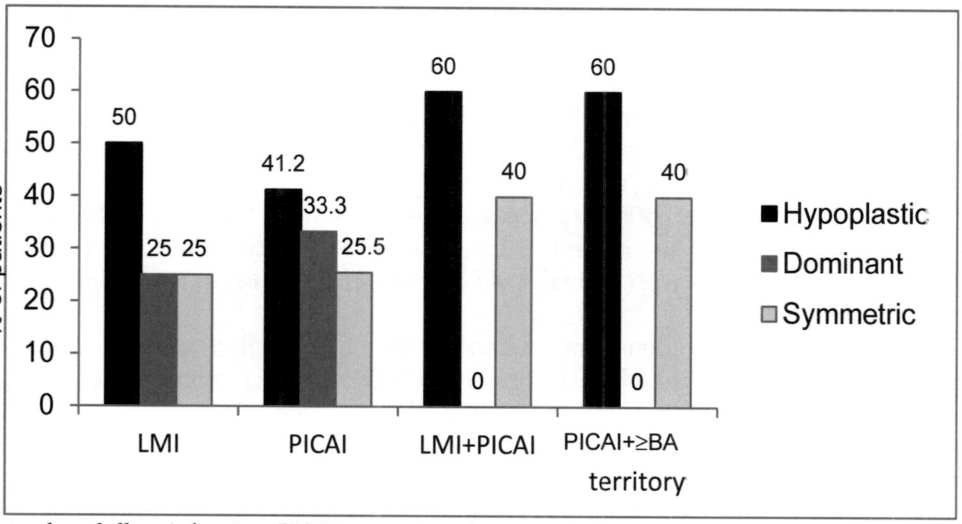

LMI, lateral medullary infarction; PICAI, posterior inferior cerebellar artery infarction; ≥BA, more than basilar artery.

Fig. 3. Lesion distribution by VA group in patients with VA territory infarction [6]

Stenosis or occlusion of the intracranial VA was significantly more prevalent in the hypoplastic group (vs. dominant or symmetric group). Taking these into account, HVA may be etiopathogenetically implicated in PCS, especially the VA territory.

In VA territory stroke, cardioembolism and artery-to-artery embolism are the two most common stroke mechanisms [9]. Most of VA territory stroke patients with ipsilateral HVA showed stenosis/occlusion and multiple ischemic lesions were dominant in the HVA group. Cardioembolic stroke was least prevalent in the HVA group. It is thought that luminal narrowing of the HVA might make it less feasible for cardiogenic emboli to pass through it. Accordingly, HVA-related ischemic stroke is based on large-artery atherosclerosis [6]. The HVA may not be an uncommon asymptomatic if there are no risk factors, but it may contribute to PCS in some patients, if additional risk factors are present [10].

3. Ischemic stroke patterns and hemodynamic features in patients with HVA or small vertebrobasilar artery

In terms of BA hypoplasia (BAH), there have been few case reports regarding an association between BAH and PCS [11, 12]. A recent study showed that BAH, defined as a diameter <2 mm was 3-fold higher in patients with PCS (vs. ACS), in which the stroke subtype was undetermined or lacunar stroke [13]. Localization of PCS was predominant in pons or cerebellar territories (71.4%). Half of PCS of BAH patients were characteristic of small infarcts by pontic-penetrating arteries [13]. The blood flow volume and velocity might be decreased in small-sized (hypoplastic artery), resulting in a higher susceptibility to pro-thrombotic or atherosclerosis processes than normal-sized artery [14].

Actually however, BAH usually accompanied by HVA which can be seen on MRA or transfemoral cerebral angiography (TFCA). Age-related atherosclerosis might gradually restrict the compliance of the vertebro-basilar artery hypoplasia. Sudden exertion or emotional stress would incur a paradoxical cerebral vasoconstriction and the following transient hemodynamic insufficiency may occur [15].

How do ischemic patterns in patients with hypoplastic VBA differ from those in subjects with a normal-sized VBA? Recently ischemic patterns, collateral features, and stroke mechanisms in 37 acute (2.3 ± 1.1 days after stroke onset) PCS patients after stroke onset with small vertebrobasilar artery (SVBA) were investigated [16]. The mean diameter of the normal BA has been reported to be 3.17 mm [17] and the HVA was defined to have a lumen diameter of less than 2–3 mm [18, 19]. Accordingly, SVBA was defined as a lumen diameter of <3 mm. The diameter of SVBA was measured in the mid-portion level of the BA and the V_2 of the largest VA by using magnified images of MRA. Thirty acute (2.2 ± 1.4 days after stroke onset) PCS patients with normal-sized BA (>3 mm in diameter) were compared as the control group.

Ischemic lesions were predominantly observed in the cerebellum and/or medulla (VA territory) [16]. All subjects had fetal posterior circulation (FPC) from the internal carotid artery to the posterior cerebral artery. Many of the patients had distal or diffuse VA stenosis/occlusion (88.9%) and long circumferential artery (77.8%). As the degree of VA disease increased (i.e., from "none" to "unilateral" to "bilateral"), the frequency of long circumferential artery (posterior/inferior/anterior cerebellar artery) prominence (i.e., "none," "one," and "two or more") tended to increase ($P<0.05$). Ischemic lesions were predominantly observed in the cerebellum and/or medulla in the VA territory (72.2%). Relatively small, scattered infarcts were observed in patients with SVBA than in those with stenotic normal-sized VBA (Fig. 4-A and 4-B). In atherothrombotic patients, infratentorial PCS might occur following artery-to-artery embolism from the low-flowed or stenotic VA to long circumferential artery. Regardless of extensive arterial lesions, relatively small infarcts may be due to previously established collaterals from the long circumferential artery (e.g. PICA, anterior inferior cerebellar artery, superior cerebellar artery), which could compensate for the defects in the infratentorial area.

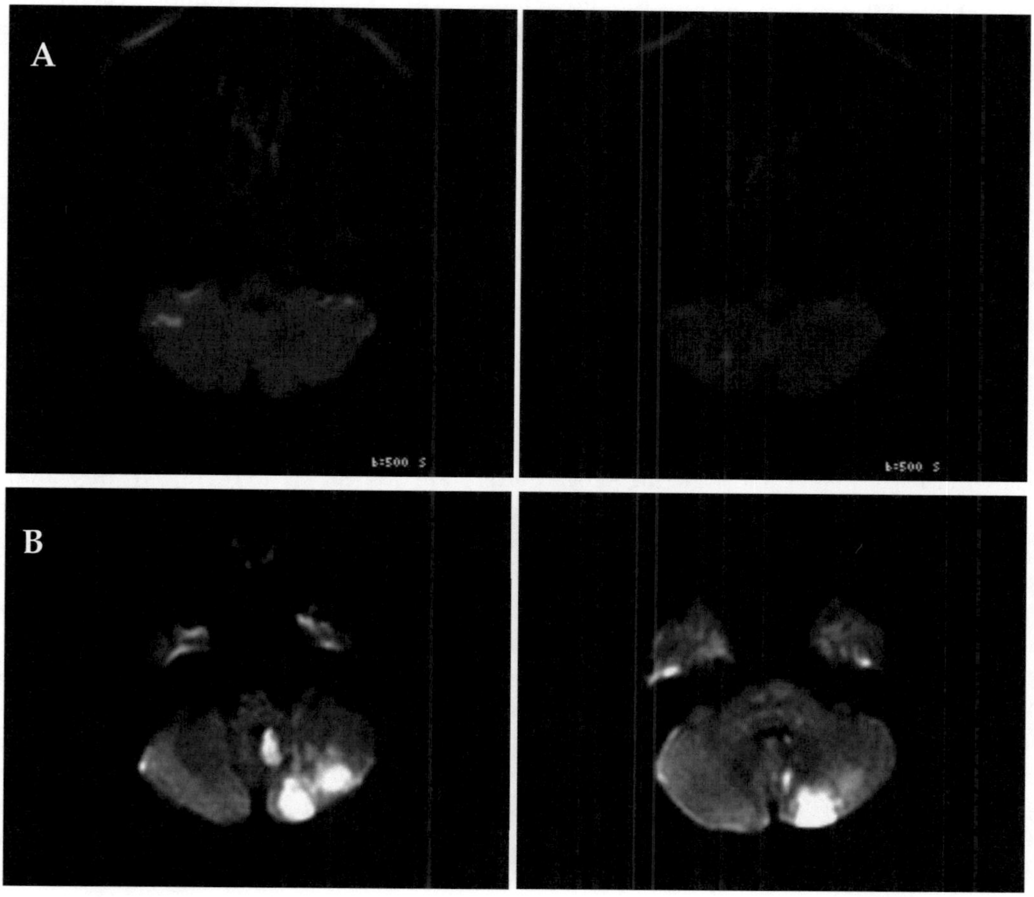

SVBA, small vertebrobasilar artery

Fig. 4. Relatively small, scattered infarcts were observed in patients with SVBAs (Fig. 4-A) than in those with stenotic normal-sized VBA (Fig. 4-B).

The stenotic normal-sized VBA group showed relatively large, conglomerate infarct patterns compared with those of stenotic SVBA group. However, the ischemic findings of some patients with normal-sized VBA were similar to those of SVBA group. They had common feature that showed extracranial focal VA lesion (below the V_3).

4. Association of fetal posterior circulation with PCS

Fetal posterior circulation (FPC) is a fetal variant of the posterior cerebral artery from the internal carotid artery. The prevalence of FPC is reported to be 32% in the general population [20]. A recent study showed the existent varieties of FPC (bilateral in 88.9% of patients), and suggested that FPC may compensate the posterior circulation zone for the hemodynamic insufficiency caused by SVBA [16]. Since the cerebellar tentorium impedes the formation of a leptomeningeal connection, FPC does not contribute to the perfusion of the infratentorial area [21]. Consequently, FPC makes the development of leptomeningeal collaterals between the internal carotid artery and the vertebrobasilar system impossible [21]. The result [16] that most of the infratentorial lesions originated from the cerebellum and/or medulla (VA territory) or the pons (BA territory) are consistent with that [21] FPC would not be able to protect the infratentorial area against PCS.

5. SVBA is of congenital origin or a consequence of multiple or longitudinal atherosclerotic narrowing?

Embryologically, if the BA does not become the main source of blood supply to the developing posterior cerebral arteries, the FPC might persist and remain large in size [22]. The observations that all the study patients had FPC and that the FPC was larger than the vertebrobasilar artery may support the hypothesis that the SVBA is congenitally small rather than acquired [16].

6. Hemodynamic mechanism of hypoplastic artery causing to ischemic stroke

Why does size matter and how the smaller artery are susceptible to occlusion? Size alone cannot be explained because many intracranial arteries are smaller than the hypoplastic arteries and they are not predisposed to occlude [14]. An interaction between blood pressure, blood constituents and the rheology and physics of blood flow at various arterial locations might affect arterial occlusion [14]. The HVA, which shows lower mean flow volume [7, 23, 24] and decreased flow velocities [24], seems to be more susceptible to pro-thrombotic or atherosclerotic processes than normal or dominant VAs. Under the decreased VA flow capacity, hypoplastic artery is prone to collapse as a result of Bernoulli's effect [25]. Therefore, it is postulated that a HVA can result in the ipsilateral occlusion of this vessel due to a direct decrease in blood flow and easy collapse of the vessel caused by the smaller VA caliber [26]. The HVA may further contribute to PCS, if additional risk factors such as hypertension, diabetes exist. Most of patients with VA territory stroke who showed VA stenosis/occlusion had HVA [6].

7. Characteristic findings of HVA or SVBA by ultrasonography

Jeng et al attempted to attain reference values for VA flow volume by color Doppler ultrasonography, analyze age and gender effects on VA flow volume and develop a definition of HVA [5]. Color Doppler ultrasonography was performed in 447 subjects free of stroke or carotid stenosis. They found significant asymmetries in diameter, flow velocities and flow volume with left-sided dominance. Diameters were different on left (0.297 ± 0.052 cm) and right (0.323 ± 0.057 cm) sides ($P<0.001$). Flow volume was different on right (83.0 ± 36.9 mL/min) and left (96.6 ± 42.4) sides ($P<0.001$). Women had significantly smaller diameters, higher flow velocities and lower resistance indexes (RIs) than men. VA flow volume did not change with aging. They defined HVA as a significant decrease in flow velocities and increase in RI for VA diameters <0.22 cm. This definition is supported by findings of an increase in ipsilateral flow resistance (RI ≥0.75), contralateral diameter (side-to-side diameter difference ≥0.12 cm), and flow volume (side-to-side flow volume ratio ≥5).

The stroke mechanism of PCS patients with SVBA was mostly large-artery atherosclerosis and they showed stenosis or poor perfusion state (from blunted to absent signal) of VA and/or BA on transcranial Doppler [16]. According to the Bernoulli's principle, the greater the flow velocity, the less the lateral pressure on the vessel wall. Therefore, if an hypoplastic artery is narrowed by atherosclerotic plaque, the flow velocity would increase through the constriction and decrease in lateral pressure.

8. Evaluation of patients with HVA or SVBA

Evaluation of the patient with presumed vertebrobasilar insufficiency or PCS should begin with a thorough clinical history and examination followed by noninvasive imaging (e.g. MRA) as for patients with carotid artery disease [27]. In case of a patient with symptomatic HVA or SVBA, which was initially seen on three-dimension time-of-flight (3D TOF) circle of Willis MRA, contrast-enhanced neck computed tomography angiography (CTA) or contrast-enhanced neck MRA is recommended.

Contrast-enhanced CTA and MRA were associated with higher sensitivity (94%) and specificity (95%) than duplex ultrasonography (sensitivity 70%), and CTA had slightly superior accuracy [28]. Because neither CTA nor MRA reliably delineates the origins of theVAs, catheter-based contrast angiography is typically required before revascularization for patients with symptomatic posterior cerebral ischemia [28].

In patient with SVBA, 3D TOF MRA can barely demonstrate VBA configuration. Even the VBA system cannot be seen entirely according to the degree of atherosclerotic burden. TFCA enables us to see collaterals from the VBA. In some patients, TFCA provides hemodynamical information that upper brainstem was supplied from retrograde filling of BA through the fetal circulation. Rarely, there can be seen some collaterals around the VBA in a patient whose VBA is nearly invisible in 3D TOF MRA. Such findings are correlated with collaterals from long circumferential arteries in TFCA. In fact, advanced arterial narrowing from the VA orifice made it difficult to access the entire VBA by TFCA. The TFCA may be actually dangerous than contrast-enhanced imaging because of catheter-induced embolization in an atherogenic small caliber.

9. Management of PCS patients with HVA or SVBA

PCS patients by stenotic HVA or SVBA is encountered very less commonly in clinical practice than those with usual PCS, and the evidence-based guideline for evaluation and management is less substantial.

9.1 Medical therapy

Therapeutic guidelines are as same as patients with VA disease [1]: antiplatelet drug therapy is recommended as part of the initial management for patients with symptomatic HVA or SVBA. Aspirin (81 to 325 mg daily), the combination of aspirin plus extended-release dipyridamole (25 and 200 mg twice daily, respectively), and clopidogrel (75 mg daily) are acceptable options. Selection of an antiplatelet regimen should be individualized on the basis of patient risk factor profiles, cost, tolerance, and other clinical characteristics, as well as guidance from regulatory agencies [31–36].

There is no consensus about anticoagulation therapy. Most of the HVA- or SVBA-related ischemic stroke is based on large-artery atherosclerosis [6, 16]. The WASID (Warfarin versus Aspirin for Symptomatic Intracranial Disease) trial found aspirin and warfarin to be equally efficacious after initial noncardioembolic ischemic stroke [37, 38]. Accordingly, anticoagulation may not be generally recommended as a rational therapeutic option in PCS patients with HVA or SVBA.

9.2 Endovascular revascularization

In terms of endovascular interventions, although angioplasty and stenting of the VAs are technically feasible, as for high-risk patients with carotid artery stenosis, there is insufficient evidence from randomized trials to demonstrate that endovascular management is superior to best medical management [1].

9.3 Surgical revascularization

When both VAs are patent and one symptomatic VA has a definite stenotic lesion with the uninvolved larger VA supplying sufficient blood flow to the BA, corrective surgery may be effective [1]. The surgical approach to atherosclerotic lesions at the origin of the VA includes trans-subclavian vertebral endarterectomy, transposition of the VA to the ipsilateral common carotid artery, and reimplantation of the VA with vein graft extension to the subclavian artery. Distal reconstruction of the VA, necessitated by total occlusion of the midportion, may be accomplished by anastomosis of the principal trunk of the external carotid artery to the VA at the level of the second cervical vertebra [39].

10. Summary

The PCS group showed a higher frequency of HVA than the ACS group and all the patients with unilateral HVA among those with VA territory stroke showed ipsilateral ischemic lesions. These findings provide evidence that HVA may be etiopathogenetically implicated in PCS [6]. Patients with SVBA showed FPC with bilateral dominance and FPC may compensate the supratentorial posterior circulation zone (e.g. temporooccipital area) for the hemodynamic insufficiency: most of the infratentorial lesions originated from the cerebellum and/or medulla (VA territory) or the pons (BA territory). Regardless of the presence of extensive arterial lesions (atherothrombotic SVBA), relatively small infarcts can be attributed to the established leptomeningeal collaterals from the long circumferential arteries that can compensate for the defects in the infratentorial area. Thus, the degree of collateral development along with a chronic process of atherothrombosis may determine the pattern (particularly, the size) of an ischemic lesion [16].

Optimum management of PCS patients with HVA or SVBA is not as well established as that for patients with carotid stenosis [1]. Considering for small-diameter vascular state, medical therapy and lifestyle modification to reduce atherosclerotic burden would be most appropriate, which is identical with patients with VA disease [29, 30]. This would be optimal measures in principle directed at reduction of atherosclerotic burden and the prevention of recurrent PCS, although none have been evaluated in randomized trials about medical versus surgical approaches.

11. References

[1] Brott TG, Halperin JL, Abbara S, Bacharach JM, Barr JD, Bush RL, Cates CU, Creager MA, Fowler SB, Friday G, Hertzberg VS, McIff EB, Moore WS, Panagos PD, Riles TS, Rosenwasser RH, Taylor AJ. 2011 ASA/ACCF/AHA/AANN/AANS/ACR/ASNR/CNS/SAIP/SCAI/SIR/SNIS /SVM/SVS Guideline on the Management of Patients With Extracranial Carotid and Vertebral Artery Disease. A Report of the American College of Cardiology Foundation/American Heart Association Task Force on Practice Guidelines, and the American Stroke Association, American Association of Neuroscience Nurses, American Association of Neurological Surgeons, American College of Radiology, American Society of Neuroradiology, Congress of Neurological Surgeons, Society of Atherosclerosis Imaging and Prevention, Society for Cardiovascular Angiography and Interventions, Society of Interventional Radiology, Society of NeuroInterventional Surgery, Society for Vascular Medicine, and Society for Vascular Surgery. *Stroke* 2011 [Epub ahead of print]

[2] Caldemeyer K, Carrico J, Mathews V. The radiology and embryology of anomalous arteries of the head and neck. *AJR Am J Roentgenol* 1998;170:197–203.

[3] Fisher CM, Gore I, Okabe N, et al. Atherosclerosis of the carotid and vertebral arteries—extracranial and intracranial. *J Neuropathol Exp Neurol* 1965;24:455–476.

[4] Cloud GC, Markus HS. Diagnosis and management of vertebral artery stenosis. *Q J Med* 2003;96:27–34.

[5] Jeng JS, Yip PK. Evaluation of vertebral artery hypoplasia and asymmetry by color-coded duplex ultrasonography. *Ultrasound in Med Biol* 2004;30:605–609.

[6] Park JH, Kim JM, Roh JK. Hypoplastic vertebral artery; frequency and associations with ischemic stroke territory. *J Neurol Neurosurg Psychiatry* 2007;78:954–958.

[7] Chuang YM, Huang YC, Hu HH, Yang CY. Toward a further elucidation: role of vertebral artery hypoplasia in acute ischemic stroke. *Eur Neurol* 2006;55:193–197.

[8] Perren F, Poglia D, Landis T, Sztajzel R. Vertebral artery hypoplasia: a predisposing factor for posterior circulation stroke? *Neurology* 2007;68:65–67.

[9] Caplan LR, Wityk RJ, Glass TA, Tapia J, Pazdera L, Chang HM, Teal P, Dashe JF, Chaves CJ, Breen JC, Vemmos K, Amarenco P, Tettenborn B, Leary M, Estol C, Dewitt LD, Pessin MS. New England Medical Center Posterior Circulation registry. *Ann Neurol* 2004;56:389–398.

[10] Giannopoulos S, Markoula S, Kosmidou M, Pelidou SH, Kyritsis AP. Lateral medullary ischaemic events in young adults with hypoplastic vertebral artery. *J Neurol Neurosurg Psychiatry* 2007;78:987–989.

[11] Szdzuy D, Lehmann R. Hypoplastic distal part of the basilar artery. *Neuroradiology.* 1972;4:118–120.

[12] Hegedus K. Hypoplasia of the basilar artery. Three case reports. *Eur Arch Psychiatr Neurol Sci* 1985;234:395–398.

[13] Olindo S, Khaddam S, Bocquet J, Chausson N, Aveillan M, Cabre P, Smadja D. Association between basilar artery hypoplasia and undetermined or lacunar posterior circulation ischemic stroke. *Stroke* 2010;41:2371–2374.

[14] Caplan LR. Arterial occlusions: does size matter? *J Neurol Neurosurg Psychiatry* 2007;78: 916.

[15] Chuang YM, Hu HH, Pan PJ. Cerebral syncope: insights from Valsalva maneuver. *Eur Neurol* 2005;54:98–102.

[16] Park JH, Roh JK, Kwon HM. Ischemic patterns and hemodynamic features of hypoplastic vertebrobasilar artery. *J Neurol Sci* 2009;287:227–235.

[17] Smoker WR, Price MJ, Keyes WD, Corbett JJ, Gentry LR. High-resolution computed tomography of the basilar artery: Normal size and position. *AJNR Am J Neuroradiol* 1986;7:55–60.

[18] Fisher CM, Gore I, Okabe N, White PD. Atherosclerosis of the carotid and vertebral arteries-Extracranial and intracranial. *J Neuropathol Exp Neurol* 1965;24:455–476.

[19] Touboul PJ, Bousser MG, LaPlane D, Castaigne P. Duplex scanning of normal vertebral arteries. *Stroke* 1986;17:921–923.

[20] Krabbe Hartkamp MJ, Van der Grond J, de Leeuw FE, de Groot JC, Algra A, Hillen B, Breteler MM, Mali WP. Circle of Willis: morphologic variation on three-dimensional time-of-flight MR angiograms. *Radiology* 1998;207:103–111.

[21] van Raamt AF, Mali WP, van Laar PJ, van der Graaf Y. The fetal variant of the circle of Willis and its influence on the cerebral collateral circulation. *Cerebrovasc Dis* 2006;22:217–224.

[22] Chaturvedi S, Lukovits TG, Chen W, Gorelick PB. Ischemia in the territory of a hypoplastic vertebrobasilar system. *Neurology* 1999;52:980–983.

[23] Schöning M, Hartig B. The development of hemodynamics in the extracranial carotid and vertebral arteries. *Ultrasound Med Biol* 1998;24:655–662.

[24] Bartels E, ed. Vertebral sonography. Color-coded duplex ultrasonography of the cerebral vessels:atlas and manual. Stuttgart: Schattauer, 1999:113–155.

[25] Binns RL, Ku DN. Effect of stenosis on wall motion. A possible mechanism of stroke and transient ischemic attack. *Arteriosclerosis* 1989;9:842–847.

[26] Hong JM, Chung JS, Bang OY, Yong SW, Joo IS, Huh K. Vertebral artery dominance contributes to basilar artery curvature and peri-vertebrobasilar junctional infarcts. *J Neurol Neurosurg Psychiatry* 2009;80:1087–1092.

[27] Blacker DJ, Flemming KD, Wijdicks EF. Risk of ischemic stroke in patients with symptomatic vertebrobasilar stenosis undergoing surgical procedures. *Stroke* 2003;34:2659–2663.

[28] Long A, Lepoutre A, Corbillon E, Branchereau A. Critical review of non- or minimally invasive methods (duplex ultrasonography, MR- and CT-angiography) for evaluating stenosis of the proximal internal carotid artery. *Eur J Vasc Endovasc Surg* 2002;24:43–52.

[29] Third Report of the National Cholesterol Education Program (NCEP) Expert Panel on Detection, Evaluation, and Treatment of High Blood Cholesterol in Adults (Adult Treatment Panel III) final report. *Circulation* 2002;106:3143–3421.

[30] Ginsberg HN, Kris-Etherton P, Dennis B, Elmer PJ, Ershow A, Lefevre M, Pearson T, Roheim P, Ramakrishnan R, Reed R, Stewart K, Stewart P, Phillips K, Anderson N. Effects of reducing dietary saturated fatty acids on plasma lipids and lipoproteins in healthy subjects: the DELTA Study, protocol 1. *Arterioscler Thromb Vasc Biol* 1998;18:441–449.

[31] Adams RJ, Albers G, Alberts MJ, Benavente O, Furie K, Goldstein LB, Gorelick P, Halperin J, Harbaugh R, Johnston SC, Katzan I, Kelly-Hayes M, Kenton EJ, Marks M, Sacco RL, Schwamm LH; American Heart Association; American Stroke Association. Update to the AHA/ASA recommendations for the prevention of stroke in patients with stroke and transient ischemic attack. *Stroke* 2008;39:1647–1652.

[32] Antithrombotic Trialists' Collaboration. Collaborative meta-analysis of randomised trials of antiplatelet therapy for prevention of death, myocardial infarction, and stroke in high risk patients. *BMJ* 2002;324:71–86

[33] CAPRIE Steering Committee. A randomised, blinded, trial of clopidogrel versus aspirin in patients at risk of ischaemic events (CAPRIE). *Lancet* 1996;348:1329–1339.

[34] Diener HC, Bogousslavsky J, Brass LM, Cimminiello C, Csiba L, Kaste M, Leys D, Matias-Guiu J, Rupprecht HJ; MATCH investigators. Aspirin and clopidogrel compared with clopidogrel alone after recent ischaemic stroke or transient ischaemic attack in high-risk patients (MATCH): randomised, double-blind, placebo-controlled trial. *Lancet* 2004;364:331–337.

[35] Diener HC, Cunha L, Forbes C, Sivenius J, Smets P, Lowenthal A. European Stroke Prevention Study 2. Dipyridamole and acetylsalicylic acid in the secondary prevention of stroke. *J Neurol Sci* 1996;143:1–13.

[36] Sacco RL, Diener HC, Yusuf S, Cotton D, Ounpuu S, Lawton WA, Palesch Y, Martin RH, Albers GW, Bath P, Bornstein N, Chan BP, Chen ST, Cunha L, Dahlöf B, De Keyser J, Donnan GA, Estol C, Gorelick P, Gu V, Hermansson K, Hilbrich L, Kaste M, Lu C, Machnig T, Pais P, Roberts R, Skvortsova V, Teal P, Toni D, Vandermaelen C, Voigt T, Weber M, Yoon BW; PRoFESS Study Group. Aspirin and extended-release dipyridamole versus clopidogrel for recurrent stroke. *N Engl J Med* 2008;359:1238–1251.

[37] Kasner SE, Lynn MJ, Chimowitz MI, Frankel MR, Howlett-Smith H, Hertzberg VS, Chaturvedi S, Levine SR, Stern BJ, Benesch CG, Jovin TG, Sila CA, Romano JG; Warfarin Aspirin Symptomatic Intracranial Disease (WASID) Trial Investigators. Warfarin vs aspirin for symptomatic intracranial stenosis: subgroup analyses from WASID. *Neurology* 2006;67:1275–1278.

[38] Benesch CG, Chimowitz MI. Best treatment for intracranial arterial stenosis? 50 years of uncertainty. The WASID Investigators. *Neurology* 2000;55:465–466.

[39] Berguer R, Bauer RB. Vertebral artery reconstruction: a successful technique in selected patients. *Ann Surg* 1981;193:441–447.

12

Hyperbaric Oxygen for Stroke

Ann Helms and Harry T. Whelan
Medical College of Wisconsin
USA

1. Introduction

The largest body of evidence involving the use of hyperbaric oxygen for neurologic illness is found in the field of cerebral ischemia. At the center of an infarct, blood flow is completely absent, causing neurons to die within a matter of minutes. This area, therefore, may not be amenable to treatment after the start of symptoms. The region of the brain that draws the most interest is the penumbra, where evidence has shown that blood flow is diminished, but not absent. The cells in this region remain viable for a prolonged period, and can be saved if adequate perfusion is restored. The only FDA approved therapies for acute ischemic stroke include tPA, and interventional intra-arterial treatments aimed at restoring blood flow to the ischemic penumbra, but must be used within the first few hours of the onset of symptoms. There is also evidence that a percentage of the cells subjected to prolonged ischemia will inevitably undergo apoptosis, either after prolonged ischemia or due to reperfusion injury in the case of temporary ischemia. As a result, there has been great interest in using HBO_2T for the added benefit of its anti-inflammatory and anti-apoptotic properties. There is reasonable evidence from animal studies, involving mice, rats, gerbils, and cats that damage from focal cerebral ischemia is ameliorated after treatment with HBO_2T. Several human trials investigating the use of HBO_2T for ischemic stroke have also been performed. Most of these lacked controls, as well as uniform standards for inclusion criteria and outcome measurement. There have been three prominent randomized controlled studies that have evaluated HBO_2T in ischemic stroke, none of which where able to demonstrate statistically significant benefit. One might conclude from this that HBO_2T is an ineffective treatment for ischemic stroke, however, it should be noted that these studies enrolled patients well after the therapeutic window of 6 - 12 hours suggested by previous animal studies. Additionally, two of the three also used lower doses of HBO_2T than was found effective in animal studies. Based on our present understanding of ischemia, one would not expect improvement in measured outcomes under these conditions.

It seems therefore reasonable to assess patients presenting for potential HBO_2T for a pattern of penumbra as this provides the strongest evidence of recoverable tissue. As the ischemic penumbra represents the area which is expected to be most salvageable, it is reasonable to determine whether a penumbra is or is not present in patients undergoing experimental treatment with HBO_2T. On MRI, penumbra is represented by perfusion-diffusion mismatch. More simply stated, we must find the area of brain which is dying in hope that HBO_2T can still save it before it is dead. This is called ischemic penumbra. In the rat model of focal ischemic stroke produced via thrombotic occlusion of the MCA, MRI revealed perfusion-diffusion mismatch which persists up to 6-12 hours after the occlusion. In patients such mismatch is usually present during the first 6 hours after stroke. Noticeably, HBO_2T was effective against experimental stroke if administered when a penumbra is typically present in the brain. HBO_2T administered at a time when penumbra is usually gone (e.g. at 23 hours) may even be harmful. The clinical trials done with HBO_2T so far did not follow this paradigm, which creates the most important discrepancy between experimental and clinical work. We propose that the evaluation of patients in any future clinical trial should include separate subgroup analyses of patients with and without confirmed penumbra as the impact on outcomes may be different in these two groups.

As the accepted standards of stroke care are paramount in treatment of any patient presenting with acute stroke, patients presenting within the therapeutic window for tPA should be treated with tPA but should be considered for HBO_2T as well if they have persistent neurologic deficits on physical examination and can be treated within the time window. This is because even in cases of temporary ischemia HBO_2T has shown benefit in animal studies through decreases in reperfusion injury.

2. Hyperbaric oxygen for stroke protocol background

This chapter discribes the protocol which we propose ulitmitaly leading to a multicenter trial, as follows.

The purpose of this study is to determine the safety of hyperbaric oxygen therapy of acute ischemic stroke at a dose of 2.4ATA for 90 minutes administered in the first 12 hours of symptoms. The data obtained will be used to determine safety and to estimate effect size in order to plan a larger, adequately powered, multicenter trial.

Presently, in the US, tPA is the only FDA approved therapy for treatment of acute ischemic stroke (AIS). Unfortunately, only around 3-5% of patients with stroke receive tPA therapy due to the strict time limitations and the high risk of bleeding associated with its use. Therefore, other modalities of treatment for acute ischemic stroke need to be investigated.

Animal studies have suggested that administration of pure oxygen at high pressure can be protective against the effects of cerebral ischemia. Some small uncontrolled studies in humans have shown benefit of HBO. However, no study has tested HBO in stroke at a time and a dose which, based on animal studies, could be expected to be effective.

HBO therapy of cerebral ischemia has been shown to be effective in numerous animal models of AIS (1). Animals treated with HBO after either temporary (2, 3, 4, 5, 6, 7, 8, 9, 10) or permanent (9, 10) cerebral arterial occlusion showed decreased infarct size versus controls. Improved survival, function and behavior in HBO treated animals were also reported (2, 3, 5, 6, 9, 10, 11, 13, 14, 15, 16, 17, 18, 19). Several of the studies used a model involving the nearly immediate institution of HBO, starting treatment immediately (2, 9, 13, 20) or within minutes (8, 11, 12, 14) of ischemia. In models more consistent with conditions in a clinical setting, however, HBO delayed until several hours after the beginning of ischemia was also been shown to be effective. (3, 4, 7, 8, 10, 15) There may, though, be an early window of opportunity after ischemia for HBO to be effective. One study found that treatment after 1 or 3 hours of ischemia decreased infarct size and improved outcome behaviorally, whereas, treatment after 4 hours had no effect on infarct size. (3) A more recent study, however, showed that HBO treatments initiated up to 24 hours after transient cerebral ischemia in rats resulted in decreased infarct size and neurologic deficits at 4 weeks (10).

Human trials of HBO for AIS have been less conclusive. Most of the early trials reported a benefit from treatment of ischemic stroke patients with HBO. (21, 22, 23, 24, 25) These trials, however, were for the most part, uncontrolled, and utilized greatly disparate criteria for inclusion as well as for evaluation of improvement. Of the three small recent randomized trials of HBO in AIS (26, 27, 28), no significant difference was seen between treatment and sham groups. Significantly, however, treatments were not limited to the hyperacute stage, as patients were enrolled up to 24 hours after symptom onset in 2 studies, and up to 2 weeks in the third. Also, in two of the studies, patients receiving sham treatment were given either hyperbaric air, or 100% O2 at slightly increased pressure, neither of which is known to be clinically insignificant. Further, these studies used a lower dose of HBO than has been shown effective in animal studies, as well as in human clinical use for other approved indications (wound healing, CO poisoning, etc.)

All but one of the studies evaluating HBO therapy of ischemic stroke have used a dose of 1.5 ATA. This was selected based upon concerns for increased risk of oxidative stress with higher doses suggested in a single study from 1977 (29). This study was limited, however, by inclusion of only 7 ischemic stroke patients (the rest had traumatic brain injury) and the administration of HBO several days after the cerebral insult. Despite concerns for increased oxidative stress, the patients who received the higher doses of HBO did not have seizures or worsening of neurologic deficits.

There is a theoretical concern that hyperbaric treatment at a higher dose could cause oxidative stress through free radical damage leading to an increase in neuronal loss and thus a worse clinical outcome. Some animal studies have shown increases in lipid peroxidation (52), a marker of free radical damage, but most have not (12, 53-55). The single study which assessed the use of HBO at 2.5 ATA in acute stroke did raise concerns of worsened stroke outcome at the higher dose, but was limited by several factors (28). First, most of the patients were treated after 12 hours. Second, the control group was subjected to 100% O2 at 1.14 ATA, which is not standard care. Third, there was no cut-off for stroke severity, such that very mild strokes were included, making evaluation of the effect of HBO difficult. Also, the differences seen were not statistically significant.

The selection of the dose for this study is based on several facts. First, HBO is approved for use by the FDA at a dose of 2.4 ATA for 90 minutes for treatment of numerous conditions and is well tolerated (30). Despite the above stated safety concerns, patients with arterial gas embolism and decompression illness, both of which commonly cause ischemia of the central nervous system, are treated with even higher doses of HBO with good efficacy and acceptable safety levels (31, 32). This cannot, however, be directly compared to ischemic stroke as the pathological mechanism of ischemia is different, and as such, a study is warranted. Second, this dose is more consistent with animal studies which have shown efficacy (see above).

The rationale for the use of HBO in cerebral ischemia centers upon increasing oxygenation to an ischemic penumbra and thus reducing the subsequent effects of hypoxia. Additionally, there may be other effects of HBO contributing to improved outcome after cerebral ischemia. Decrease in cerebral blood flow caused by oxygen induced vasoconstriction, has been shown in humans (35) as well as animals (5, 36) treated with HBO, and may produce a decrease in cerebral edema. Also, HBO may have benefit in the treatment of stroke by exerting an indirect neuroprotective effect. Decreased neuronal shrinkage and edema as well as decreased necrotic damage have been described histologically in animals treated with HBO after ischemia. (13, 19, 20, 37) Additionally, and perhaps more importantly, far fewer neurons show evidence of having undergone subsequent apoptosis after ischemia in animals treated with HBO. (15, 37, 38) HBO exposures in the first few minutes or hours after ischemia must, therefore, effect a lasting physiologic change which interrupts the subsequent cell death cascade.

It is felt that this effect may be mediated through inhibiting the inflammatory response to ischemia. Neutrophil accumulation and adhesion have been identified in ischemic brain tissue (39) and are correlated with poor clinical outcome (40, 41). Elevated serum levels of selectin and immunoglobulin-type adhesion molecules have been described after acute stroke (42, 43, 44). In other studies, elevated serum levels of ICAM-1 seen at 12 and 24 hours after symptom onset were shown in humans to be directly related to infarct size on diffusion weighted imaging (45). In the same group of studies matrix mettaloproteinases were also shown to be elevated in ischemia and presentation levels of MMP-9 were correlated with eventual infarct size (45).

Previous studies have shown that administration of antibodies to ICAM-1 after transient cerebral ischemia in animals decreased leukocyte adhesion and limited infarct size as well as the number of apoptotic cells (46, 47, 48) suggesting there is a neuroprotective effect of decreasing ICAM-1 activity after reperfusion. Hyperbaric oxygen therapy may exert its antiapoptotic effects through this pathway, since decreased leukocyte adherence and neutrophil accumulation were seen after cerebral ischemia in HBO treated animals (5, 9). ICAM-1 levels have also been shown to be decreased in ischemic tissues in HBO treated animals (49), as well as in human tissue cultures (50) Interestingly, this effect was not seen in non-reperfused tissue (22, 47). Also, in healthy human volunteers, HBO treatment caused reductions in leukocyte adherence that was seen at 2.8 and 3.0 ATA but not at 1.0 or 2.0 ATA (51).

The outcomes scales selected for the study includes the NIH stroke scale (NIHSS), the modified Rankin scale (mRS), the Barthel index, and the Glasgow Outcome scale. These have been used and validated in numerous stroke studies. As they are non-linear scales, they have been utilized for binary outcomes, good versus poor. Good outcome designations are usually understood to be NIHSS ≤ 1, mRS ≤ 1, Barthel 95-100, Glasgow Outcome scale= 5. (33, 34)

3. Hypothesis and objectives

Hyperbaric oxygen therapy administered within twelve hours of symptom onset to patients with acute ischemic stroke at a dose of 2.4 ATA for 90 minutes is safe.

Specific Aim 1: Safety

We will determine whether patients presenting with acute ischemic stroke with a National Institute of Health Stroke Scale score of ≥ 4 given one treatment of hyperbaric oxygen at 2.4 ATA for 90 minutes initiated within 12 hours of symptom onset do not have a significantly higher rate of adverse events, or a singificantly increased infarct size by MRI.

Specific Aim 2: Pilot data for a larger study

This study will provide pilot data to be used to estimate effect size of the use of HBO on functional outcome of ischemic stroke as stated above in order to determine sample size to adequately power a larger multicenter study to determine efficacy of the treatment.

Specific Aim 3: Pilot data on mechanism of HBO

3a. Perfusion:

We will gather pilot data on the effect of treatment with HBO as described above on perfusion of the ischemic territory evaluated by pre- and post-treatment perfusion MRI scanning of the brain (in the first 20 patients). This will be used to gain insight into whether a protective effect of HBO is mediated through altered perfusion to the ischemic penumbra, or if, as is expected, perfusion is not directly affected, but poorly perfused brain territory is protected by other mechanisms.

3b. Leukocyte adhesion:

We will test the hypothesis that the mechanism of neuroprotection provided by hyperbaric oxygen therapy exerts itself through changes in leukocyte adhesion. Using MMP-9 levels at presentation, known to be correlated with eventual infarct size, as a standard for stroke severity, we will determine whether the normally exhibited increase in serum levels of ICAM, VCAM and SELAM after onset of acute ischemic stroke, also correlated with infarct size, is attenuated in patients receiving HBO therapy as described above, and if the decrease in leukocyte adhesion factors correlates with decreased infarct size and improved neurologic outcome.

This is how we determined the number of participants necessary to conduct the study:

1. To evaluate efficacy, the first 10 subjects in each group - HBO and non-HBO - will have in addition to their NIHSS, Barthel index and Rankin scale score, an MRI with diffusion and perfusion weighted imaging, which will be performed pre and post treatment (for the first 20 patients and 72 hours post enrollment for the control group). If there is no differential effect between the controls and the HBO on outcome, the study will be terminated for lack of efficacy.
2. To evaluate safety, 36 subjects in each of the HBO and non-HBO stroke treatments would allow a difference of 20% in aspiration pneumonia Adverse Events to be detected with a power of 80% and a type I (alpha) error of 5%. This would also allow detection of a 20% increase in the rate of post-treatment seizures.

The acute stroke team will make first contact when they are consulted for patients with acute ischemic stroke. Patients will be recruited from all emergency room and inpatient consults for acute stroke called to the stroke team. Women and minorities will be included as they present.

Patients and/or involved family members will be presented with the study and the informed consent will be obtained after all questions/concerns are addressed completely. If the patient is unable to give informed consent themselves, then the LAR will give informed consent on their behalf. If the patient does not have a LAR (Living adult relitive), then we will solicit consent from a next of kin (in the following order): the spouse, adult child, parent, adult sibling, grandparent, or adult grandchild. If none of these options are available then we will be unable to consent the patient and they will not be considered for enrollment in the study. If patient's become able to give consent during the study period they will be reconsented at that time.

Potential subjects and their families will be told that this is an emergency treatment study. We will explain that time is of the essence and that if they feel they are unable to make an informed decision in a timely fashion (approx. 20 minutes), they will be unable to participate in the study. We had several people with no medical background who are not involved with the study read the consent form and on average it took them about 20 minutes to read and understand the consent and fill out the consent questionnaire.

The consent questionnaire is used to evaluate the consent process and document the understanding of the patient and/or LAR of his/her obligations as a patient and the obligation of the PI. If the patient or LAR failed to answer more than 50% of the questions we will offer them the opportunity to rereview the consent forms. If they continue lack of understanding of the research study we will no longer consider them for participation.

Exclusion criteria:

1. Neuroimaging evidence of ICH, intraventricular or subarachnoid blood, tumor, encephalitis or diagnosis other than stroke.
2. Posterior circulation infarction.
3. Active pulmonary disease, pneumothorax, intubation or possible necessity for intubation. ABG findings of pH < 7.32 or pCO2 >49.
4. Active cardiac disease.
5. Decreased level of consciousness (score > 0 on NIHSS item #1a).
6. Inability to lie flat.
7. Claustrophobia.
8. Life expectancy less than 6 months.
9. Pregnancy or breast feeding.
10. Treatment with any other experimental stroke therapy since symptom onset.
11. Patients requiring continuous IV treatment for elevated or depressed blood pressure.
12. Inability to undergo MRI (pacemaker, AICD, etc.)
13. History of seizure.
14. Diabetic patients with a blood glucose <110
15. A GFR blood test resulting in a value of <30 because then the patient would be unable to undergo MRI with contrast.
16. History of inner or middle ear surgery (other than tube placement)
17. History of pneumothorax.
18. History of exposure to Bleomycin.
19. Presently taking steroids.
20. Presently taking Doxorubicin, cis-platinum or disulfiram.

The target enrollment will be 72 patients. Subjects arriving in the emergency department with a presumptive diagnosis of acute stroke will be evaluated by the on-call neurologist. If the time since symptom onset is less than 12 hours and the subject has no known exclusion criteria, a certified examiner will evaluate them using the NIHSS.

Subjects with at least a score of 4 on the NIHSS who are determined to have anterior circulation ischemia as determined by the clinical judgment of the examiner will be enrolled. The NIHSS will be conducted by a study team member, all of whom are NIHSS certified by the American Heart Association and the National Stroke Association. If a subject is determined to have a NIHSS of less than 4, they will not be considered eligible for the study. Also, if a patient is non-responsive when exmained, they will also be excluded from the study. A copy of the NIHSS is included in the source documents which are attached to section 52 of the study smartform. A pregnancy test will be performed on all women of child-bearing age who have a uterus and ovaries. Premorbid mRS score will be discerned through discussion with the patient or family/friends. If this information if not available in time for randomization, the subject will be excluded. If treatment cannot be started within 12 hours from symptom onset, the subject is excluded. Patients deemed candidates for thrombolytic therapy will be treated accordingly and if the patient is randomized to treatment, the HBO will not begin until the tPA infusion has ended.

A noncontrast head CT is done routinely on all patients presenting to the emergency department with acute stroke. This CT scan will be reviewed for evidence of ICH or other exclusionary pathology prior to randomization.

As part of the normal standard of care for these patients, anyone presenting with a possible stroke has an acute stroke panel blood work-up done. A creatinine test is done as part of this panel. Patient's need to have normal kidney functions in order to have gadolinium given with their MRI. If a patient has a GFR of < 30, then they will be exlcuded from the study. This would indicate abnormal kidney functions and they would be unable to undergo MRI with contrast.

In all patients enrolled, NIHSS assessment will be repeated at 7 days or at discharge from the hospital, whichever is first. Rankin scale, Barthel index, and Glasgow outcome scale will be assessed at the same time. Subjects will have a follow-up clinic visit at 90 days with repeat NIHSS testing as well as mRS score, Barthel index, and Glasgow outcome scale assessment. (see Appendix A)

If the subject agrees to participate, an arterial blood gas will be drawn for evaluation. Patients exhibiting blood gas abnormalities consistent with underlying pulmonary disease (pH <7.32 or >7.48 or pCO2 > 49) will be excluded. Eligible patients will be randomized in equal numbers to receive HBO treatment or standard of care treatment.

If no exclusions exist, the subjects randomized to HBO therapy will receive one treatment of 100% O2 at 2.4ATA for 90 minutes in a monoplace hyperbaric chamber.

Prior to treatment an MRI of the brain with diffusion weighted imaging will be performed. Infarct size will be estimated by selecting the image with the largest area of restricted diffusion. This will be measured by length x width x slice thickness to estimate infarct volume in that slice as an estimate of infarct size. If more than one area of infarction exists, they will be evaluated separately and added together. The first twenty patients randomized will undergo further testing. In those patients, 10 HBO, 10 control, MRI with diffusion and perfusion weighted imaging will be performed within 72 hours following treatment or randomization for the control patients. A liquid containing gadolinium contrast agent will be innjected into a vien prior to the MRI scan. This agent increases the ability of the MRI scan to show abnormal tissues in the brain or elsewhere in the body.

Blood will also be drawn at randomization and at 12 and 24 hours from stroke onset (if different from randomization). These will undergo enzyme-linked immunosorbent assays on plasma for MMP-9 and serum for ICAM-1, VCAM-1, and sELAM-1. Additionally, PFA-100 platelet function tests will be run on blood drawn at enrollment and 24 hours.

Our primary outcomes will be rates of adverse events and infarct size on MRI diffusion weighted imaging (DWI). Adverse events will include pneumonia, seizures, and infarct increase. An infarct increase will be defined as an increase in the area of restricted diffusion on DWI over pretreatment baseline of greater than 10% for patients with no diffusion-perfusion mismatch, or a final DWI lesion size which is greater than 10% larger than the baseline perfusion deficit for patients with a perfusion-diffusion mismatch. The rate of adverse events will be compared between treatment and control groups. If the rate of AEs is not statistically significantly larger in the treatment group, the treatment will be considered safe.

Secondary outcomes will include modified Rankin scale score, NIHSS score, Barthel index score, length of hospital stay, intracerebral hemorrhage and symptomatic intracerebral hemorrhage rates and discharge location. Patients will be categorized as having a good outcome (NIHSS 0 or 1, Rankin 0 or 1) or not. The number of patients in treament and control groups achieving a good outcome will be compared. If there is a significant increase in good outcome in the treatment group, the treatment will be considered effective.

Data collected specifically for research purposes will include: NIHSS scores at 7 days or discharge, and at 30 days, as well as mRS scores, Barthel index, and Glasgow outcome scores at 7 and 30 days.

These are the risks we will explain to patients:

Common:

1. Claustrophobia during HBO treatment or MRI (reversible, treat by terminating HBO or MRI)
2. Ear pain during HBO treatment (reversible, treat by terminating HBO)

Uncommon:

1. Hematoma or bleeding from blood draws (reversible or treatable with transfusion)
2. Infection from blood draws (treatable with antibiotics)
3. Increased likelihood of aspiration pneumonia (treatable with antibiotics)

Very uncommon:

1. Seizure from HBO (reversible, treat by terminating HBO)
2. Barotrauma from HBO including pneumothorax, ruptured eardrum, (usually reversible/treatable)
3. Breach of confidentiality/loss of privacy
4. Allergic reaction to MRI contast medium (treatable with antihistamines, epinephrine). Side effects, such as mild headache, nausea and local burning at the IV site can occur. Patients are occasionally allergic to gadolinium contrast resulting most commonly in hives and itchy eyes, and in very rare cases, a bee-sting type of severe allergic reaction (anaphylactic shock). Use of a gadolinium contrast agent may be linked to a rare but sometimes fatal condition (nephrogenic systemic fibrosis or NSF) in people with severe chronic kidney disease or acute kidney problems. Therefore, before you are given a contrast agent for MRI, your risk factors for kidney disease will be reviewed and a blood test for kidney function will be done to exclude severe kidney disease

Patients will be screened by a physician with specialized training in hyperbaric medicine to exclude patients at higher risk of adverse affects from HBO. Trained technicians will monitor treatment under the supervision of this physician to assess patients during treatment and terminate treatment if necessary. Patients will be monitored through constant verbal and visual contact and if deemed necessary, through continuous pulse oximetry and blood pressure measurements. Blood draws will be performed under usual precautions against infection and bleeding.

All patient data will have most identifiers removed (except age, which may include those >89 years old) and will be stored on a password-protected computer database. Additionally a checklist for side effects and their severity will be filled out at completion of the HBO treatment and at discharge or 7 days whichever is earlier. In the case of ear pain which does not resolve after return to normal pressure, ENT will be consulted for evaluation and quantification of any damage using the Teed Scale for quantification.

Patients will be monitored clinically while receiving hyperbaric treatment by the technician and the physician. Patients will be monitored by constant visual and verbal contact and when deemed necessary by the treating physician, by continuous pulse oximetry and blood pressure monitor. Patients will be monitored while inpatient by one of the study physicians or nurses for AEs or SAEs. AEs or SAEs occurring after discharge will be assessed at the follow-up visit. Any adverse events or serious adverse events will be reported to the PI immediately.

The potential benefit to the subject is improved outcome in terms of neurologic function by limiting the damage to the brain from ischemia. Other patients and society could benefit by the development of an additional therapy to limit brain damage from acute ischemic stroke, particularly in patients who are not thrombolytic candidates. Data will be kept on a password-protected database. Only participating study team members will have access to the database. Specimins of serum and plasma will be kept in a locked freezer prior to analysis. Only study team members will have access to the freezer.

4. Conclusions

Hyperbaric oxygen (HBO) therapy of cerebral ischemia has been evaluated in a number of human and animal studies; however, there is presently no consensus on its efficacy. We performed a systematic review of the literature searching Medline database from 1966-2005 using the terms: hyperbaric, hyperbaric oxygenation, cerebrovascular accident, stroke, ischemia, and infarction. We identified 603 articles and selected 89 as relevant. Animal studies of HBO have shown promise by reducing infarct size and improving neurologic outcome. Early reports in humans also suggested benefit in stroke patients treated with HBO. Recent randomized, controlled human studies, however, have not shown benefit. All but one of the studies evaluating HBO therapy of ischemic stroke have used a dose of 1.5 ATA, based upon concerns for increased risk of oxidative stress with higher doses suggested in a single study from 1977. Despite concerns for increased oxidative stress, the patients who received the higher doses of HBO did not have seizures or worsening of neurologic deficits. The single study which assessed the use of HBO at 2.5 ATA in acute stroke did raise concerns of worsened stroke outcome at the higher dose, but was limited by several factors. First, most patients were treated after 12 hours. Second, the control group was subjected to 100% O2 at 1.14 ATA, which is not standard care. Third, there was no cut-off for stroke severity, such that very mild strokes were included, making evaluation of the effect of HBO difficult. Important differences between animal and human studies suggest HBO might be more effective in stroke within the first few hours and at a pressure of 2 to 3 ATA. Therefore, clinical trials of HBO in acute ischemic stroke should be designed to evaluate treatment administered earlier and in higher doses to more clearly address its efficacy. We propose such a clinical trial, in this chapter.

5. References

[1] Helms AK, Torbey MT, Whelan HT. Hyperbaric oxygen therapy of cerebral ischemia. Cerebrovasc Dis 2005;20:417-426.

[2] Chang CF, Niu KC, Hoffer BJ, et al. Hyperbaric oxygen therapy for treatment of postischemic stroke in adult rats. Exper Neurol 166:298-306.2000.

[3] Weinstein PR, Anderson GG, Telles DA. Results of hyperbaric oxygen therapy during temporary middle cerebral artery occlusion in unanesthetized cats. Neurosurg 20:518-24. 1987.

[4] KawamuraS, Yausi N, Shirasawa M. et al. Therapeutic effects of hyperbaric oxygenation on acute focal cerebral ischemia in rats. Surg Neurol 34:101-6.1990.

[5] Atochin DN, Fisher D, Demchenko IT. Neutrophil sequestration and the effect of hyperbaric oxygen in a rat model of temporary middle cerebral artery occlusion. Undersea & Hyperbar Med 27:185-90.2000.

[6] Veltkamp R, Warner DS, Domoki R, et al. Hyperbaric oxygen decreases infarct size and behavioral deficit after transient focal cerebral ischemia in rats. Brain Res 853:68-73.2000.
[7] Badr AE, Yin W, Mychaskiw G, et al. Effect of hyperbaric oxygen on striatal metabolites: a microdialysis study in awake freely moving rats after MCA occlusion. Brain Research 916:85-90.2001.
[8] Yin W, Badr AE, Myechaskiw G, et al. Down regulation of COX-2 is involved in hyperbaric oxygen treatment in a rat transient focal cerebral ischemia model. Brain Res. 926:165-71.2002.
[9] Miljkovic-Lolic M, Silbergleit R, Fiskum G et al. Neuroprotective effects of hyperbaric oxygen treatment in experimental focal cerebral ischemia are associated with reduced brain leukocyte myeloperoxidase activity. Brain Res 971:90-4.2003.
[10] Yin D, Zhang JH. Delayed and multiple hyperbaric oxygen treatments expand therapeutic window in rat focal cerebral ischemic model. Neurocrit Care 2:206-11.2005.
[11] Burt JT, Kapp JP, Smith RR. Hyperbaric oxygen and cerebral infarction in the gerbil. Surg Neurol. 28:265-8.1987.
[12] Sunami K, Takeda Y, Hashimoto M, et al. Hyperbaric oxygen reduces infarct volume in rats by increasing oxygen supply to the ischemic periphery. Crit Care Med 28:2831-6.2000.
[13] Weinstein PR, Hameroff SR, Johnson PC, et al. Effect of hyperbaric oxygen therapy or dimethyl sulfoxide on cerebral ischemia in unanesthetized gerbils. Neruosurg 18:528-32. 1986.
[14] Reitan JA, Kien ND, Thorup S, et al. Hyperbaric oxygen increases survival following carotid ligation in gerbils. Stroke 21:119-23. 1990.
[15] Yin D, Zhou C, Kusaka I, et al. Inhibition of apoptosis by hyperbaric oxygen in a rat focal cerebral ischemic model. J Cereb Blood Flow Metab 23:855-64. 2003.
[16] Takahashi M, Iwatsuki N, Ono K, et al. Hyperbaric oxygen therapy accelerates neurologic recovery after 15-minute complete global cerebral ischemia in dogs. Crit Care Med 20:1588-94.1992.
[17] Iwatsuki N, Takahasi M, Ono K, et al. Hyperbaric oxygen combined with nicardipine administration accelerates neurologic recovery after cerebral ischemia in a canine model. Crit Care Med 22:858-63. 1994.
[18] Krakovsky M, Rogatsky G, Zarchin N, et al. Effect of hyperbaric oxygen therapy on survival after global cerebral ischemia in rats. Surg Neurol 49:412-6.1998.
[19] Rosenthal RE, Silbergleit R, Hof PR, et al. Hyperbaric oxygen reduces neuronal death and improves neurological outcome after canine cardiac arrest. Stroke 34:1311-6.2003.
[20] Yang Z, Camporesi C, Yang X, et al. Hyperbaric oxygenation mitigates focal cerebral injury and reduces striatal dopamine release in a rat model of transient middle cerebral artery occlusion. Eur J App Physiol 87:101-7.2002.
[21] Neubauer RA, end E. Hyperbaric oxygenation as an adjunct therapy in strokes due to thrombosis. Stroke 11:297-300.1980.
[22] Kapp JP. Neurological response to hyperbaric oxygen - a criterion for cerebral revascularization. Surg Neurol 15:43-6.1981.
[23] Holbach K-H, Wassmann H. Neurological and EEG analytical findings in the treatment of cerebral infarction with repetitive hyperbaric oxygenation. Proc sixth Int Cong Hyperbaric Med Aberdeen, Scotland, : Aberdeen University Press 1977, 205-10.

[24] Hart GB, Thompson RE. Treatment of cerebral ischemia with hyperbaric oxygen. Stroke 2:247-50.1971.

[25] Smith G, Lawrence DD, Renfrew S, et al. Preservation of cerebral cortical activity by breathing oxygen at 2 ATA pressure during cerebral ischemia. Surg Gynecol Obstet 113:13-6.1961.

[26] Anderson DC, Bottini AG, Jagiella WM, et al. A pilot study of hyperbaric oxygen in the treatment of human stroke. Stroke 22:1137-42.1991.

[27] Nighoghossian N, Trouillas P, Adelaeine P et al. Hyperbaric oxygen in the treatment of acute ischemic stroke: a double-blind pilot study. Stroke 26:1369-72.1995.

[28] Rusyniak DE, Kirk MA, May JD, et al. Hyperbaric oxygen therapy in acute ischemic stroke results of the hyperbaric oxygen in acute ischemic stroke trial pilot study. Stroke 34:571-4.2003.

[29] Holbach KH, Caroli A, Wassmann H. Cerebral energy metabolism in patients with brain lesions at Normo-and hyperbaric oxygen pressures. J Neurol 217:17-30.1977.

[30] *Hyperbaric Medicine Practice*. Kindwall EP and Whelan HT eds. Best Publishing, Flagstaff , AZ. 1999.

[31] Elliott DH, Kindwall EP. Decompression Sickness. in *Hyperbaric Medicine Practice*. Kindwall EP and Whelan HT eds. Best Publishing, Flagstaff , AZ. 1999.

[32] Kindwall EP. Gas Embolism. In *Hyperbaric Medicine Practice*. Kindwall EP and Whelan HT eds. Best Publishing, Flagstaff , AZ. 1999.

[33] The national institute of neurological disorders and stroke rt-PA stroke study group. Tissue plasminogen activator for acute ischemic stroke. NEJM 333:1581-7. 1995.

[34] Broderick JP, Lu M, Kothari R, et al. Finding the most powerful mesures of the effectiveness of tissue plasminogen activator in the NINDS tPA stroke trial. Stroke 31:2335-41. 2000.

[35] Omae T, Ibayashi S, Kusuda K, et al. Effects of high atmospheric pressure and oxygen on middle cerebral blood flow velocity in humans measured by transcranial doppler. Stroke 29:94-7.1998.

[36] Zhilyaev SY, Moskvin AN, Platonova TF, et al. Hyperoxic vasoconstriction in the brain is mediated by inactivation of nitric oxide by superoxide anions. Neurosci Behav Phys 33:783-7.2003.

[37] Konda A, Baba S, Iwaki T, et al. Hyperbaric oxygenation prevents delayed neuronal death following transient ischaemia in the gerbil hippocampus. Neruopath Appl Neurobiol 22:350-60.1996.

[38] Calvert JW, Yin W, Patel M, et al. Hyperbaric oxygenation prevented brain injury induced by hypoxia-ischemia in a neonatal rat model. Brain Res 951:1-8.2002.

[39] Kataoka H, Kim S-W, Plasnila N. Leukocyte-endothelium interactions during permanent focal cerebral ischemia in mice. J Cereb Blood Flow Metab 24: 668-676. 2004.

[40] Jean W, Spellman SR, Nussbaum ES, Low WC. Reperfusion injury after focal cerebral ischemia: the role of inflammation and the therapeutic horizon. Neurosurg 43: 1382-1396. 1998.

[41] Pozzilli C, Lenzi GL, Argentino C, Bozzao L, Rasura M, Giubilei F, Fieschi C. Peripheral white blood cell count in cerebral ischemic infarction. Acta Neurol Scan 71:396-400. 1985.

[42] Lindsberg, PJ, Carpen O, Petau A, Karjalainen-Lindsberg M-L, Kaste M. Endothelial ICAM-1 expression associated with inflammatory cell response in human ischemic stroke. Circulation 94:939-945.1996.

[43] Fassbender K, Massner R, Motsch L, Kischka U, Grau A, Hennerici M. Circulating selectin-and immunoglobulin-type adhesion molecules in acute ischemic stroke. Stroke 26:1361-1364.1995.
[44] Montaner J, Alvarez-Sabin J, Molina C, Angles A, Abilleira S, Arenilla J, Gonzalez M, Monasterio J. Matrix metalloproteinase expression after human cardioembolic stroke. Stroke 32:1759-1766.
[45] Montaner J, Rovira A, Molina CA, Arenillas JR, Ribo M, Chacon P, Monasterio J, Alvarez-Sabin J. Plasmatic level of neuroinflammatory markers predict the extent of diffusion-weighed image lesions in hyperacute stroke. J Cereb Blood Flow Metab 23:1403-1407. 2003.
[46] Chopp M, Li Y, Jiang N, Zhang RL, Prostak J. Antibodies against adhesion molecules reduce apoptosis after transient middle cerebral artery occlusion in rat brain. J. Cereb Blood Flow Metab 16:578-584. 1996.
[47] Zhang Rl, Chopp M, Jiang N, Tang WX, Prostak J, Manning AM, Anderson DC . Antiintercellular adhesion molecule-1 antibody reduces ischemic cell damage after transient but not permanent middle cerebral artery occlusion in the wistar rat. Stroke 26:1438- 1443.1995.
[48] Bowes M, Zivin J, Tothlein R. Monoclonal antibody to the ICAM-1 adhesion site reduces neurological damage in a rabbit cerebral embolism stroke model. Exp Neurol 119:215-219. 1993.
[49] Hong JP, Kwon J, Chung YK, Jung SH. The effect of hyperbaric oxygen on ischemiareperfusion injury. Ann Plast Surg 51:478-487.2003.
[50] Buras JA, Stahl GL, Svoboda KH, Reenstra WR. Hyperbaric oxygen downregulates ICAM-1 expression induced by hypoxia and hypoglycemia: the role of NOS. Am J Physiol Cell Physiol 278:C292-302. 2000.
[51] Thom SR, Mendiguren I, Hardy K, Bolotin T, Fisher D, Nebolon M, Kilpatrick L. Inhibition of human neutrophil beta2-integrin –dependent adherence by hyperbaric O2. Amer J Physiol 272:C770-C777. 1997.
[52] Noda Y, MeGeer PL, McGeer EG. Lipid peroxide distribution in brain and the effect of hyperbaric oxygen. J. Neurochem 40:1329-1332.1983.
[53] Hjelde A, Hjelstuen M, Haraldseth O, Martin JD, Thom SR, Brubakk AO. Hyperbaric oxygen and neutrophil accumulation/tissue damage during permanent focal cerebral ischaemia in rats. Eur J Appl Physiol 86:401-405.2002.
[54] Mink RB, Dutka AJ. Hyperbaric oxygen after global cerebral ischemia in rabbits does not promote brain lipid peroxidation. Crit Care Med 23:1398-1404.1995.
[55] Schäbitz, W-R, Schade, H, Heiland S, Kollmar R, Bardutsky J, Henninger N, Müller H, Carl U, Toyokuni S, Sommer C, Schwab S. Neuroprtoection by hyperbaric oxygenation after experimental focal cerebral ischemia monitored by MRI. Stroke 35:1175-1179.2004.
[56] Mohr JP, Caplan LR, Melski JW, et al. The Harvard Cooperative Stroke Registry: a prospective registry. Neurol 28:754-62. 1978.
[57] Marti-Vilalta JL, Arboix A. The Barcelona Stroke Registry. Eur Neurol. 41:135-42. 1999.
[58] Yamamoto H, Bogousslavsky J, van Melle G. Different predictors of neurological worsening in different causes of stroke. Arch neurol 55:481-6. 1998.
[59] Johnston SC, Leira EC, Hanse, MD et al . Early recovery after cerebral ischemia risk of subsequent neurological deterioration. Ann Neurol 54:439-44.2003